Hazardous Materials for EMS

Practices and Procedures

Hazardous Materials for EMS Practices and Procedures

Phil Currance, EMT-P, RHSP

Operations Officer, U.S. Public Health Service–Central U.S. National Medical Response Team for Weapons of Mass Destruction

Coordinator, Hazardous Materials Emergency Response Training
Front Range Community College
Denver, Colorado

Alvin C. Bronstein, M.D., FACEP

Assistant Professor of Surgery, Division of Emergency Medicine

Director, Occupational Medicine and Toxicology Clinic
University of Colorado Health Sciences Center

Attending Faculty, Rocky Mountain Poison and Drug Center
Denver, Colorado

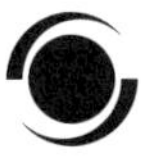

Original photography by Phil Currance

with 153 illustrations

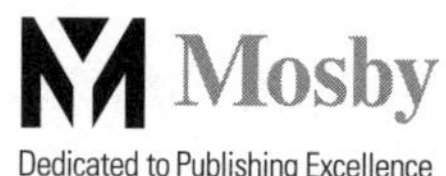

Dedicated to Publishing Excellence

Developmental Editor: Tamara Myers
Project Manager: Mark Spann
Senior Production Editor: Anne Salmo
Book Design Manager: Judi Lang
Manufacturing Supervisor: Linda Ierardi
Cover Design: Teresa Breckwoldt

A NOTE TO THE READER: Information contained in this text in no way authorizes anyone to perform any of the procedures or protocols that are listed. Operating protocols, standing, and/or verbal orders must be established by local Emergency Medical Service Physician control.
To the best of our knowledge, drug indications, dosages, and precautions are current as of publication. The reader is urged to consult the package information provided by the manufacturer for the latest changes.
Do not enter hazardous environments or carry out decontamination procedures without proper protective equipment. It is beyond the scope of this text to advise the exact type of protective equipment needed. Other resources and chemical compatibility charts must be checked. Training in the proper use of protective equipment is essential to your safety. The authors, publisher, and their agents shall not be held responsible for any adverse effects resulting directly or indirectly from the suggested protocols, from any errors or omissions, or from the reader's misunderstanding of the text.

Composition by Clarinda Company
Printing/binding by Maple-Vail Book Manufacturing Group

Mosby, Inc.
11830 Westline Industrial Drive
St. Louis, Missouri 63146

Library of Congress Cataloging-in-Publication Data
Currance, Phillip L.
Hazardous materials for EMS : practices and procedures / Phil Currance, Alvin C. Bronstein.
p. cm.
Includes bibliographical references and index.
ISBN 0-8151-1984-4
1. Hazardous substances. 2. Medical emergencies. 3. Emergency medical personnel. I. Bronstein, Alvin C. II. Title.
RC87.3.C87 1999
616.02'5—dc21 98-56388
CIP

99 00 01 02 03 / 9 8 7 6 5 4 3 2 1

Reviewers

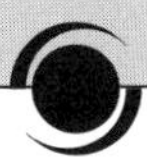

Lt. Ross E. Dinkel
BA Fire Service, NFPA-FO II, Instructor IV, HM Tech, HM I/C
Instructor, Anne Arundel EMS/Fire/Rescue
P.O. Box 276
Millersville, Maryland 21108

Lt. Steve Kidd
Company Officer, Orange County Fire/Rescue Division
Orlando, Florida

Steven V. Rinehart
AS Fire Science, EMT, NFPA-FO I, Instructor III, HM Tech
Associate Instructor, Fire and Rescue Training Institute
University of Missouri
Columbia, Missouri
Battalion Chief/Training Officer, West Alton Volunteer Fire Department
West Alton, Missouri

To Lana, for your patience and love.

Phil Currance

To Ted Hirsch—the last of the old ones—a real mensch.

Alvin C. Bronstein, M.D., FACEP

Preface

It seems that almost everybody has a different idea about where the responsibility of hazardous materials incident mitigation rests. This especially is true when discussing the subject of patients involved in a hazardous materials incident. Personnel from the fire department or hazardous materials (HAZMAT) response team often feel that the responsibility of patients rests with EMS responders. EMS responders commonly do not want anything to do with these patients until they have been completely decontaminated by the fire department or HAZMAT team. Emergency department personnel often cringe at the thought of contaminated patients showing up on their doorstep without the benefit of field decontamination. In a perfect world, patients would be rescued by the HAZMAT team, thoroughly decontaminated by fire/HAZMAT units on the scene, and then stabilized and transported by EMS personnel to a prepared hospital for definitive management.

Unfortunately, we do not live in this mythical world. EMS responders may arrive at the scene long before other responders. In fact, occupational/industrial medical departments are on scene when the incident occurs. Trained and equipped HAZMAT response teams may have an extended response time, delaying patient rescue, decontamination, and patient management. Field responders may quickly be overcome with the number of patients involved in the incident, and patients may scatter and make their way to local hospitals even as responders are arriving at the scene. In some cases, patient involvement may be delayed. Exposure to some hazardous materials may result in a delayed onset of symptoms, causing patients to self-refer to their private physicians, clinics, and hospital emergency departments hours after an incident.

Clearly, EMS personnel at all levels can become involved with hazardous materials. Although this always has been a threat, the frightening reality of terrorist attack is increasing the risk. EMS personnel must be able to recognize the presence of hazardous materials and have an understanding of the types of damage that they are capable of inflicting. An understanding of how to safely respond and protect yourself is vital. Patient decontamination and management procedures must be established and practiced.

In 1989 the Occupational Safety and Health Administration enacted legislation mandating training for personnel who respond to hazardous materials emergencies. This training is established for five different levels of responder involvement: awareness, operations, technician, specialist, and incident command. Unfortunately, most training programs and texts that are available are directed toward hazardous materials responders who will control the scene and mitigate the response. So far, little attention has been paid to the unique concerns of EMS personnel who must respond to these incidents and care for contaminated patients. Recently, specific training programs have been established, and the National Fire Protection Association developed a voluntary training standard. NFPA 473 is specifically designed to meet the needs of EMS personnel who respond to hazardous materials incidents. This text has been designed to assist those responders in meeting this vital training goal.

It is the intention of the authors that this text will provide EMS personnel with an informed view of potential hazardous materials problems and a logical approach to safe response. Our hope is that the contribution of this text will make a difference in the management of patients exposed to hazardous materials. Most importantly we hope that its concepts will assist in improving the safety of EMS personnel at all levels who are responsible for the provision of this essential emergency care.

Phil Currance, EMT-P, RHSP

Alvin C. Bronstein, M.D., FACEP

Acknowledgments

Many people have contributed to the development of this text. Although it is impossible to acknowledge all of them, I would like to pass on special thanks to the following: the personnel and staff of the West Metro Fire Department (formerly the Lakewood Fire Department), where I learned what it means to be a part of a dedicated emergency response agency. Since leaving the fire department and becoming an instructor, I have learned that the process of learning never ends. I will forever be in debt to all of the students whom I have ever had the honor of instructing. It seems that I always come away from a class with more knowledge and information than when it started. A thank you is due to Mosby. Over the past 10 years, Mosby editors have given us the opportunity to publish several of our ideas on medical/hazardous materials response. A special thanks to Tamara Myers, the developmental editor who has taken this project and managed to guide it through the maze of publishing problems that always seem to appear out of thin air. Steve Berry, whose work always reminds me that there is a place for humor in everything you do. You just have to look for it. Thank you for allowing us to use your work to improve ours. A group that deserves mention is the fire-rescue departments from Marion County, Florida, and Ocala, Florida, and the EMS staff from Munroe Regional Medical Center who let us use their talents as actors, as well as responders, for a related video project. They served as the models for many of the illustrations included in this text. A thank you also is due to the team members of the Central U.S. National Medical Response Team for Weapons of Mass Destruction. They continually allow me to use them as test subjects for new curriculum and instructional techniques. Last, but most definitely not least, I thank my wife, Lana, for putting up with me during this project and all the other projects that I just can't seem to say no to. She deserves credit for all of the good things that have occurred since she entered my life.

Phil Currance, EMT-P, RHSP

The letters and reviews from practicing EMS providers of our first text, *Emergency Care for Hazardous Materials Exposure,* were instrumental in the genesis of this work. Books take a toll on the authors, their associates, and families. Many individuals contributed in diverse ways to this project's success. The expertise of Tamara Myers and, in particular, Anne Salmo's perseverance and attention to detail, made this book a reality. I would like to acknowledge Georgia Bedwell for her continuous support and for keeping the home together and the dogs and cats fed; my secretary, Jeanne Johnson, for her kind assistance; and Kristin Lee, R.N., who constantly adjusted my schedule. I also would like to acknowledge Richard C. Dart, medical director of the Rocky Mountain Poison and Drug Center; Kathy Wruk, managing director of the RMPDC; the RMPDC toxicology fellows (past and present), who affectionately call me the "old guy"; and Barry H. Rumack, my first toxicology mentor.

Alvin C. Bronstein, M.D., FACEP

Illustration Credits

Figs. 1-1, 1-2, 1-3, 1-4, 1-5, 1-6, 1-7, 2-1, 2-2, 2-3, 2-4, 2-5, 3-1, C, 3-4, 3-5, 3-6, 3-7, 3-9, 3-11, 3-12, 3-13, 3-18, 3-20, 3-22, 3-23, 3-24, 3-25, 4-1, 4-2, 4-4, 4-8, 4-10, 4-12, 5-1, 6-1, 6-2, 6-3, 6-4, 6-5, 8-1, 8-2, 8-3, 8-4, 8-5, 8-6, 8-7, 8-8, 8-9, 8-10, 8-11, 8-12, 8-13, 8-14, 8-15, 8-16, 8-17, 8-18, 8-19, 9-1, 9-2, 9-3, 9-4, 9-6, 9-8, 9-9, 9-10, 9-11, 9-12, 9-13, 9-15, 9-16, 9-17, 9-18, 9-19, 9-20, 10-1, 10-2, 10-3, 10-5, 10-6, 10-7, 10-8, 10-9, 10-10, 11-1, 11-2, 11-3, 11-4, 11-5, 12-1, 12-2, 14-1, 14-2, 14-3, 14-4, 14-5, 14-6, 17-1, 17-2, 17-3, 17-4, 18-1, 18-2, 18-3, 20-1, 20-2, 20-3, 20-4, 20-5, 20-6, 20-7, and 20-8: Courtesy Phil Currance.

Fig. 4-3: Courtesy Dennis Terpin.

Figs. 3-1, A and B, 3-2, 3-3, 3-8, 3-10, 3-14, 3-15, 3-16, 3-17, 3-19, 3-21, 3-26, 4-6: Courtesy National Audio Visual Center.

Fig. 7-1: From Perry AG, Potter PA: *Clinical nursing skills and techniques,* ed 4, St. Louis, 1998, Mosby.

Fig. 15-1, A and B: ACEP: *Paramedic field care,* St. Louis, 1997, American College of Emergency Physicians.

Unnumbered figures 2-1, 3-1, 8-1, 10-1, 11-1, 13-1, 18-1, 20-1: From Steve Berry's *I'm Not an Ambulance Driver* cartoon book series.

Inside back cover: Reprinted with permission from NFPA 704-1990, *Identification of the fire hazards of materials,* Quincy, Mass, 1990, National Fire Protection Association. This reprinted material is not the complete and official position of the National Fire Protection Association on the referenced subject, which is represented only by the standard in its entirety.

CONTENTS

SECTION ONE

SECTION TWO

SECTION THREE

SECTION FOUR

SECTION FIVE

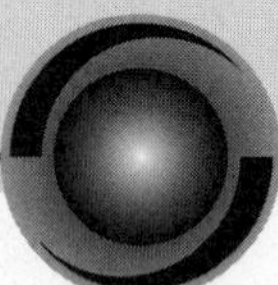

SECTION ONE

Hazardous Materials Overview

1

Introduction and Training Requirements

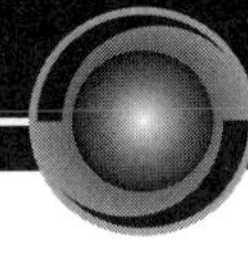

Phil Currance

CHAPTER OBJECTIVES

At the conclusion of this chapter the student will be able to:

- Identify training regulations regarding Emergency Medical Services (EMS) and hazardous materials response and contact agencies that may provide additional information.
- Describe EMS involvement at hazardous materials incidents.
- Identify possible hazards that may be encountered at hazardous materials incidents.
- Discuss Occupational Safety and Health Administration (OSHA) regulations regarding emergency response to hazardous materials incidents.
- Discuss National Fire Protection Association (NFPA) standards regarding emergency response to hazardous materials incidents, especially NFPA 473.

CASE STUDY

EMS and fire responders are called to the scene of a possible man down at a local farm. EMS personnel are the first to arrive on scene and find an apparently unconscious victim lying next to a tractor and pesticide sprayer unit. A strong, unusual odor is present, and the victim's clothes appear to be wet (Fig. 1-1).

- ◆ Are hazardous chemicals involved?
- ◆ Can EMS personnel safely approach the patient?
- ◆ What type of hazardous materials training is required for EMS personnel?
- ◆ What types of injury or exposure may be present?

Although what constitutes a hazardous material has been defined many ways, the most basic one is probably the best. A *hazardous material* is a solid, liquid, or gas substance that, when released from a container, is capable of harming people, the environment, and property. Hazardous materials may be found nearly everywhere, including in industrial locations, swimming pools, hospitals, agricultural areas, and homes. Hazardous materials also are transported by rail, boat, truck, and, in limited quantities, air.

Incidents involving hazardous materials may occur during transportation or at any location where hazardous materials are stored or used. They may occur in residential areas with commonly used household cleaning chemicals or pesticides. Incidents involving illegal drug laboratories are becoming increasingly commonplace, and terrorist activities involving chemicals are now a frightening reality. Incidents may involve a single patient or multiple casualties or, in the event of a disaster, may involve a large segment of the community.

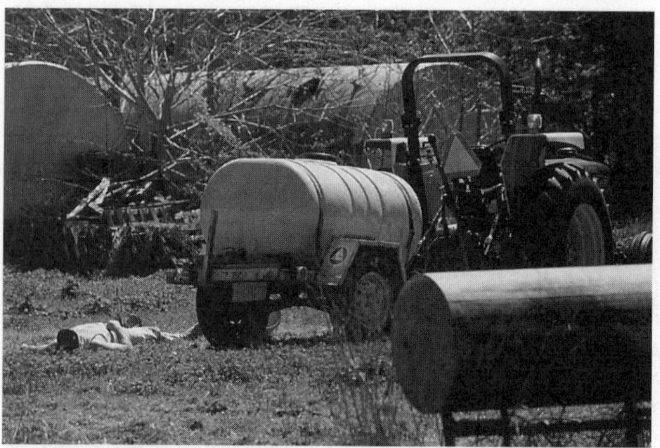

FIG. 1-1 Potential chemical exposure.

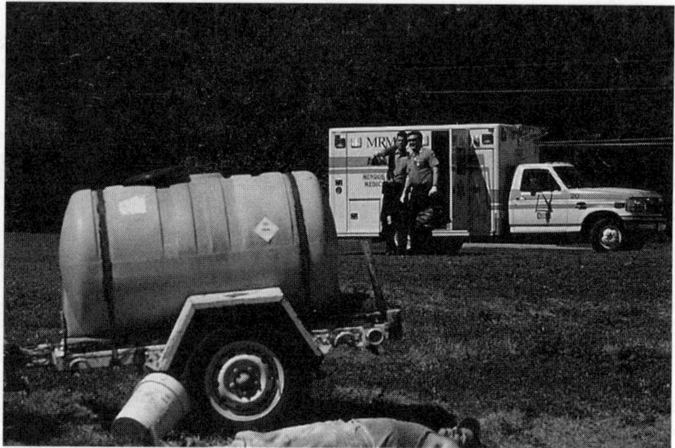

FIG. 1-2 EMS responders may be on the scene before the hazardous materials team.

EMS Responders

When these incidents occur, EMS responders may come into contact with patients exposed to or contaminated by hazardous materials. EMS personnel may be dispatched to a situation in which the presence of hazardous materials has not been recognized. They must understand what hazardous materials are and what they can do.

Willingly or not, EMS responders often become active players at hazardous materials incidents. Involvement may include:

- Optimally, receiving "clean patients" from a hazardous materials (HAZMAT) team
- Being called to incidents not involving fire department response (i.e., "sick" buildings, synergistic exposures, sensitive individuals)
- Being the first to recognize that the incident involves hazardous materials
- Because of delayed onset of symptoms or repeated secondary contamination exposures, encountering patients hours or days after exposure
- At large incidents, when patients may scatter, encountering contaminated patients some distance from the scene and organized response
- At incidents in which multiple casualties are involved and the number of trained HAZMAT responders is limited, encountering patients who have received less than adequate decontamination
- Being on the scene long before the arrival of the HAZMAT team, whose response may take considerably longer (Fig. 1-2)

The adequate management of patients exposed to hazardous materials may require changes in your normal response practices. Toxic materials may affect the way the body responds to trauma and medical conditions, necessitating triage protocol changes. Standard treatment protocols may need to be modified to provide effective patient management. Decontamination protocols must be developed to limit injury to contaminated patients and reduce the likelihood of secondary contamination to emergency responders and hospital personnel.

BOX 1-1

Physical Hazards

Heavy containers (drums weigh approximately 500 lbs)
Heavy equipment
Electrical hazards
Safety hazards (holes, ditches, slippery surfaces, sharp objects, improperly stacked material)

Hazardous materials may cause harm in multiple ways. They may be flammable, corrosive, toxic, radioactive, or reactive, or may be any combination of these. Exposed patients may exhibit various problems. Besides the chemical threat, many other hazards may be present at the scene of a hazardous materials incident. Chemical releases usually occur because the container has been damaged. The physical cause of the incident may have resulted in trauma to individuals. The response process itself will generate some physical risks and psychological stress (Box 1-1).

Another hazard to responders in protective equipment at hazardous materials incidents is heat stress. When responders wear chemical-protective equipment, they are at high risk for heat-induced injuries. EMS personnel often are called on to monitor and treat HAZMAT team members for heat-stress–related problems.

Training Requirements

Occupational Safety and Health Administration and Environmental Protection Agency

Response to hazardous materials incidents is inherently dangerous, and EMS personnel must be trained to respond safely and effectively. The Occupational Safety and Health Administration (OSHA) and the Environmental Protection Agency (EPA) have established mandatory safety procedures for personnel who deal with problems involving hazardous materials. These safety procedures were first mandated in 1986 by EPA's Superfund Amendment and Reauthorization Act (SARA). SARA was designed to update the original Comprehensive Environmental Response, Compensation and Liability Act (CERCLA). CERCLA, more commonly called *Superfund,* was written to oversee the cleanup of uncontrolled hazardous waste sites and the response to large hazardous materials emergencies. SARA reauthorized the Superfund law and included sections on community emergency planning and worker protection. It mandated that both OSHA and the EPA pass worker protection standards within 5 years.

OSHA took the lead and in 1989 enacted OSHA 29 CFR 1910.120. Commonly called the *HAZWOPER standard* (*H*azardous *W*aste *Op*erations and *E*mergency *R*esponse), this law provides for the safety of personnel who work on hazardous waste cleanup sites or hazardous waste treatment storage and disposal sites, or who respond to hazardous materials emergencies no matter where they occur. The provisions of HAZWOPER include:

- Training
- Hazard identification and characterization
- Personal protective equipment (PPE)
- Decontamination procedures
- Safe work or response practices
- Medical monitoring of personnel

Because federal and local government personnel are exempted from federal OSHA standards, the EPA enacted EPA 40 CFR 311. This "mirror standard" was designed to protect these workers. Because of the federal OSHA exemptions, many states have enacted their own OSHA regulations, which cover all workers in the state no matter for whom they work.

The HAZWOPER and specific state standards require training for all personnel who respond to any emergency hazardous materials incident. For emergency responders, the standards require that the training should be based on their expected activities. The regulations break the training down into five levels: awareness, operations, technician, specialist, and incident command. EMS responders, at a minimum, must be trained to the awareness level. Some states require that EMS personnel be trained to the operations level, since they respond to protect life and safety at a hazardous materials emergency. In some areas, EMS agencies have decided to take an active role in hazardous materials response and have trained their responders to the technician level.

Awareness level

First responders at the awareness level are likely to witness or discover a release of hazardous materials and are trained to initiate an emergency response (Fig. 1-3). No hourly training requirement is listed in either OSHA 29 CFR 1910.120 or EPA 40 CFR 311 for this level. First responders at this level must have sufficient training or

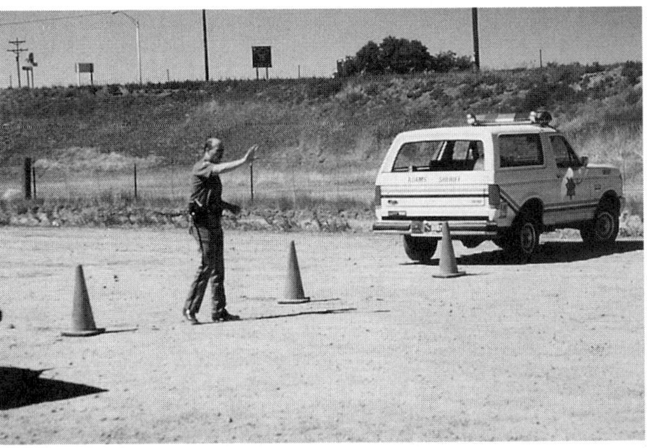

FIG. 1-3 Awareness level responder at a hazardous materials incident.

experience to demonstrate competency in the following areas:

- An understanding of what hazardous materials are and their risks
- An understanding of potential outcomes when hazardous materials are present during an emergency
- The ability to recognize the presence of hazardous materials
- An understanding of the first responder's role and use of the *North American Emergency Response Guidebook*
- The ability to recognize the need for additional resources and knowledge of the procedure to make appropriate notifications

Operations level

First responders at the operations level respond to releases, or potential releases, as part of the initial response to protect people, property, and the environment from the effects of the release (Fig. 1-4). Operations-level first responders are trained to take defensive actions rather than try to stop the release. Their function is to contain the release from a safe distance, keep it from spreading, and prevent exposures. OSHA 29 CFR 1910.120 requires that first responders at the operations level receive at least 8 hours of training or have sufficient experience to demonstrate competencies objectively. First responders must have the knowledge of awareness-level competencies, and they are required to:

- Know basic hazard and risk assessment
- Know how to select and use available protective equipment
- Understand basic terms related to hazardous materials
- Know how to perform basic control, containment, and confinement operations within the capabilities of their resources and protective equipment
- Know basic decontamination procedures

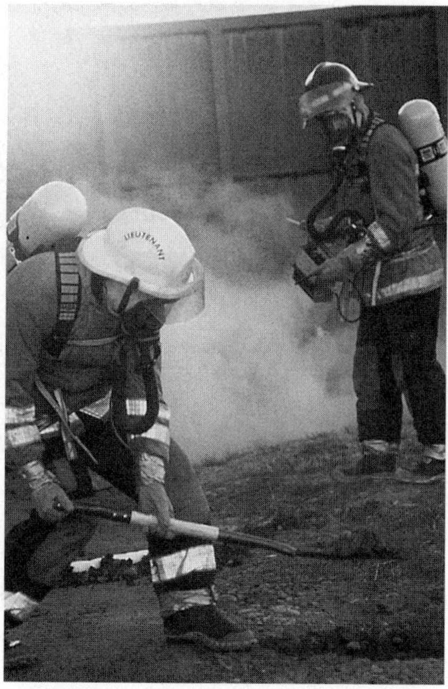

FIG. 1-4 Operations level hazardous materials responders.

- Understand relevant standard operating procedures (SOPs) and termination procedures
- Although the entire operations level curriculum may not be appropriate for medical responders, certain tasks in this level are appropriate for EMS field activities. It is advisable to train EMS responders to the operations level with a program that is specialized to medical needs.

Technician level

Hazardous materials technicians respond to releases or potential releases to stop the release (Fig. 1-5). This level requires at least 24 hours of training at the operations level, training equal to the competencies at the technician level, and certification by the employer. Hazardous materials technicians assume a more aggressive role than first responders at the operations level. They approach the point of release to plug, patch, or otherwise stop the release of a hazardous substance. They must be trained at the first responder operations level, and they are required to:

- Know how to implement the employer's emergency response plan
- Know how to identify materials by using field survey instruments
- Be able to function in an assigned role in the incident command system
- Know how to select and use specialized PPE
- Understand hazard and risk assessment techniques
- Be able to perform advanced control and containment operations within the resources and equipment available

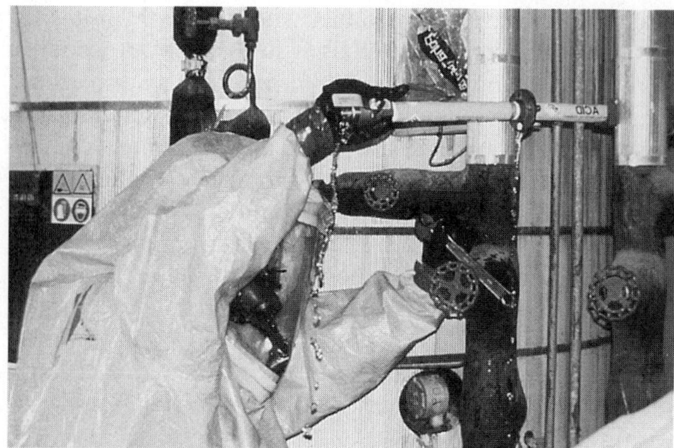

FIG. 1-5 Hazardous materials technician at a hazardous materials incident.

- Understand and implement decontamination procedures

Like the operations level, the technician level will include some competencies, such as advanced control and containment practices, that may not be appropriate for the EMS responder. A program can be designed that will parallel the technician level and give specific medical and hazardous materials information.

Specialist level

Hazardous materials specialists are those senior, experienced individuals who respond with and support hazardous materials technicians. Their duties parallel those of hazardous materials technicians, but specialists are required to have more direct or specific knowledge of the various substances they may be called on to contain. They also act as senior leaders of HAZMAT teams and may act as site liaisons with federal, state, and local government authorities with regard to site activities according to OSHA CFR 1910.120. OSHA regulations also require that specialists be certified by their employers. Hazardous materials specialists should receive at least 24 hours of training equal to the technician level, and they must:

- Know how to implement the local emergency response plan
- Be able to use advanced survey instruments
- Have knowledge of their state's emergency response plan
- Be able to select and use proper specialized protective equipment
- Understand in-depth hazard and risk assessment techniques
- Be able to perform specialized control and containment operations with the available equipment and resources
- Be able to implement decontamination procedures

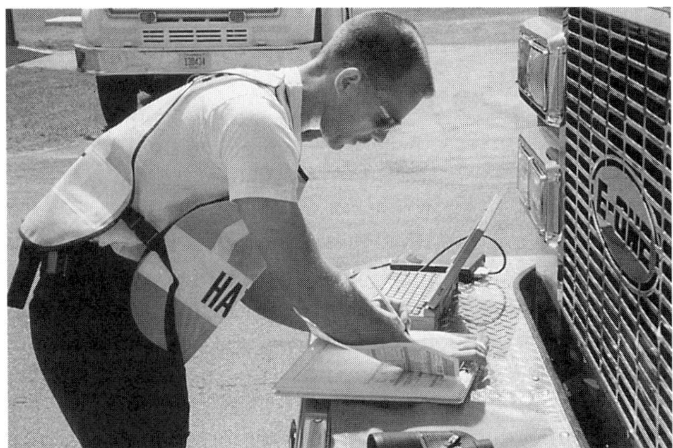

FIG. 1-6 An incident commander at a hazardous materials incident.

- Be able to develop a site safety plan
- Understand chemical, radiological, and toxicological terminology and behavior

Incident command level

Incident command level responders who assume control of the incident scene beyond the first responder awareness level should receive at least 24 hours of training equal to the first responder operations level (Fig. 1-6). In addition, the employer must certify that personnel in this position:

- Are able to implement their employer's incident command system
- Are able to implement their employer's emergency response plan
- Understand the risks associated with working in chemical-protective clothing
- Know how to implement the local emergency response plan
- Have knowledge of their state's emergency response plan and the federal regional response team
- Understand the importance of decontamination

National Fire Protection Association

In addition to OSHA and EPA regulations, the National Fire Protection Association (NFPA) has developed voluntary training competencies for personnel who respond to hazardous materials incidents. NFPA 471 sets competency standards for hazardous materials emergency response. NFPA 472 sets training standards for emergency response personnel. The NFPA 472 standards parallel the OSHA/EPA regulations while adding more detail and description.

Of special interest to EMS responders is NFPA 473 (see Appendix A). This standard is designed for EMS personnel who respond to hazardous materials incidents. It designates two levels of training, Level 1 and Level 2.

EMS/HM level 1

Emergency medical services personnel at EMS/Hazardous Materials (HM) Level 1 may, in the course of their normal duties, be called on to perform patient care activities in the "cold zone" at a hazardous materials incident. The *cold zone* contains the command post and other support functions. It also is referred to as the *clean,* or *support, zone.* This zone should be free of contamination, and response activities in this area represent a minimal risk. The role of the EMS/HM Level 1 responder is to provide care only to those individuals who no longer pose a significant risk of secondary contamination (i.e., a risk of contaminating others, including those providing care).

The NFPA standard suggests that as a minimum these EMS personnel be trained to meet the requirements of the OSHA first responders awareness level, as well as the specific requirements listed in NFPA EMS/HM Level 1. In addition, EMS responders must meet all applicable local and state training requirements. **EMS/HM Level 1** responders should be able to demonstrate the following competencies:

- Assessing incident scene hazards and risks of patient secondary contamination
- Incident scene response planning, including determining PPE needs and defining roles and responsibilities of the EMS/HM Level 1 responders
- Ability to perform EMS/HM Level 1 patient preparation, care, and preparation for transport
- Ability to perform postincident EMS reporting, documentation, and follow-up

EMS/HM level 2

EMS personnel at the EMS/HM Level 2 may, in the course of their normal duties, be called on to perform patient care activities during decontamination procedures in the *warm zone,* (the area where personnel and equipment decontamination takes place) at hazardous materials incidents. Personnel in this zone have a greater chance of being exposed to the hazardous material and are at higher risk than personnel in the cold zone. The EMS/HM Level 2 response personnel may provide care to individuals who still pose a significant risk of secondary contamination. Using EMS responders trained in hazardous materials activities to assist in decontamination procedures will result in a higher level of care and the ability to provide effective and efficient patient assessment and prehospital care to exposed and contaminated patients (Fig. 1-7).

EMS/HM Level 2 responders should be able to analyze hazardous materials incidents to determine the magnitude of problem areas. In addition, they are expected to plan a response and provide the appropriate level of emergency care and decontamination to patients involved in the incident. They must be able to select and use appropriate PPE. Personnel at this level should also be able to coordinate EMS activities at a hazardous materials in-

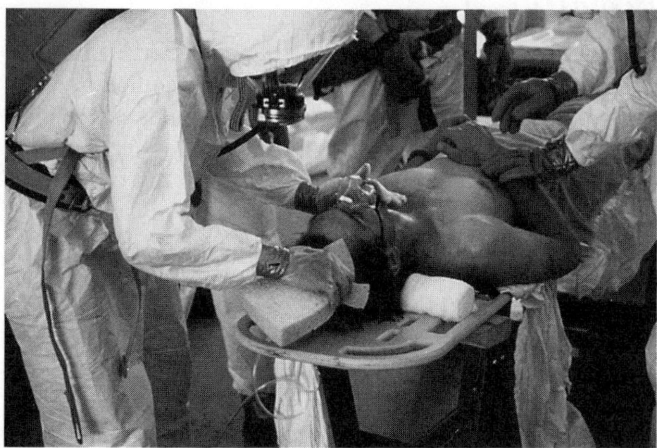

FIG. 1-7 EMS/HM Level 2 responders in protective equipment decontaminate an injured patient.

cident and provide medical support for hazardous materials response personnel.

EMS/HM Level 2 responders should meet all requirements listed for **EMS/HM Level 1,** and all applicable local and state training requirements. In addition, they must be able to demonstrate the following competencies:

- Assessment of incident scene hazards and risks of patient secondary contamination
- Incident scene response planning, including determining PPE needs, and defining roles and responsibilities of the EMS/HM Level 2 responder
- Ability to perform EMS/HM Level 2 patient decontamination and treatment in the warm and hot zones of an incident scene
- Ability to perform postincident EMS reporting, documentation, and follow-up

Because of the detailed competencies and requirements expected of the EMS/HM Level 2 responder, it is advised that candidates attend specially designed training that will parallel the basic duties of the hazardous materials technician.

Summary

Medical personnel who may respond to hazardous materials incidents or who may come into contact with contaminated patients may place themselves at great risk. In addition, patients who are exposed to hazardous materials may require special treatment modalities to reduce the chance of morbidity and mortality. Training and regular continuing education to maintain competency in both emergency medical technology and hazardous materials response procedures can result in a safer and more effective response.

This text is designed to provide a training tool for EMS personnel who respond to hazardous materials incidents. It will assist you in meeting the competencies of the awareness, operations, and specific parts of the technician levels of the OSHA standard, and the EMS/HM Level 1 and EMS/HM Level 2 competencies of NFPA 473.

Hazardous materials incidents are among the most dangerous and complicated to which you will respond. Please keep these points in mind. This text is intended to be used as a supplemental resource, not a replacement for any part of your training. It was produced to share information, but it is up to you to judge the merits of the philosophies and techniques. Always follow your SOPs. They were developed for your specific problems, equipment, and personnel. Remember that personnel should never attempt to carry out procedures unless they have received specific training for those procedures. In the field, decisions should be based on everything that the responder has learned and experienced. Never rely on just one source of information.

CHAPTER REVIEW QUESTIONS

1. List four ways that EMS responders may encounter contaminated patients.
2. Describe the hazards that may be found at the scene of a hazardous materials emergency.
3. Identify the levels of hazardous materials response training listed in OSHA 29 CFR 1910.120, and describe the differences.
4. Explain the differences between EMS/HM Level 1 and EMS/HM Level 2 responders as described in NFPA 473.
5. List five locations at which hazardous materials emergencies may be encountered.

Suggested Reading

Two references that you may find useful are the *Hazardous Materials Response Handbook, Third Edition,* available from the National Fire Protection Association, and the *Guidelines for Public Sector Hazardous Materials Training,* developed under the Hazardous Materials Emergency Preparedness Grant Program and available from the National Emergency Training Center ([301] 447-1009). The *Hazardous Materials Response Handbook* explains all of NFPA 471, 472, and 473. The *Guidelines for Public Sector Hazardous Materials Training* is a free publication that details both required and recommended training competencies for all levels of responders, including EMS.

BIBLIOGRAPHY

Agency for Toxic Substances and Disease Registry: *Managing hazardous materials incidents, emergency medical services: a planning guide for the management of contaminated patients,* Atlanta, Ga, 1992, USDHHS.

Andrews LP, editor: *Emergency responder training manual for the hazardous materials technician,* New York, 1992, Van Nostrand Reinhold.

Bronstein AC, Currance PL: Module 4: emergency medical operations. In Ayers S, Christopher J, editors: *Medical response to chemical emergencies,* Washington, DC, 1994, Chemical Manufacturers Association.

Coleman RJ, Williams KH: *Hazardous materials dictionary,* Lancaster, Pa, 1988, Technomic Publishing.

Currance PL: *Hazmat for EMS,* St Louis, 1995, Mosby (videotape and guidebook).

EPA: *EPA standard safety operating guidelines,* Washington, DC, 1984, US Government Printing Office.

Guidelines for public sector hazardous materials training. 1998 ed, HMEP Curriculum Guidelines, Emmitsburg, Md, 1998, National Emergency Training Center.

Hazardous materials response training program, New Jersey/New York, 1988, Hazardous Materials Worker/Training Program.

National Fire Protection Association: *NFPA 471, Recommended practice for responding to hazardous materials incidents,* Quincy, Mass, 1992, The Association.

National Fire Protection Association: *NFPA 472, Standard for professional competence of responders to hazardous materials incidents,* Quincy, Mass, 1992, The Association.

National Fire Protection Association: *NFPA 473, Standard for professional competence of EMS responders to hazardous materials incidents,* Quincy, Mass, 1992, The Association.

Noll GG, Hildebrand MS, Yvorra JG: *Hazardous materials: managing the incident,* ed 2, Stillwater, Okla, 1995, Fire Protection Publications.

OSHA: 29 CFR 1910.120, Hazardous waste operations and emergency response; Final rule, March 6, 1989; Washington, DC, US Government Printing Office.

Strong CB, Irvin TR: *Emergency response and hazardous chemical management: principles and practices,* Delray Beach, Fla, 1996, St. Lucie Press.

Tokle G, editor: *Hazardous materials response handbook,* ed 2, Quincy, Mass, 1993, National Fire Protection Association.

2

Hazardous Materials Preplanning and the Incident Management System

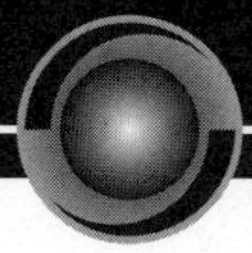

Phil Currance

CHAPTER OBJECTIVES

At the conclusion of this chapter the student will be able to:

- Discuss the importance of preplanning in safely and effectively responding to hazardous materials incidents.
- Identify common functional areas of an Incident Management System (IMS) and their activities.
- Identify the functional areas of an IMS to which Emergency Medical Services (EMS) responders will report.
- Discuss the need and function of staging areas at a hazardous materials response.
- Identify common areas of concern in planning the EMS/hazardous materials response.
- Explain the need for an emergency response plan.
- List items that should be included in an emergency response plan.
- Identify community information resources available to the EMS responder.
- Discuss the importance of identifying preexisting health concerns in the EMS responder.

CASE STUDY

A fire at a chemical plant is burning out of control. Health department officials have determined that the smoke cloud is toxic. Approximately 4000 residents downwind from the plant are being evacuated, and 50 workers from the plant and four firefighters are complaining of shortness of breath and chest pain. Numerous agencies are present at the site: fire and police department personnel, EMS responders, local and state health officials, a private hazardous materials cleanup contractor, and a county hazardous materials (HAZMAT) response team (Fig. 2-1).

- ◆ Who is in charge?
- ◆ Where does EMS fit into this response?
- ◆ Who is responsible for safety on the scene?
- ◆ What types of chemicals are used at the plant?
- ◆ What types of resources are available in the community to assist in patient care activities?

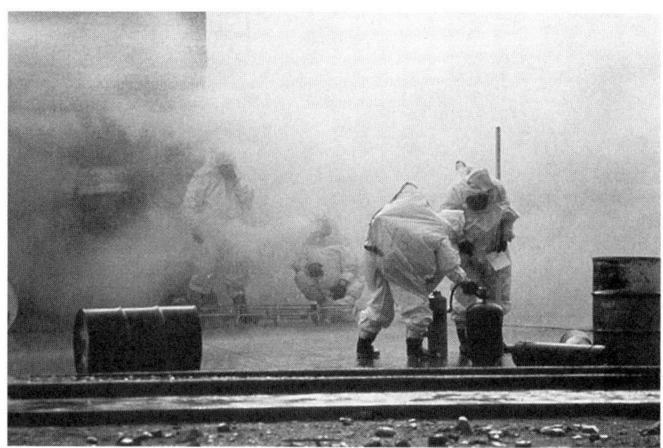

FIG. 2-1 Hazardous materials technicians attempt to control the incident.

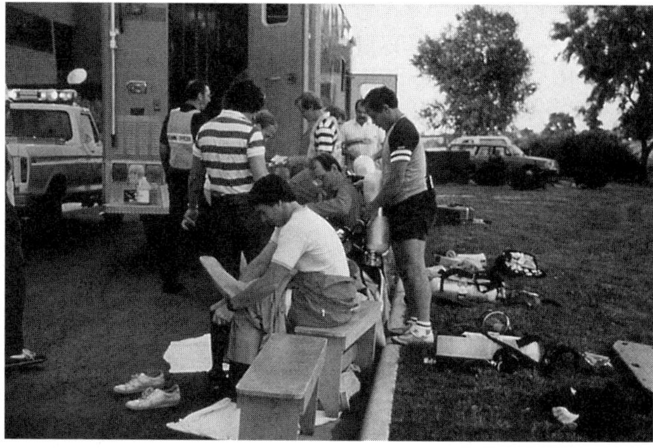

FIG. 2-2 Many agencies can become involved in a hazardous materials emergency.

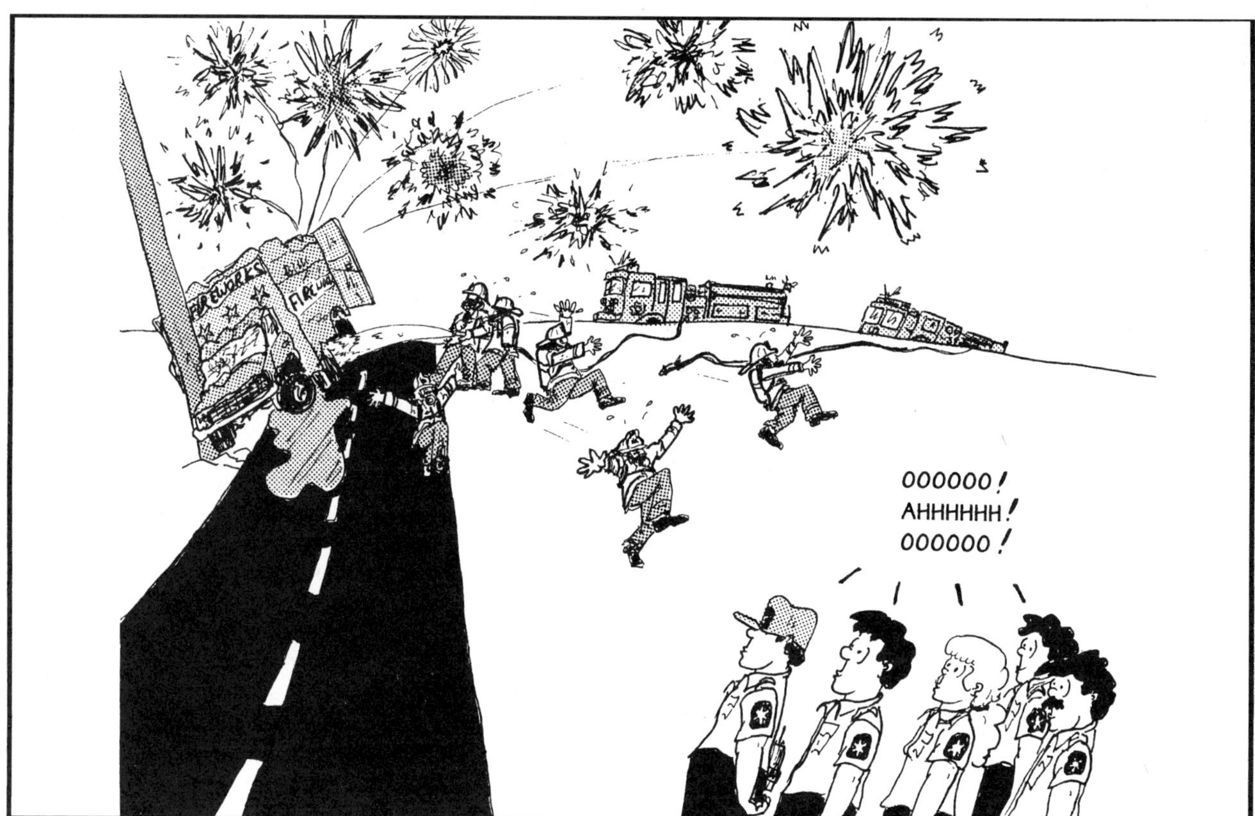

Reprinted with permission from Steve Berry's *I'm Not an Ambulance Driver* cartoon book series.

Preplanning is a vital part of safe and effective response to hazardous materials incidents. Many aspects of a hazardous materials response must be determined far in advance of an actual emergency. Response to these types of incidents is a team effort, and many agencies are likely to become involved (Fig. 2-2). In a typical incident, EMS responders; fire, police, and highway department personnel; local or state health department representatives; the EPA; the county HAZMAT team; and private hazardous materials cleanup contractors all may be present. The chain of command and communication structure at an incident must be followed.

Medical responders must have an idea of who will be in charge. What resources are available in the area, and how are they accessed? Who can provide consultation on patient management concerns? Other concerns are equipment availability, knowledge of hazards commonly present in the area, and the responder's health status.

The Incident Management System

Federal regulations (OSHA 29 CFR 1910.120 and EPA 40 CFR 311) mandate that emergency response to all incidents involving hazardous substances be managed under an incident management system (IMS). This system is designed to focus the actions of all responders on safely and efficiently mitigating the incident. EMS responders must be able to function under the local IMS.

An IMS is a management tool consisting of procedures for organizing personnel, facilities, equipment, and communications at the scene of an emergency. It is organized in a modular format. It should be a "top-down" organizational structure that can be used for any incident. Modules typically are organized according to function, with six primary functional areas, or sections, established as follows:

- Command
- Operations
- Safety
- Planning
- Logistics
- Finance or administrative support

Each functional area will be recognized in any implementation of the IMS; however, each area does not require independent staffing. In a small incident, one person may be responsible for several functions. As the incident expands, so does the IMS, with an individual in charge of each area.

Command

The command function involves directing, ordering, and/or controlling resources. The senior person at the scene is usually considered to be the incident commander (Fig. 2-3). The incident commander may change at various stages of the incident as more qualified personnel arrive on scene. The incident commander has the primary authority for the overall control of the emergency event. All response operations are to be conducted under the control of this person. Laws or policies in force at different locations may specify the individuals to be designated the incident commander at hazardous materials incidents. In some locations the fire chief may be the incident commander, whereas in other places the police chief or emergency operations officer may be in charge. To minimize confusion, the agency having jurisdiction must be identified before an incident takes place.

Operations

The operations function is responsible for managing all tactical operations at the incident. This section is coordinated by the operations officer, who reports to the incident commander. Tasks may be organized into sectors or groups under the control of operations. Depending on the incident, fire control, police operations, and EMS and HAZMAT team activities may all report to the operations officer.

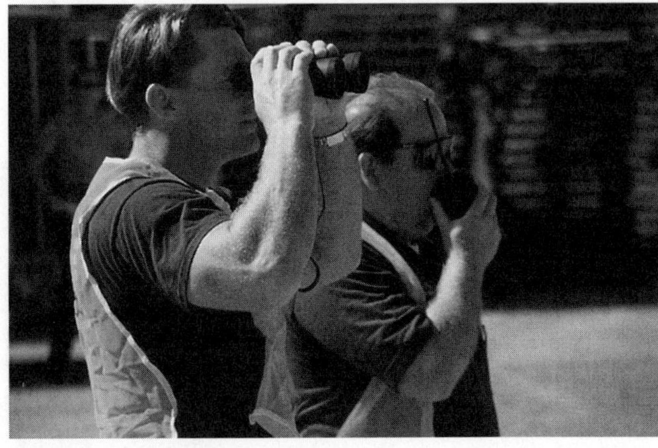

FIG. 2-3 Incident commander and safety officer at the scene of a hazardous materials emergency.

Safety

The incident commander must appoint an incident safety officer at hazardous materials emergencies. This officer reports to the incident commander. He or she is responsible for seeing that all operations are conducted safely. The incident safety officer is authorized to stop any unsafe act and correct the problem.

Planning

Responsibilities of the planning section include collecting and evaluating information about the response. The planning section also is responsible for developing a suggested action plan for approval by the incident commander. At smaller incidents the planning function is often combined with the operations function.

Logistics

The logistics function is responsible for locating, organizing, and providing facilities, services, and materials needed for mitigation of the incident. The logistics officer reports to the incident commander.

Finance or Administrative Support

The finance or administrative support function is responsible for tracking all incident costs and evaluating the financial considerations of the incident. They may also be responsible for securing resources that are unavailable to the logistics officer.

Depending on local jurisdiction and their activity at the scene, EMS providers may fall into many of these functional areas. For example, the EMS providers managing injuries that occurred at the incident will most likely be assigned to a medical sector or group under the operations function. The senior EMS provider on the scene may be assigned to be the medical sector officer. EMS providers supporting the HAZMAT team may be assigned to the hazardous materials sector or the logistics function.

The incident commander must be informed of all activities that deviate from the established plan. Final approval of any actions must come from the incident commander. Finally, hazardous materials medical specialists may be assigned to the planning function to help develop the medical aspects of the action plan. It is vital that medical responders determine their actions under the local IMS in preplanning, before an incident takes place.

An IMS also will help to organize response activities and ensure that safety procedures are followed at the scene. It suggests a range of control, defined as the number of subordinates one supervisor can manage effectively, to ensure that the safety of every responder is maximized. The guidelines delineate a desirable range of from three to seven persons reporting to a supervisor, with an optimal number of five.

As previously mentioned, an IMS is a top-down structure. There will always be an incident commander; the remaining functional areas are added as needed. The first arriving responder will assume the role of the incident commander. Communication between the first arriving unit to the dispatcher is essential to ensure that the proper resources are sent to the emergency. An arrival report should include the type of problem, a brief description of the scene, a request for appropriate resources, the safest route of approach, and the location of the command post. As more qualified personnel arrive on the scene, the person assuming the role of incident commander may change, but the responsibilities remain the same. It is vital that the person relinquishing command and the person assuming command communicate. Information regarding the status of the response and resources available must be passed on to the new commander.

Staging Areas

For EMS responders, an important concept of the IMS is the staging area. A staging area is a resource marshaling area to which units report while awaiting specific assignments and direction. Only those resources that are needed immediately at the scene of the emergency should be on the site. Different personnel and resources are needed at different times and in different locations. In addition, when they are needed, they must be available to respond in a controlled, organized, and effective manner. Above all, the safety of the responders must be ensured. The way to achieve these goals is to use staging areas (Fig. 2-4).

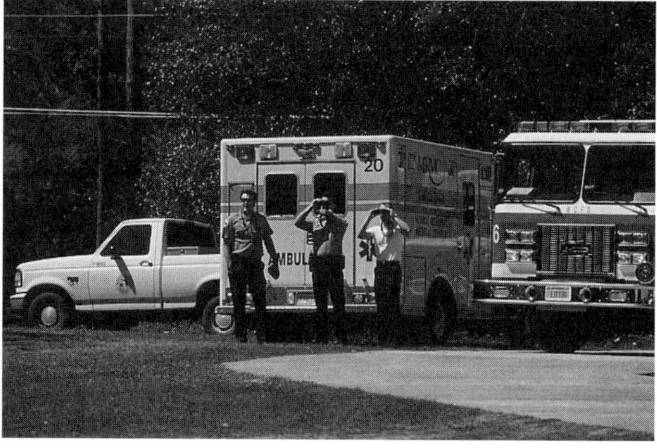

FIG. 2-4 EMS units at the staging area.

Depending on the size and nature of the incident, one or more staging areas may be established. The staging area provides a safe location where personnel and resources may wait until needed, prevents the freelancing of incoming units, and provides accountability for the units on scene and their status. Key considerations for selecting a site to be the staging area include:

- Proximity to the incident scene
- Easy access in and out
- Parking areas and storage space
- Security for equipment and supplies

Staging areas are under the control of a staging area manager, who must be in direct contact with the operations officer. The operations officer must be kept fully informed as to what resources are available for deployment.

Response Capabilities

In many places, EMS responders believe that all hazardous materials responsibilities belong to the fire department. Although this often is the case, the hazardous materials response capabilities of all agencies must be assessed. Hazardous materials operations are expensive and require long training hours. Some fire departments have decided to train their personnel to the operations level and limit their response to defensive actions only. In these cases, a county, state, or private hazardous materials agency usually is available. Although this may be a cost-effective use of budget and resources, it may prolong the response time of technician-level trained personnel and specialized equipment, thereby directly affecting the time that it takes to reach and rescue victims who are incapacitated or trapped. The capabilities of all primary response agencies (i.e., police, fire, hazardous materials) must be assessed and developed into a response plan. The roles of other agencies, such as the local health department and utility company, must also be ascertained and included in a response plan.

Hospital capabilities must also be determined before an incident occurs. Not every hospital is equipped to handle patients from a hazardous materials incident. Patient needs must be matched with the destination hospital. Because absolute decontamination is sometimes difficult to achieve in the field, the hospital should be equipped with the proper facilities, trained personnel, and protective equipment to carry out decontamination procedures. Patient treatment considerations also must be addressed. The destination facility should have consultation support from a medical toxicologist and local or regional poison center to guide patient care and decontamination decisions. Equipment, such as a hyperbaric chamber and special physiological antagonists (antidotes), also should be available.

Response Planning

One of the most important tools to help ensure the safety of personnel in an emergency is an emergency response plan. This plan should be developed, rehearsed, modified as necessary, and rehearsed again (Box 2-1). It should establish the response agency's actions when faced with a hazardous materials emergency. At a minimum the plan should include:

- Local hazard assessment
- Preemergency planning and coordination with outside agencies and private parties
- Personnel roles, lines of authority, training, and communications
- Emergency recognition and prevention
- Emergency alerting and response procedures
- Safe distances and places of refuge
- Site security and control
- Evacuation routes and procedures
- Personal protective equipment (PPE) and emergency equipment
- Decontamination procedures
- Emergency medical treatment
- Incident termination procedures, including postincident analysis of response and follow-up
- Responder exposure reporting and tracking

Emergency response organizations may use the local emergency response plan or the state emergency response plan as a model to avoid duplication. If the local or state plan is used, it still must be modified to be specific to the emergency response organization.

A comprehensive response plan must address the hazards that may be encountered in the area. This information will allow the response agency to plan training, protective equipment, and resource needs. Although it is not possible to identify all potential problems in the area, information should be gathered on as many hazards as possible (Box 2-2). Types of chemicals commonly manufactured, used, or stored in the response area should be identified and included in response planning and training. In addition to chemicals used in the community, products that are transported through the area also must be identified and included.

The Superfund Amendment and Reauthorization Act

In 1986 the Environmental Protection Agency (EPA) developed legislation known as the *Superfund Amendment and Reauthorization Act (SARA).* A vital part of this legislation is Title III, also known as *Community Right to Know.* Under this legislation, each state was mandated to form a State Emergency Response Commission (SERC). These commissions formed Local Emergency Planning Committees (LEPC) in local communities. These planning committees were charged with obtaining local company inventory lists of chemicals or Material Safety Data Sheets (MSDS) of chemicals that were on the SARA list of extremely hazardous substances (EHS) above threshold planning quantities. Because EHS chemicals are the focus of the law, reporting may not include complete inventories, and many facilities may not be in compliance. The LEPC can request that all hazardous substances on site, whether or not they are considered an EHS, be re-

BOX 2-1

Preplanning Questions

Who has jurisdiction?
What is the local type of incident management system (IMS) structure? How does EMS fit in?
Capabilities of local responders?
- Fire
- Hazardous materials
- Police
- Health department
- Public utilities

Agency response time?
Local hospital capabilities?
- Decontamination capabilities
- Medical toxicology support
- Special drug/equipment availability (e.g., physiological antagonists, hyperbaric chamber)

Types of hazards that may be found in the area
Types of hazards transported through the local and surrounding community
From whom is decontamination advice available?

BOX 2-2

Information Sources

Local Emergency Planning Committee (LEPC)
SARA Title III reports
Fire department inspections
Fire department reports (previous product releases and problems)
Police or state patrol records
Local industry representatives

ported. Contingency plans also must be developed and provided to the LEPC. Industries also are required to provide inventories or MSDSs to local emergency response agencies. Under this legislation, industries are required to file a report of all chemical releases to the LEPC and SERC. This mandated reporting of inventory and releases is an ideal information source for emergency responders. In addition, this law requires that emergency responders and hospitals be included in the contingency planning process. Committee meetings are held, and direct contact can be made with representatives of the local companies.

The Process Safety Management Standard

Another recent OSHA law, the Process Safety Management Standard (29 CFR 1910.119) will also assist emergency personnel who may respond to fixed-facility emergencies. This standard lists chemicals that, when released, may cause a sitewide problem. The standard requires that facilities conduct emergency planning, failure mode analysis, and training, and have process diagrams and emergency shutdown procedures. Adherence to this standard should reduce chemical releases and help control the releases that do happen. However, only certain chemical processes are covered, and all facilities may not be in compliance.

Additional information regarding chemicals found at local industries can be obtained from fire department inspections and reports concerning prior releases and incidents. The local police department, county sheriff, and state patrol can be excellent sources of information regarding which chemicals are routinely transported through the area.

Responder Health Status

One of the most important preplanning concerns centers on the health status of the responders. Unlike workers who are exposed to relatively few hazardous materials, EMS responders may find themselves in contact with various substances from day to day. An understanding of how different chemicals may affect the responders' health is vital. An example of this principle is exposure to a sensitizer such as an isocyanate. Isocyanates are chemicals that are commonly used in paints, the manufacture of varnishes, and as mediators in chemical reactions. Exposure to a chemical sensitizer may cause an allergic-type reaction in the responder when they subsequently are exposed to other products. In addition, many preexisting medical conditions may be aggravated by exposure to chemicals. Preexisting cardiac, respiratory, nervous system, or skin conditions all may be aggravated by chemical exposure. For example, exposure to ethylene oxide, used in the production of many industrial chemicals and in hospital sterilizers, may aggravate preexisting respiratory system, nervous system, or skin disorders.

The reproductive system also is at risk from certain exposures. Chemicals may interfere with development or maturation of the sperm or egg, cause sterility, a reduced capacity to fertilize, or abnormal development of the fetus. Examples include metals, chlorinated organic compounds, and anesthetics. Some chemicals are considered mutagens. They are able to change the genetic (DNA) structure of the fertilizing sperm or egg in exposed individuals, resulting in birth defects in their offspring. Examples include mercury, lead compounds, mustard gas, hydrazine, and ethylene oxide. Embryo-toxic or fetotoxic products can cause damage to or death of the developing fetus. Other chemicals may be teratogens, which are able to cross the placental membrane and affect the developing embryo, resulting in abnormal development. Examples include methyl mercury, lead compounds, alcohol, and certain insecticides, pesticides, and solvents. Teratogens are most dangerous when the pregnant responder is exposed during the first and second trimesters.

These concepts must be considered when responding to events that include hazardous substances (Box 2-3). Even though EMS responders usually will stay in relatively safe areas, the possibility of exposure is always present. Wind conditions may change, or patients may not be adequately decontaminated, resulting in responder exposure. A knowledge of potential exposure outcomes will allow the responder to institute proper safety procedures.

BOX 2-3

Health Status of the Medical Responder

Previous exposure to poisons
Preexisting medical conditions
Reproductive hazard exposure concerns

Equipment Needs

A major preplanning concern is equipment needs. Inventory check lists should be developed to guide equipment needs. Locations of extra supplies should be identified. Equipment must be compatible with the hazards found in the response area. Protective equipment concerns must be addressed before any response activity. Decisions about protective equipment must be based on responder involvement. Protective equipment commonly used for body substance isolation will be adequate for providing care to patients who have been completely decontaminated. It will not be adequate for use in contaminated areas or for use during primary decontamination activities. In these areas, chemical-protective equipment is needed. The use of this equipment requires special training and selection by a knowledgeable, experienced person. Protective equipment selection and use will be covered in depth in Chapter 8, which discusses personal protective equipment (PPE).

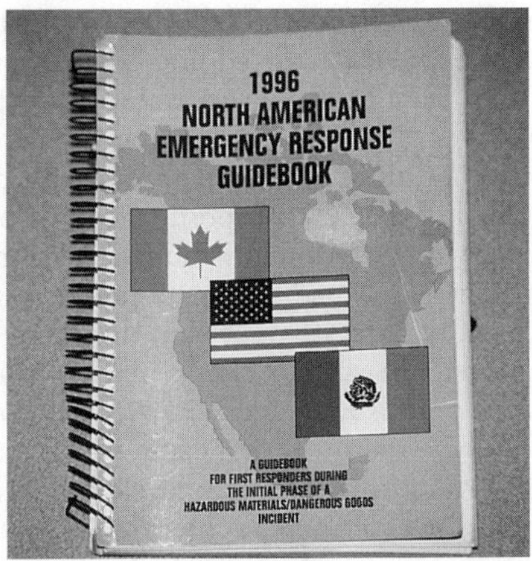

FIG. 2-5 *North American Emergency Response Guidebook.*

Appropriate reference sources also are needed. EMS responders should have access to references that will supply information on safe response activities and detailed hazardous materials medical references to identify patient symptoms and guide treatment. The most commonly used reference by first responders is the *North American Emergency Response Guidebook* (Fig. 2-5).

This convenient reference combines emergency information from the United States, Canada, and Mexico. It will assist the responder in identifying hazardous materials and provides emergency information on potential hazards associated with the chemical. It also provides information on public safety, protective equipment, evacuation, firefighting procedures, spill and leak procedures, and basic first aid. The guide also provides initial isolation and protection distances for many chemicals. This reference, as well as many others, is discussed in detail in Chapter 6.

In addition, special equipment, such as disposable diagnostic/patient care instruments and decontamination equipment, may need to be added to the inventory. A detailed discussion of all equipment concerns will follow in Chapter 10.

Operating Procedures

Operating procedures also must be developed in preplanning. All responders should be trained beforehand to the level of action that they would be expected to take during a response. Specific training needs should be guided by area hazards. Response procedures should be developed to guide safe scene operations. Checklists can be a valuable addition to standard operating procedures (SOPs). Special patient decontamination, treatment, medication, and destination protocols will have to be developed by your local medical adviser.

Summary

Response activities at hazardous materials incidents can be complicated and dangerous. To simplify these responses and ensure responder safety, the use of an IMS is mandatory. The size and organization of the IMS will depend on the specific conditions present at the incident. Another key element of safe response practices is preplanning. Potential problems and solutions need to be identified far in advance of the emergency. A comprehensive emergency response plan will also help to ensure the safety of responders at a hazardous materials emergency. Response to hazardous materials incidents often will require specialized equipment and resources, which need to be identified and made available to responders. Finally, the health status of responders must be considered. Preexisting medical conditions that may be aggravated by chemical exposure must be identified, and appropriate precautions must be taken.

CHAPTER REVIEW QUESTIONS

1. List the six functional areas that are commonly established in an incident management system.
2. Describe the individual tasks of each of the six functional areas in an incident management system.
3. List at least four things that should be identified in assessing a hospital's ability to care for patients exposed to hazardous materials.
4. List at least eight items that should be included in an emergency response plan.
5. List at least four sources of information about hazardous materials that may be found in your response area.
6. Give at least three examples of how hazardous materials may affect preexisting medical conditions.

BIBLIOGRAPHY

Agency for Toxic Substances and Disease Registry: *Hospital emergency departments: a planning guide for the management of contaminated patients,* Atlanta, Ga, 1992, USDHHS.

Agency for Toxic Substances and Disease Registry: *Managing hazardous materials incidents, emergency medical services: a planning guide for the management of contaminated patients,* Atlanta, Ga, 1992, USDHHS.

Andrews LP, editor: *Emergency responder training manual for the hazardous materials technician,* New York, 1992, Van Nostrand Reinhold.

Bowen JE: *Emergency management of hazardous materials incidents,* Quincy, Mass, 1995, National Fire Protection Association.

Bronstein AC, Currance PL: *Emergency care for hazardous materials exposure, ed 2, 1994,* St Louis, Mosby.

Bronstein AC, Currance PL: Module 4: Emergency medical operations. In Ayers S, Christopher J, editors: *Medical response to chemical emergencies,* Washington, DC, 1994, Chemical Manufacturers Association.

Brunancini AV: *Fire command,* Quincy, Mass, 1985, National Fire Protection Association.

Chemical Manufacturers Association: *Crisis management planning for the chemical industry,* Washington, DC, 1991, The Association.

Currance PL: *Hazmat for EMS,* St Louis, 1995, Mosby (videotape and guidebook).

Fire Protection Publications: *Incident command system,* Stillwater, Okla, Fire Protection Publications, 1983, Oklahoma State University.

Guidelines for public sector hazardous materials training. 1998 ed, HMEP Curriculum Guidelines, Emmitsburg, Md, 1998, National Emergency Training Center.

Haddad LM, Shannon MW, Winchester JF: *Clinical management of poisoning and drug overdose,* ed 3, Philadelphia, 1998, WB Saunders.

Hazardous material emergency planning guide. In Tokle G, editor: *Hazardous materials response handbook,* ed 2, Quincy, Mass, 1993, National Fire Protection Association.

Keffer WJ: So you want to start a haz mat team! In Tokle G, editor: *Hazardous materials response handbook,* ed 2, Quincy, Mass, 1993, National Fire Protection Association.

National Fire Protection Association: *NFPA 471, Recommended practice for responding to hazardous materials incidents,* Quincy, Mass, 1992, The Association.

National Fire Protection Association: *NFPA 1561, Technical standard on fire department incident management,* Quincy, Mass, 1990, The Association.

NIOSH/OSHA/USCG/EPA: *Occupational safety and health guidance manual for hazardous waste site activities,* Washington, DC, 1985, DHHS (NIOSH) Publication No 85-115, US Government Printing Office.

Noll GG, Hildebrand MS, Yvorra JG: *Hazardous materials managingthe incident,* ed 2, Stillwater, Okla, 1995, Fire Protection Publications.

Olson KR, editor: *Poisoning and drug overdose,* ed 2, East Norwalk, Conn, 1994, Appleton & Lange.

OSHA: 29 CFR 1910.120, Hazardous waste operations and emergency response; Final rule, March 6, 1989; Washington, DC, US Government Printing Office.

Strong CB, Irvin TR: *Emergency response and hazardous chemical management: principles and practices,* Delray Beach, Fla, 1996, St. Lucie Press.

Sullivan JB, Kreiger GR, editors: *Hazardous material toxicology, clinical principles of environmental health,* Baltimore, 1992, Williams & Wilkins.

Teele BW, editor: *NFPA 1500 Handbook,* Quincy, Mass, 1993, National Fire Protection Association.

Tokle G, editor: *Hazardous materials response handbook,* ed 2, Quincy, Mass, 1993, National Fire Protection Association.

3

Recognition and Identification of Hazardous Materials

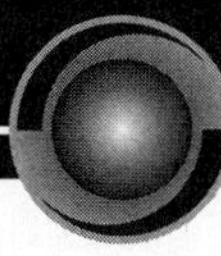

Phil Currance

CHAPTER OBJECTIVES

At the conclusion of this chapter the student will be able to:

- Discuss the importance of recognizing and identifying hazardous materials that may be present during an emergency response.
- Identify possible hazardous materials groups by their transportation containers.
- Discuss the information that may be found on hazardous materials shipping papers.
- Identify the location of shipping papers in commonly encountered transportation means.
- Identify the International/DOT hazard classes.
- Match placards and labels with the appropriate hazard class.
- Discuss how storage containers can be used to identify the type of hazardous materials that they contain.
- Identify various marking/labeling systems that can be found in industrial settings.
- Discuss limitations of industrial marking systems.
- Discuss how planning and reporting requirements can assist in the recognition and identification of hazardous materials in industrial settings.
- Identify commonly used recognition and identification clues.
- Discuss the limitations of each of the recognition clues.

CASE STUDY

A tractor with a semitrailer is being unloaded at a business. The worker unloading the truck starts to complain of nausea, then collapses and has a seizure. Other workers drag the victim onto the dock, and Emergency Medical Services (EMS) is called. As EMS personnel approach the victim and first responders, they notice an unusual odor and a very small amount of grayish vapor inside the truck. First responders also are complaining of nausea. Numerous containers are visible inside the trailer.

- What is the mechanism of injury/illness?
- Could hazardous materials be involved?
- How can the hazardous materials be identified?

The presence of hazardous materials may not always be apparent at the scene of an incident. EMS personnel may be dispatched to a situation at which the presence of hazardous materials has not yet been recognized.

Certain indicators may suggest the presence of hazardous materials at an emergency scene. The types of re-

I dunno... Call me crazy, but somthin' isn't right here.

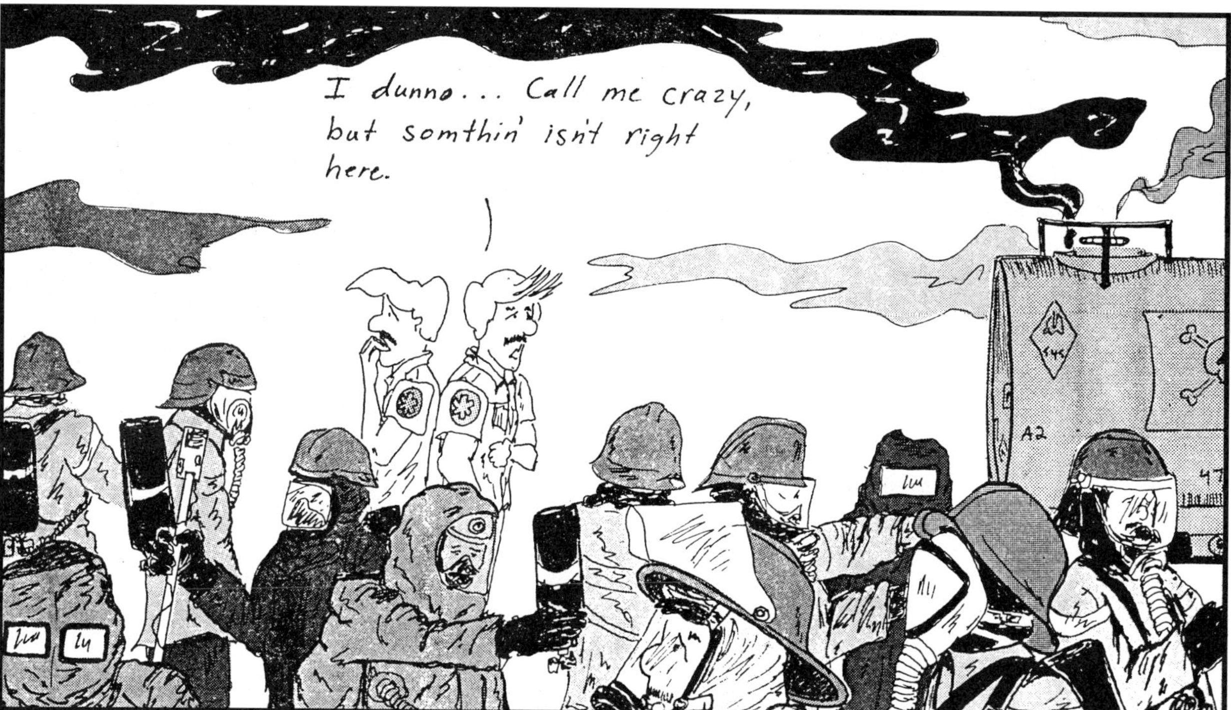

Reprinted with permission from Steve Berry's *I'm Not an Ambulance Driver* cartoon book series.

ported injuries may be an indication of hazardous materials involvement. The presence of multiple patients with similar complaints, such as difficulty breathing, seizures, nausea, disorientation, eye irritation, blisters, or rashes, is a common example.

Dead animals, birds, fish, and insects may be an indication of chemical release. Areas that look different in appearance, such as dead vegetation or lawns that are discolored or withered, or low-lying cloud/foglike conditions that are not explained by normal surroundings are signs of possible chemical presence. Numerous surfaces exhibiting oily droplets/film or numerous water surfaces that have an oily film may be present. Responders may sense unexplained odors or symptoms of irritation. Obviously, by the time responders can determine if some of these indicators are present, they will be in close proximity to the release and probably exposed. The sooner that responders realize that hazardous materials are present and take appropriate precautions, the safer they will be. Personnel must always be aware of their surroundings and be on the lookout for the presence of hazardous materials.

An understanding of how chemicals are transported, stored, and handled will assist responders recognizing and identifying hazardous materials at an incident scene. The recognition and identification of hazardous materials involvement at an emergency scene is the most important element of the response. Safe operating procedures, protective equipment needs, response techniques, and patient care all will depend on this step!

Transportation of Hazardous Materials

Hazardous materials transportation is governed by the Department of Transportation (DOT) regulation known as the *Hazardous Materials Transportation Act (HMTA)* under Chapter 49 of the Code of Federal Regulations. This standard regulates the types of containers used, the markings of those containers, the mode of transportation used, and the types of documentation needed. Recent updates to the HMTA, known as *HM-181,* are bringing United States regulations into international compliance.

Transportation Containers

Containers are used to transport hazardous and nonhazardous materials. They include bulk and nonbulk containers. Nonbulk containers are smaller, individual packages (Fig. 3-1, *A* to *C*). Bags and sacks are used mainly for solid materials. Bottles are used for solids and liquids. Boxes are used for outside packaging for other nonbulk packages. Drums may be used for solids and liquids. Fiber drums and open-top drums commonly are used to contain solids. Tight, or closed-head, drums with bung openings commonly are used to transport liquids. Drums can be made from plastic (commonly used for corrosives) or steel (commonly used for solvents/fuels). Carboys are glass or plastic bottles that may be encased in outer packaging. These commonly are used to transport corrosive products.

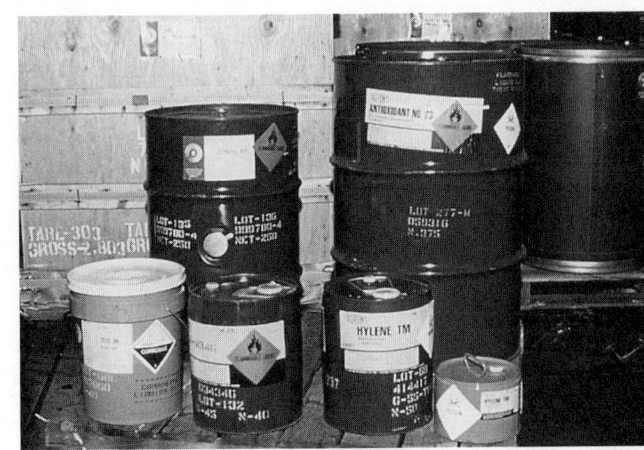

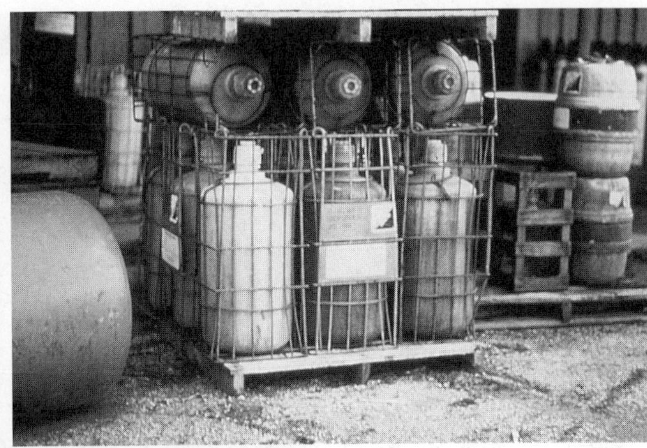

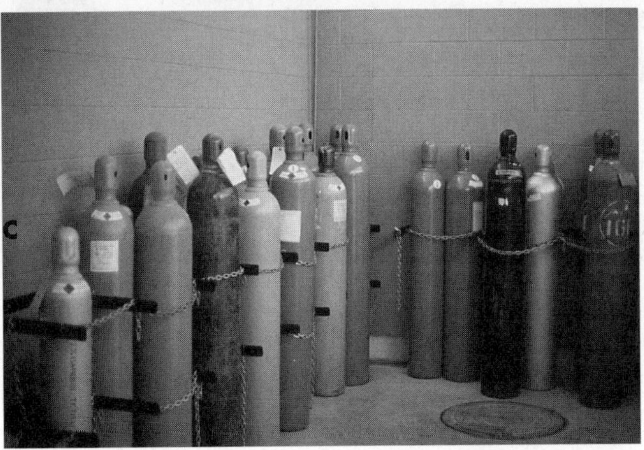

FIG. 3-1 Various types of nonbulk containers. **A,** Drums and pails. **B,** Carboys. **C,** Uninsulated cylinders.

Cylinders are nonbulk containers that normally contain liquified gases, nonliquified gases, or mixtures under pressure. Cylinders may also contain liquids or solids. Typical cylinder types include aerosol containers, uninsulated cylinders, and cryogenic (products cooled to less than −130° F [−90° C]) cylinders. Service pressures can range from a few pounds per square inch (psi) to several thousand pounds psi.

Bulk containers are larger containers and tanks used to transport large quantities of hazardous materials. Large bulk bags are used for transporting solids such as pesticides and fertilizers. Palletized, nonbulk packages consisting of nonbulk packages, such as drums or boxes, that have been placed on a pallet and fastened together with a band or plastic also are considered bulk packages (Fig. 3-2).

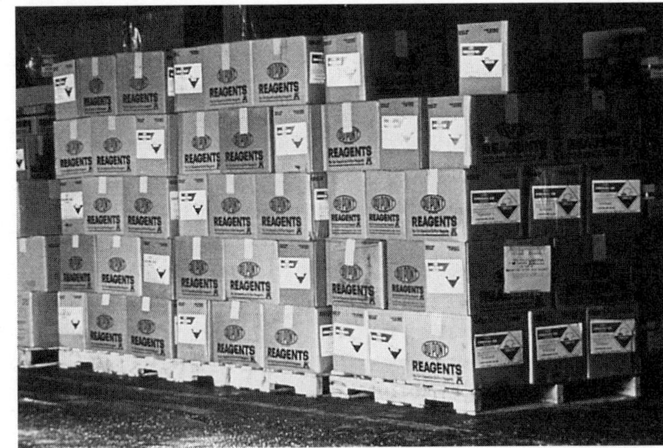

FIG. 3-2 Palletized boxes.

Portable tanks, often called *intermodal tank containers,* are enclosed in a metal supporting frame (Fig. 3-3). These tanks are bulk containers that can be transported by highway, rail, or water. Intermodal tank containers may be of the following types: nonpressure, pressure, refrigerated tank container, or high-pressure tube module.

Portable bins are portable tanks used to transport bulk solids. Ton cylinders are pressure tanks approximately 3 feet by 8 feet that transport liquified gases such as chlorine, sulfur dioxide, and phosgene (Fig. 3-4).

Protective packaging for radioactive materials includes boxes, overpacks, and casks. Shipping boxes are used for low-level shipments (Fig. 3-5). Overpacks may be cylindrical or boxlike. Casks are rigid metal packagings that

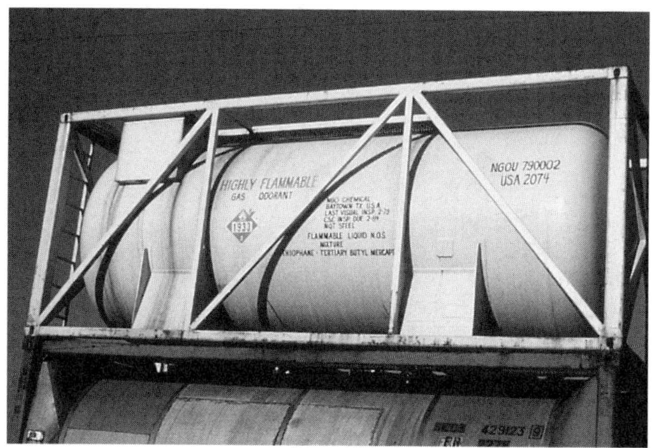

FIG. 3-3 Intermodal container.

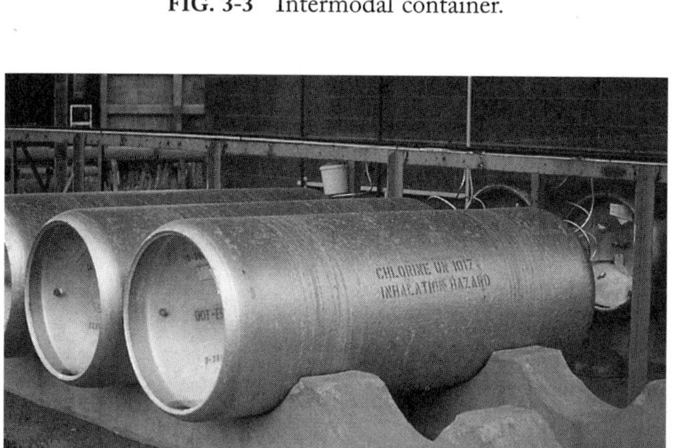

FIG. 3-4 Ton cylinders of chlorine.

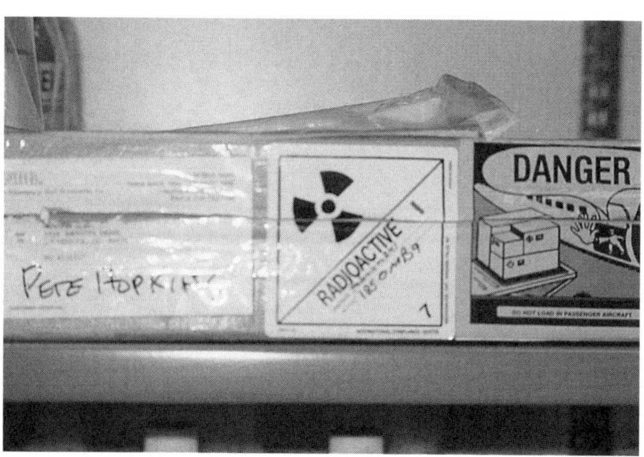

FIG. 3-5 Radioactive shipping box.

range in size up to 10 feet in diameter and 50 feet in length.

Cargo tanks transport bulk liquified or compressed gases, liquids, solids, or molten materials. They may be nonpressurized, pressurized, or of specialized design.

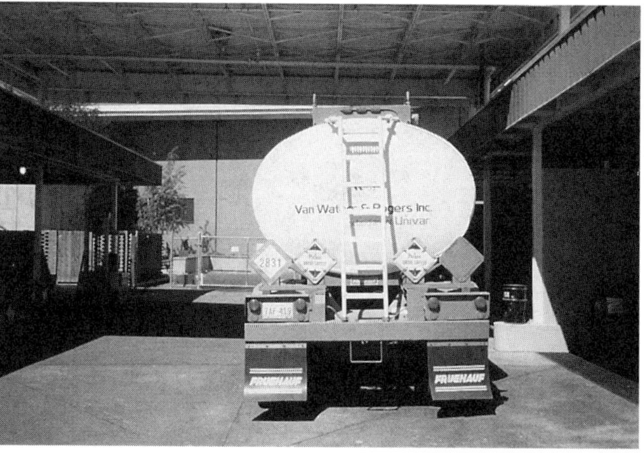

FIG. 3-6 MC 306 tank trailer.

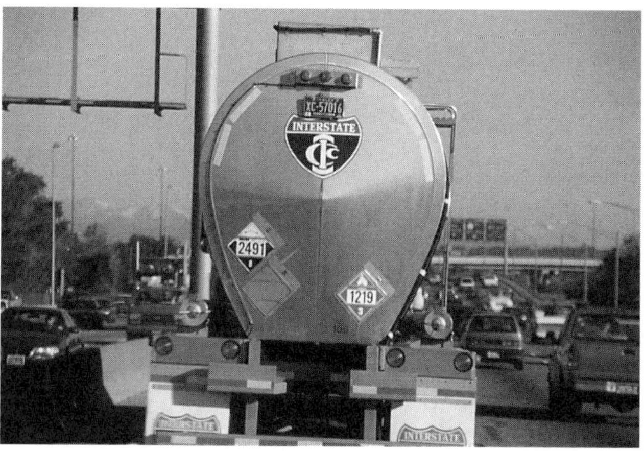

FIG. 3-7 MC 307 tank trailer.

Nonpressurized cars transport liquids. The design of the tank is indicative of the types of products that they transport. Tank trailers designated as Motor Carrier (MC) 306/DOT 406 are commonly seen on the highway (Fig. 3-6). These trailers have an elliptical-shaped cross section with flat ends and commonly are constructed from aluminum. They usually are compartmentalized and hold up to 9000 gallons of a product that is lighter than water, such as hydrocarbon products (gasoline or diesel fuel).

MC 307/DOT 407 tank trailers have a circular type cross section and flat ends and are general-purpose chemical carries (Fig. 3-7). MC 311 and 312/DOT 412 tank trailers have a smaller, rounded cross section with visible supporting rings and flat ends (Fig. 3-8). Occasionally the supporting rings are concealed by an outside jacket. These trucks commonly carry 5000 to 6000 gallons of a product that is heavier than water, such as corrosive products.

Pressurized tank trailers transport liquified and compressed gascs. MC 331 tank trailers have rounded cross sections and rounded ends and carry liquified gas such as liquified petroleum gas (LPG) or anhydrous ammonia (Fig. 3-9).

Specialized cargo tanks include cryogenic carriers,

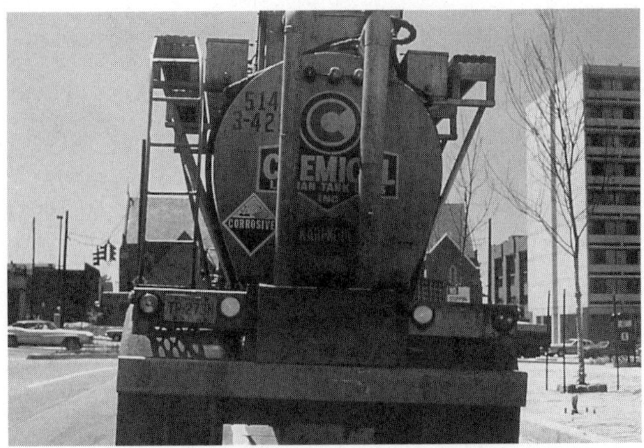

FIG. 3-8 MC 311 tank trailer.

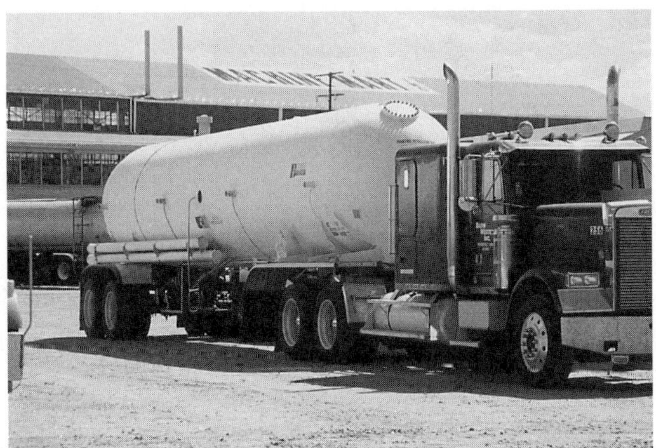

FIG. 3-9 MC 331 tank trailer.

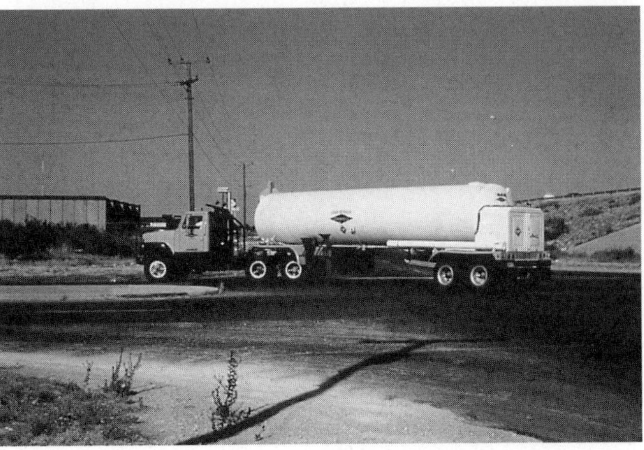

FIG. 3-10 MC 338 tank trailer.

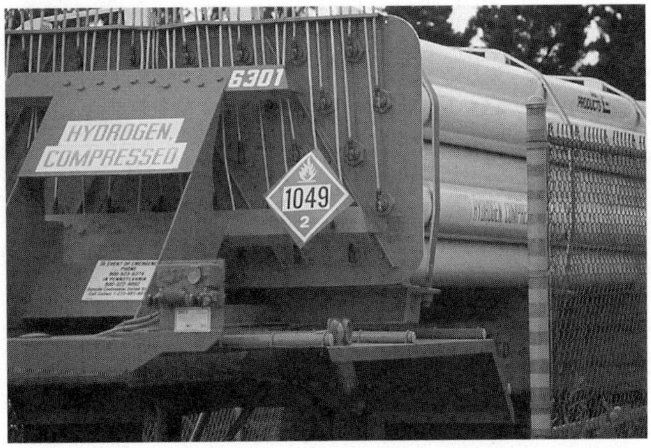

FIG. 3-11 Tube trailer.

tube trailers, and hopper trailers. MC 338 trailers are heavily insulated, cylindrical tanks with a characteristic wagonlike structure on the rear end. These trailers are used to transport cryogenic products (Fig. 3-10). Cryogenic products (i.e., liquid oxygen and nitrogen) are stored and transported in an extremely cold state. Normal, gradual warming of the product causes pressure to build inside the tank. A pressure relief valve then opens, allowing excess pressure to be released. This release of pressure is what causes the vapors that can be regularly seen coming from the relief valve on MC 338 tanks. Tube trailers are trailers carrying multiple cylinders of pressurized gases (Fig. 3-11). Pneumatic hopper trailers have V-shaped compartments with bottom openings and commonly are used to transport dry solids (Fig. 3-12).

Trucks and semitrailers include flatbed and box designs. Flatbed trailers can carry intermodal containers, ton cylinders, or nonbulk containers. Box semitrailers may carry any type of nonbulk container.

Rail freight cars can be nonpressure type; pressure type; specialized types, such as hopper and gondola cars; flatcars; and boxcars. Nonpressure cars transport liquid products (Fig. 3-13). Even though these containers are

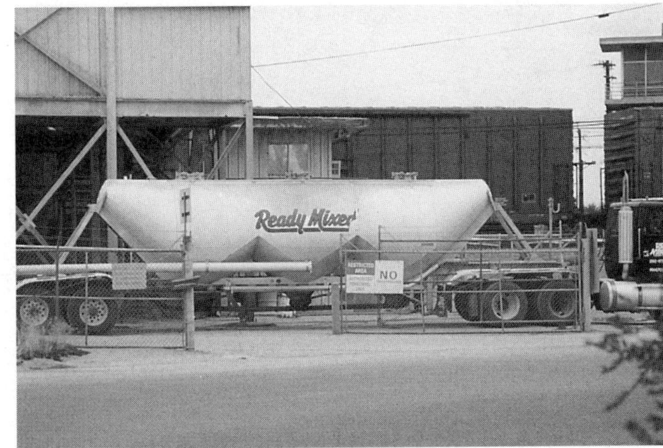

FIG. 3-12 Pneumatic hopper trailer.

classified as nonpressure, they may hold vapor pressure up to 100 lbs psi. They may be insulated or thermally protected. Most nonpressure cars can be identified by visible fittings on the top of the car and unloading valves on the bottom of the car.

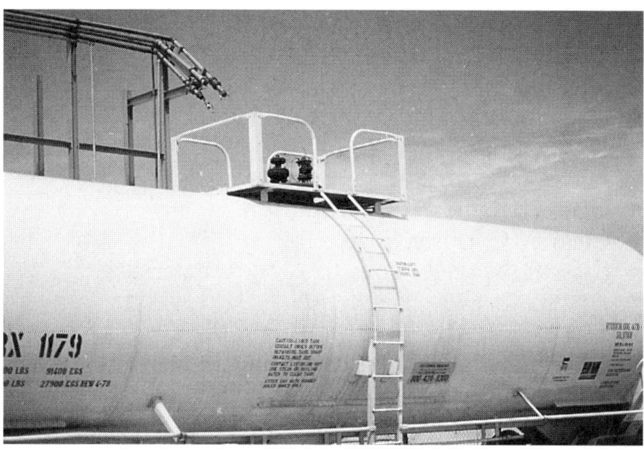

FIG. 3-13 Nonpressurized railcar.

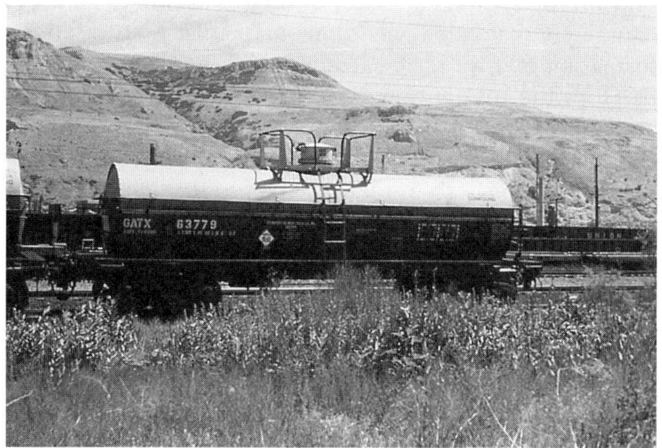

FIG. 3-14 Pressurized railcar.

Pressurized tank cars transport liquified gases (Fig. 3-14). Some of these cars are thermally protected. These tanks typically are identified by the presence on the top of the car of a single protective housing (dome), which contains all of the valves and fittings. Occasionally, nonpressure cars, such as those used to transport nitric acid, will have a protective housing similar to those found on pressure type cars.

Specialized tank cars include cryogenic and high-pressure (tube) cars. Cryogenic cars transport extremely cold (cryogenic) liquids. These are heavily insulated tanks within a tank and are usually identified by the lack of fittings on the top of the car. Another type of cryogenic tank is built inside a boxcar (Fig. 3-15). High-pressure (tube) tank cars are multiple, seamless, steel cylinders mounted horizontally in a frame with open sides. All of the cylinders on a given car will contain the same material.

Hopper cars transport bulk solids (Fig. 3-16). They have two or more sloping sided bays on the bottom. They may be open top, closed top, or pneumatically unloaded. Gondolas are similar to hopper cars in that they transport bulk ores and other solid materials. They have solid floors

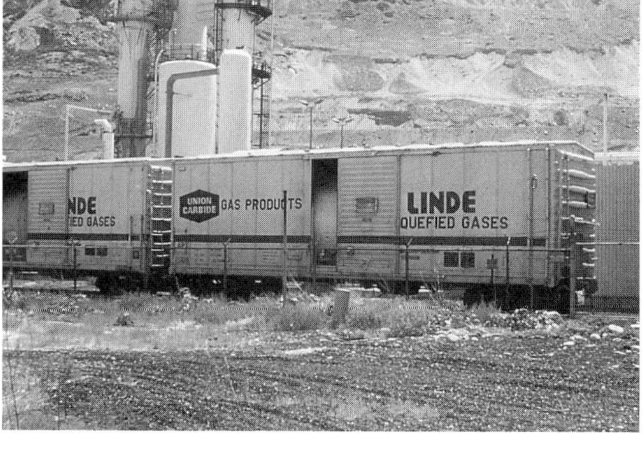

FIG. 3-15 Cryogenic car.

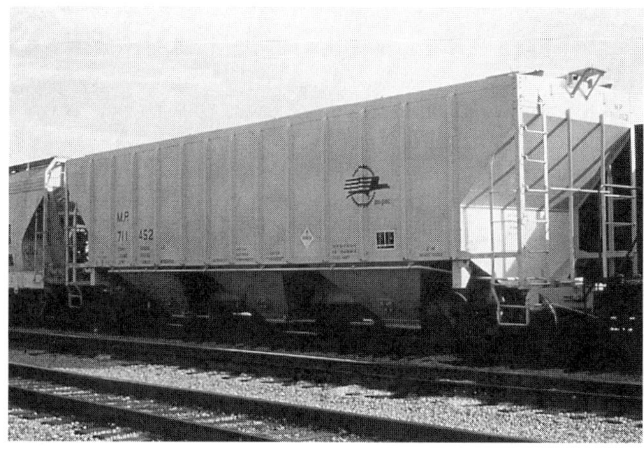

FIG. 3-16 Hopper car.

and sides and may have a removable top for weather protection. Flatcars are commonly used to transport intermodal containers and van trailers. Boxcars are enclosed rail freight cars with doors. They are used to transport nonbulk containers.

Pipelines also are transport containers. Pipelines should be marked with the product, owner, and emergency telephone number (Fig. 3-17). The emergency telephone number will connect the caller with a control room, where an operator monitors pipeline operations and can initiate shutdown procedures in case of an emergency. Many pipeline systems are monitored through a computerized program that logs the time and date a product was injected into the pipeline and its estimated delivery date and time. Although most pipelines are dedicated to a single product, in some cases pipelines can carry different materials at different times.

Transportation Identification Systems

Under DOT 49 CFR, containers carrying hazardous materials must be identified. To assist with identification of hazardous materials, the DOT organizes hazardous materials according to the international hazard classes. This classification system comprises nine classes of hazardous materials. Many of these classes are further divided into divisions to represent various degrees or types of hazards. An understanding of these classifications and the types of hazards that they represent will allow responders to anticipate the potential harm if the hazardous materials are released from their container. To assist responders in remembering the different hazard classes and placards, they are listed in the *North American Emergency Response Guidebook.*

The nine classes of hazardous materials

The nine classes of hazardous materials are as follows:

- Class 1 (Explosives)
  Division 1.1: Mass detonation hazard
  Division 1.2: Mass detonation hazard with fragments
  Division 1.3: Fire hazard with minor blast or projectile hazard
  Division 1.4: Explosive substances that present no significant hazard
  Division 1.5: Very insensitive explosives
  Division 1.6: Extremely insensitive explosives
- Class 2 (Gases)
  Division 2.1: Flammable gases
  Division 2.2: Nonflammable gases
  Division 2.3: Poisonous gases
- Class 3 (Flammable/combustible liquids)
  Division 3.1: Liquids with flash points < 0° F
  Division 3.2: Liquids with flash points from 0° F to 73° F
  Division 3.3: Liquids with flash points from 73° F to 141° F
  Combustible liquids
- Class 4 (Flammable solids)
  Division 4.1: Flammable solids
  Division 4.2: Spontaneously combustible or pyrophoric solids/liquids
  Division 4.3: Dangerous when wet

WARNING
PETROLEUM
PIPELINE
BEFORE EXCAVATING OR IN EMERGENCY CALL COLLECT
COLONIAL PIPELINE COMPANY
ATLANTA, GEORGIA
404-261-1471

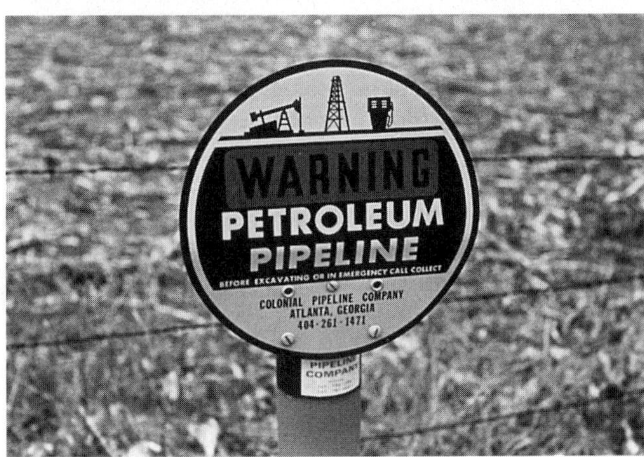

FIG. 3-17 Pipeline identification sign.

- Class 5 (Oxidizing substances)
  Division 5.1: Oxidizing substances
  Division 5.2: Organic peroxides
- Class 6 (Poisonous and infectious substances)
  Division 6.1: Poisons
  Division 6.2: Infectious substances
- Class 7 (Radioactive substances)
- Class 8 (Corrosive materials)
- Class 9 (Miscellaneous hazardous materials)

DOT placarding and labeling system

The DOT has adopted a placarding and labeling system to assist emergency responders in identifying hazardous materials involved in an incident. These placards are a valuable clue in determining the presence and preliminary identification of hazardous materials. Placards are diamond-shaped, 10¾-inch square, point-to-point signs that are placed on the sides and ends of bulk transport containers that carry hazardous materials. They relay information by four means: color background, a symbol on the top, the international class number on the bottom, and the hazard class wording or a four-digit identification number, known as the *ID number,* in the center. This number can be used to identify the product, using several resources such as the *North American Emergency Response Guidebook.*

DOT and international labels are 4-inch square versions of the placards. They are used on individual containers such as barrels, boxes, and bags. Regulations require that a product that fits into multiple hazard classes be labeled for each class that is appropriate.

- Explosive placards/labels are orange and have a symbol showing an exploding ball with fragments on the top and a division number (1.1 to 1.6) on the bottom. The word "Explosive" or a four-digit ID number appears in the center of the symbol.
- Compressed or liquified gas placards/labels are red (flammable), green (nonflammable), or white (poison); have a fire symbol, gas cylinder symbol, or a skull and crossbones on the top; and a division number (2.1 to 2.3) on the bottom. These symbols will have either "Flammable Gas," "Nonflammable Gas," or "Poison Gas" wording or a four-digit ID number in the center.
- Flammable/combustible liquids placards/labels are red, have a flame symbol on the top, and a division number (3.1 to 3.3) on the bottom. They will have the wording "Flammable Liquid" or "Combustible Liquid," or a four-digit ID number in the center.
- Flammable solid placards/labels are red and white striped (flammable solids), red over white (spontaneously combustible solids and liquids, or blue (dangerous when wet); have a flame symbol on the top; and a division number (4.1 to 4.3) on the bottom. They will have the wording "Flammable Solid," "Spontaneously Combustible," or "Dangerous When Wet" or a four-digit ID number in the center.

- Oxidizing substances placards/labels are yellow, have a symbol showing an O with flames on the top, and a division number (5.1 to 5.2) on the bottom. They will have the wording "Oxidizer" or "Organic Peroxide" or a four-digit ID number in the center.
- Poison liquid and solid material and infectious material placards/labels are white, have either a skull and crossbones, biomedical symbol, or grain stock with an X through it (depending on material) on the top; and a division number (6.1 to 6.2) on the bottom. These symbols will have the wording "Poison," "Infectious Material," "Keep Away From Foodstuffs" or a four-digit ID number in the center.
- Radioactive materials placards/labels are yellow over white, have the radioactive "propeller" symbol on the top, and the number 7 on the bottom. Labels must identify the radionuclide and the amount of activity in the package. They will have the Roman numerals I, II, or III in the center to identify the level of hazard and type of container and space to write in specific information. The I, II, or III numbering designates the amount of radiation that is detectable from outside the package. The labels will have the wording "Radioactive Material" or a four-digit ID number in the center.
- Corrosive material placards/labels are white over black, have a symbol showing a test tube spilling liquid onto a human thumb and a piece of steel on the top, and have the number 8 on the bottom. The word "Corrosive" or a four-digit ID number appears in the center.
- Miscellaneous hazardous materials placards/labels are black and white striped over white and have the number 9 on the bottom. They will have a four-digit ID number in the center.

Certain hazardous materials, regardless of the quantity, must always be placarded when transported. These materials include most explosive products, poisonous gases, water-reactive flammable solids, and most radioactive substances. Other products do not have to be identified by a placard unless more than 1001 lbs gross weight is carried. Under certain circumstances, when a mixed load is carried, a placard that reads "Dangerous" may be used. Many products can fit into multiple hazard classes (i.e., flammable and poison). In most cases the DOT has determined that only one placard (the greatest hazard) is needed on the outside of the bulk container. Empty tank trucks must remain placarded until they are cleaned. Empty rail tanks may be placarded as "Residue." These tanks may contain up to 3% of the tank's capacity.

Four-digit identification numbers

Four-digit ID numbers, also known as *United Nations (UN), North American (NA),* or *Product Identification numbers (PIN),* often can be found on the sides and ends of bulk transport containers. These numbers often are found on the placard or on an orange panel located adjacent to the placard (Fig. 3-18). They are used to identify the product, using the *North American Emergency Response Guidebook, Emergency Response for Hazardous Materials Exposure,* or other reference. They also may be found in the center of a placard-sized white panel for hazardous substances and wastes not requiring a placard.

Transportation Documentation

Under DOT regulations, shipments of hazardous materials must be accompanied by shipping papers or proper documentation to identify the materials being transported (Fig. 3-19). Shipping papers will contain the proper shipping name, hazard classification, ID number, number and type of packages, packing group, and correct weight.

The packing group number (I, II, or III) will identify the relative degree of danger associated with the material. Packing group number I is the most dangerous; group number III is the least dangerous. Shipping papers will identify hazardous materials in the shipment either by listing them first on the manifest, listing them in a contrasting color, or by check marks placed in a hazardous

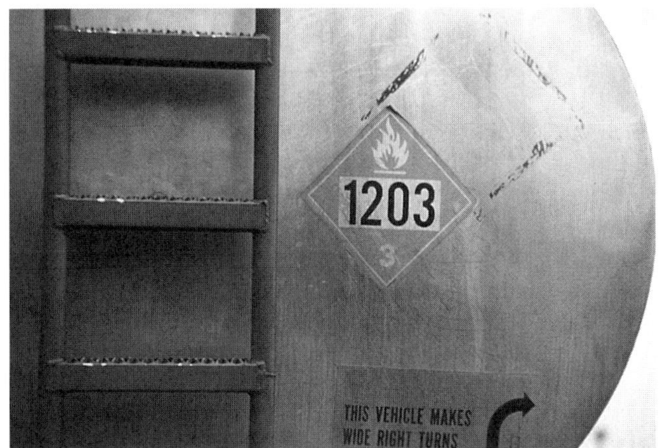

FIG. 3-18 Placard and four-digit ID number.

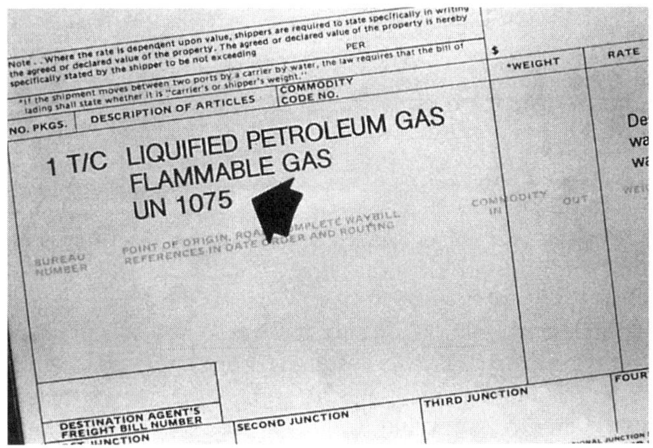

FIG. 3-19 Shipping papers.

materials identifying column. If a notation of "RQ" is listed, it identifies that chemical as having a reportable quantity listed in EPA regulations. If a specified quantity of an RQ chemical is released, the party responsible for the release must immediately notify the National Response Center in Washington, D.C., by calling 1-800-424-8802. The National Response Center (NRC), which is operated by the United States Coast Guard, receives reports when dangerous goods or hazardous substances are spilled. After receiving notification of an incident, the NRC will immediately notify the appropriate federal on-scene coordinator and concerned federal agencies.

Shipping papers for radioactive materials must identify the radionuclide and the amount of activity in the packages. Additional information for radioactive materials includes the physical and chemical form of the material. The terms *special form* and *Type B* indicate that radioactive materials are contained in packages that have been designed and tested to withstand accidents.

In truck shipments, papers can be found in the cab. Most often they are in a plastic envelope attached to the inside of the drivers door. For trains that still have a caboose, papers will be there. If no caboose is present, they will be in the lead engine. For air shipments, they can be found in the cockpit. On ships, papers are found on the bridge or wheelhouse. Under new DOT regulations, shipping papers must have a 24-hour emergency contact telephone number. Regulations also state that written emergency response information must accompany the shipment.

Another type of shipping paper is the Uniform Hazardous Waste Manifest, which is required by the Environmental Protection Agency (EPA) for all hazardous waste shipments. Similar to a shipping paper, it will identify the name and type of waste, number, and weight of containers, and the name of the waste generator.

Storage and Handling of Hazardous Materials

Just as in transportation, the way that hazardous materials are stored and handled will provide information to emergency response personnel. Understanding the types of containers and marking systems in use at fixed facilities can assist in hazard assessment and decision making.

Storage Containers

Chemicals are stored at fixed facilities in nonbulk and bulk containers. Bulk storage tanks include both pressure and nonpressure containers. Nonpressure, or atmospheric, storage tanks include aboveground vertical tanks with various types of roof designs, horizontal tanks, and underground storage tanks (Fig. 3-20). Low-pressure tanks include spheroid (round) and noded, spheroid tanks. High-pressure tanks include spheres and rounded-end pressure vessels (Fig. 3-21).

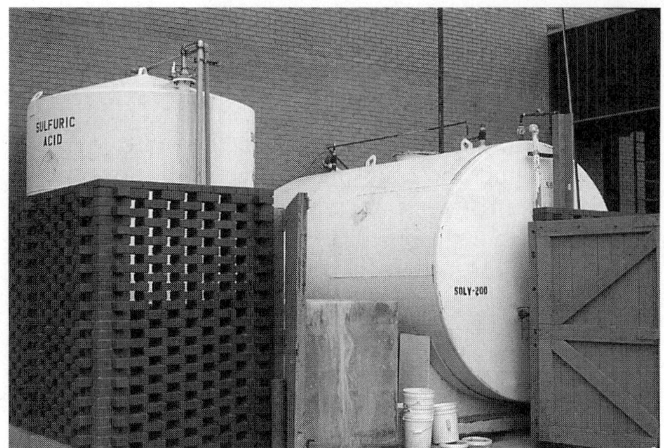

FIG. 3-20 Nonpressure tanks.

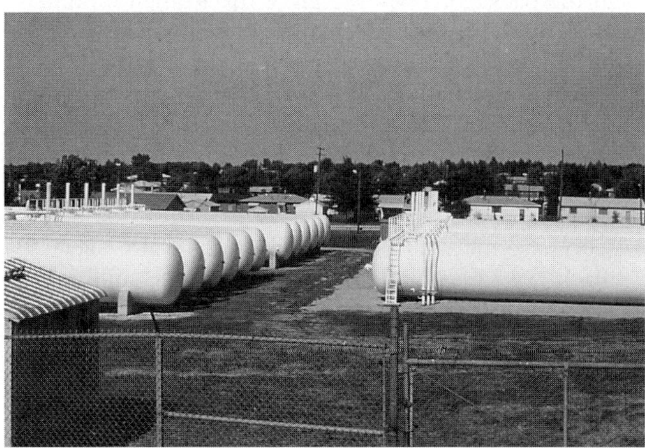

FIG. 3-21 Pressurized tanks.

Bulk containers may display marking systems, ID numbers, or the name of the product. Many bulk containers also may be marked with the storage capacity. Some pipelines at facilities may be marked to show the chemical that they transport, but it is not required by federal law.

Fixed Facility Marking and Labeling Systems

Various hazardous materials marking systems are used at facilities. One of the most popular is the National Fire Protection Association (NFPA) 704 system (Box 3-1). This system is designed to provide responders with information regarding the material inside the tank, building, or laboratory. This system uses a diamond-shaped sign that is divided into color-coded quadrants (Fig. 3-22). The red quadrant on top indicates fire hazard, the blue quadrant on the left indicates health hazard, the yellow quadrant on the right indicates reactivity, and the white quadrant on the bottom is for special information. Numbers in the red, blue, and yellow quadrants indicate the degree of hazard. These numbers range from 0 to 4 and

BOX 3-1

NFPA 704 System

RED SECTION/FLAMMABILITY HAZARD

4: Materials that will rapidly or completely vaporize at atmospheric pressure and normal ambient temperature, or that are readily dispersed in air and that will burn readily
3: Liquids and solids that can be ignited under almost all ambient temperature conditions
2: Materials that must be moderately heated or exposed to relatively high ambient temperatures before ignition can occur
1: Materials that must be preheated before ignition can occur
0: Materials that will not burn

BLUE SECTION/HEALTH HAZARD

4: Materials that on very short exposure could cause death or major residual injury
3: Materials that on short exposure could cause serious temporary or residual injury
2: Materials that on intense or continued, but not chronic, exposure could cause temporary incapacitation or possible residual injury
1: Materials that on exposure would cause irritation but only minor residual injury
0: Materials that on exposure under fire conditions would offer no hazard beyond that of ordinary combustible material

YELLOW SECTION/REACTIVITY HAZARD

4: Materials that in themselves are readily capable of detonation or of explosive decomposition or reaction at normal temperatures and pressures
3: Materials that in themselves are capable of detonation or explosive decomposition or reaction but require a strong initiating source or that must be heated under confinement before initiation or that react explosively with water
2: Materials that readily undergo violent chemical change at elevated temperatures and pressures or that react violently with water or that may form explosive mixtures with water
1: Materials that in themselves are normally stable but that can become unstable at elevated temperatures and pressures
0: Materials that in themselves are normally stable, even under fire exposure conditions, and that are not reactive with water

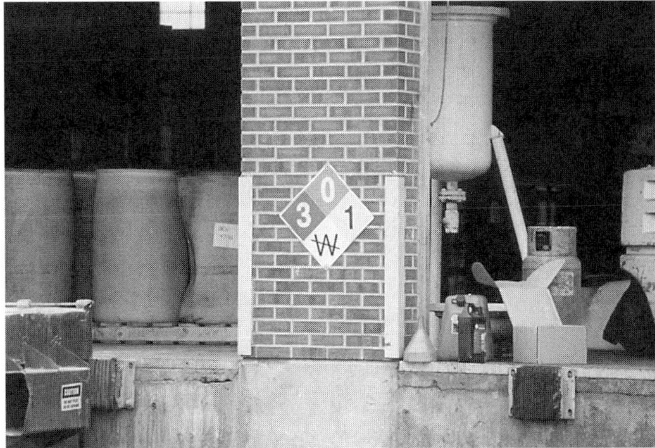

FIG. 3-22 The NFPA 704 system.

indicate specific levels of hazard. In general, a minimal hazard is indicated by the number 0 and a severe hazard by the number 4.

Special information symbols, such as OXY for an oxidizing product or a W with a slash indicating a product that is dangerous when wet, may be found in the white quadrant. Although this system provides useful information, it does have its limitations. When used on the outside of a building or laboratory, it will tell you that the structure contains hazards that meet the marking criteria. It does not specify exactly what the material is, the quantity, or the exact location. When used on a single container, such as a tank, the information is specific. The system is designed under strict criteria and sometimes is not interpreted properly. For example, the health hazard is often based on acute toxicity and may not reflect chronic toxicity. The reactivity hazard is based on the susceptibility of materials to release energy either by themselves or in combination with water. Water reactivity, fire exposure, shock, and pressure were factors considered. This system may not identify reactivity with other chemicals. For example, chlorine is highly reactive with almost everything, but it carries a zero reactivity hazard in the NFPA 704 system.

Other markings may be present. The military uses distinctly shaped markings and signs to designate certain hazards (Fig. 3-23). Both explosion/fire and chemical hazard symbols are used.

Labels often are found on hazardous-substance containers. The Occupational Safety and Health Administration (OSHA) Hazard Communication Standard (29 CFR 1910.1200), commonly referred to as *HAZCOM*, requires that containers of hazardous substances be labeled so that workers are informed of their respective hazards. Many types of labels are used to accomplish this. Manufacturers usually include a label on their containers that specifies the name of the manufacturer, name of the chemical, major hazards associated with the chemical, and a telephone number to call for additional information. A common method is to supplement the manufacturers label with Hazardous Materials Identification System (HMIS) or Hazardous Materials Identification Guide (HMIG) labels (Fig. 3-24).

These two systems use a label that is similar to the NFPA 704 system just discussed. These labels contain

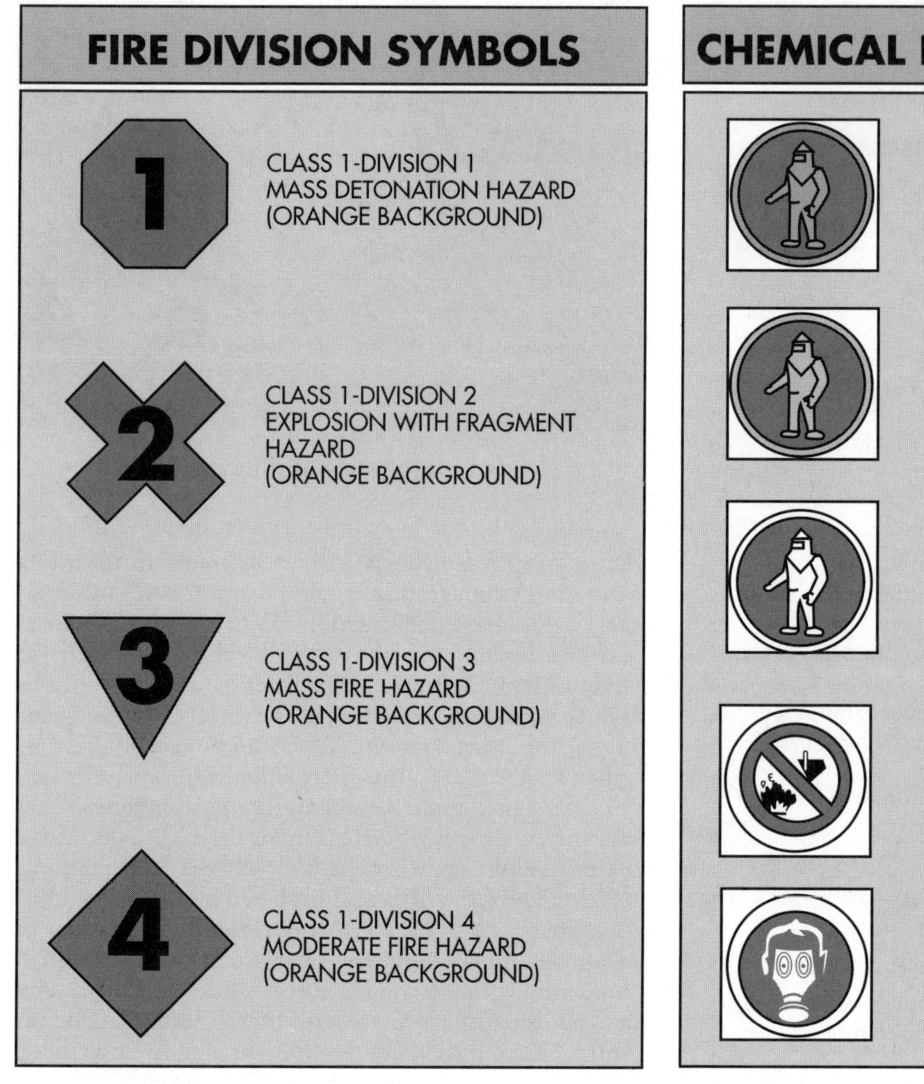

FIG. 3-23 Various military marking systems.

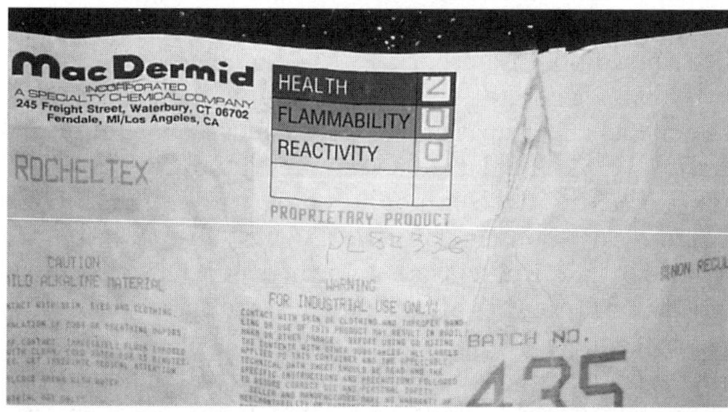

FIG. 3-24 Container with HAZCOM and HMIS labels.

the product name and protective equipment needs, and use a system similar to the NFPA system to supply information on the health, flammability, and reactivity hazards of the substance. Another label that responders may encounter is the EPA Hazardous Waste Label (Fig. 3-25). This label contains the name of the waste, ID numbers, the name of the generator of the waste, and the accumulation start date (the date when the waste first was placed in the container).

Under EPA regulations, specific information must be available on a label for pesticide containers (Fig. 3-26). This information must include the name of the pesticide, a signal word indicating toxicity (Danger—High, Warning—Moderate, Caution—Low), the EPA registration number, a precautionary statement, hazard statement, and the names of the active ingredient(s).

The United States National Bureau of Standards has developed a suggested standard for color-coding cylinders, but the standard is not required. Currently the only uniform coloring system being used is for gases intended for medical use. The color code for medical cylinders (in the United States) includes:

- Carbon dioxide: gray
- Carbon dioxide/oxygen: gray and green

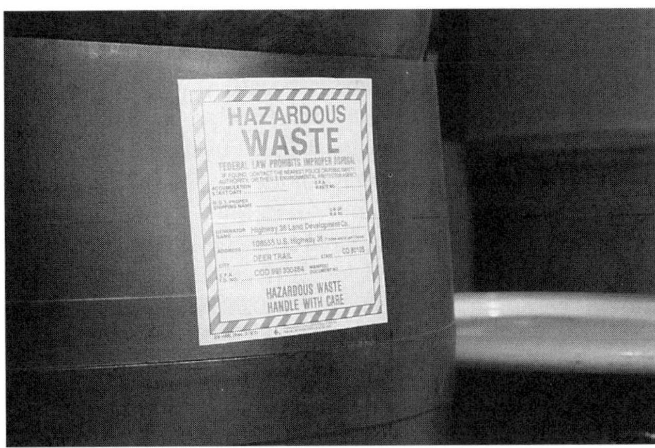

FIG. 3-25 EPA hazardous waste label.

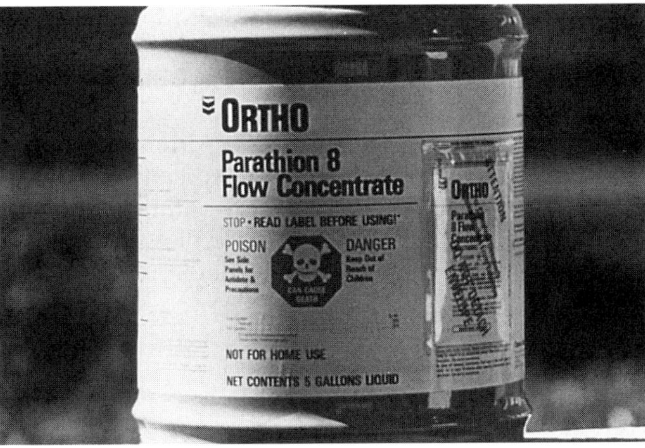

FIG. 3-26 Pesticide label.

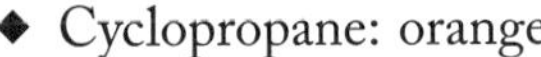

- Cyclopropane: orange
- Ethylene: red
- Helium: brown
- Helium/oxygen: brown and green
- Nitrogen: black
- Nitrous oxide: blue
- Oxygen: green
- Air: yellow

Use of Recognition and Identification Clues

An understanding of how chemicals are stored, used, and transported will assist EMS responders in recognizing and identifying hazardous materials, however, the concept must be used in an organized manner. The National Fire Academy/National Emergency Training Center manual, *Recognizing and Identifying Hazardous Materials,* outlines six clues that may confirm the presence of hazardous materials. They are as follows:

- Occupancy/location
- Container shape
- Markings and colors
- Placards and labels
- Shipping papers/manifests
- Use of senses

These clues are based on increasing risk, that is, as emergency responders approach the scene they can gather more information but the risk increases. It must be understood that these clues provide limited pieces of information, which then must be used with other sources to provide a clear picture of the situation. In many ways, they are like pieces of a jigsaw puzzle. With only one or two pieces, it is impossible to visualize what the completed puzzle will look like. The more pieces that are added, the more complete the picture will look. Although these clues provide valuable information, they have their benefits and limitations.

Occupancy and Location

The first and safest clue to hazardous substance involvement is knowledge of the types of materials that may be present in the community. Manufacturing facilities, refineries, laboratories, construction sites, hazardous waste sites, and agricultural areas are examples of locations where hazardous substances commonly are found. Responders should be aware of the hazards in their response area before a problem occurs. Inspections and Superfund Amendment and Reauthorization Act (SARA) Title III reporting data will assist responders with this clue. Obviously this clue has some major limitations. Inspections will provide information only on the chemicals that were present on the day and time of the inspection. This may change daily. SARA reporting requirements usually involve only extremely hazardous substances as defined by the law and then only in certain quantities. In an emergency situation, other chemicals may prove to be extremely dangerous. The accuracy of this clue depends on the adequacy of the inspection or report. Many things can be overlooked or missed. Another concern is the transportation of hazardous materials through the area. Information may be available from area users, transporters, and local police agencies. However, these sources will not be able to track all of the chemicals moving through the area.

Containers

Containers will be one of the first clues to look for when responding to a hazardous materials incident. The presence of hazardous materials containers at an incident is an indication that chemicals may be involved, and the shape of the containers may assist in determining the type of hazardous material(s) present. Containers also will provide information on the state of matter that may be released. In most cases solids, liquids, and gases are packed in distinctive containers. The type of material that the container is made from may provide additional information. For example, plastic drums usually contain a corrosive material. Fixed-facility tanks also are an indicator of the type of chemical contained within. Some containers are indicative of certain types of hazardous materials. Truck trailers are excellent examples. Tank shape can be an important clue in some cases, whereas in others, such as a boxcar or standard cargo truck, the individual containers that they carry are not visible. Although the container shape may not identify the exact chemical involved, it may provide preliminary information with which to assess the scene. For example, pressurized products usually present a greater hazard during a release than do liquid products.

Markings and Colors

As responders move closer to the scene, certain markings and colors may be apparent, possibly providing an indication of the product located inside the container. At fixed facilities, the four-color NFPA 704 system commonly is used. The American Association of Railroads requires that railcars that carry certain substances have the name of the substance stenciled on the side of the car. Colors may also be used to relay information. Although it is not totally reliable, an industry standard of colors for medical compressed-gas cylinders is often used. In addition to these markings, company names, ID numbers, and telephone numbers often are found on containers. The license number of the vehicle can be used to identify the owner and eventually the cargo.

Placards and Labels

Although placards are a valuable source of information, they may not always be present. Legally, only certain hazardous materials must be placarded, no matter what the quantity. Many hazardous materials do not have to be placarded unless a gross weight of more than 1001 lbs is carried. A placard with the word "Dangerous" can be used on certain mixed loads of hazardous materials. DOT regulations require that nonbulk containers be labeled for each hazard class that they fit, but in most cases, only one placard (the DOT determines the most significant hazard) will be required on the outside of the vehicle that is carrying those containers. An excellent example is nitric acid. Drums of nitric acid must be labeled as corrosive, oxidizer, and poison. Tank trucks transporting nitric acid must be placarded as corrosive. Many chemicals will present multiple hazards (e.g., flammable and poison), but will require only one label or placard. The exact label and placard needed is specified in DOT regulations. Remember that placards and labels may not always be present, or that the container/vehicle may be improperly labeled or placarded.

Shipping Papers

Shipping papers are usually an extremely accurate source for determining the identity of hazardous cargos. They can clarify what is labeled as dangerous on placards. Shipping papers should accompany all shipments of hazardous substances. Under new DOT regulations, shipping papers must list a 24-hour emergency information telephone number. The problem with shipping papers is their location. In most cases, responders will come into close proximity with the hazardous substances when retrieving shipping papers. Responders should never attempt to enter a hazardous materials scene to obtain shipping papers unless they have received proper training and are wearing appropriate protective equipment. Although shipping papers usually are accurate, they may be improperly filled out or missing.

Senses

Senses include any personal physiological reactions. Visual signs, such as visible vapor clouds, visible liquid or solid products; dead or incapacitated people or animals, dead vegetation, or odor and irritation to the skin or eyes, can signal the presence of hazardous materials. Because the use of most senses requires that responders be near the incident, relying on senses may result in exposure and therefore is not recommended. The use of sight, preferably aided by binoculars, can provide valuable information from a safe distance. Determine if anybody that was on site at the time of the release noted any unusual sights, sounds, or smells.

Some substances do not have adequate warning properties. Many are colorless, odorless, and tasteless. Many are not detectable until a toxic level has been reached. Some are able to impair the sense of smell. An example is hydrogen sulfide. It is detectable at low concentrations, but at higher levels causes olfactory fatigue (desensitization of the sense of smell). The odor will disappear, leading responders to believe that they are in a safe area. Radioactive materials are not detectable by the senses.

Summary

When responding to an emergency, first responders must be able to detect the presence of hazardous materials. The effectiveness and safety of response practices depends on the rapid recognition and identification of hazardous materials involved in the incident. An understanding of how hazardous materials are transported, stored, and used will assist responders in this vital task.

CHAPTER REVIEW QUESTIONS

1. List at least four types of nonbulk containers and the type of hazardous material that they may contain.
2. List at least four types of bulk containers and the type of hazardous materials that they may contain.
3. Describe the differences among MC 306, 307, 311, 331, and 338 cargo tanks.
4. Describe how to determine if a railcar is of the pressure or nonpressure type.

5. List the nine international hazard classes.
6. Identify the colors and symbols used on each of the nine international hazard classes.
7. Identify the locations at which hazardous materials shipping papers may be kept.
8. Describe the NFPA 704 hazardous materials classification system, and discuss its limitations.
9. Identify two types of hazardous materials labels, and list the information on each.
10. List the six commonly used hazardous materials recognition and identification clues.

BIBLIOGRAPHY

Agency for Toxic Substances and Disease Registry: *Managing hazardous materials incidents, emergency medical services: a planning guide for the management of contaminated patients,* Atlanta, Ga, 1992, US-DHHS.

Andrews LP, editor: *Emergency responder training manual for the hazardous materials technician,* New York, 1992, Van Nostrand Reinhold.

Bowen JE: *Emergency management of hazardous materials incidents,* Quincy, Mass, 1995, National Fire Protection Association.

Bronstein AC, Currance PL: *Emergency care for hazardous materials exposure, ed 2, 1994,* St Louis, Mosby.

Coleman RJ, Williams KH: *Hazardous materials dictionary,* Lancaster, Pa, 1988, Technomic Publishing.

Currance PL: *Hazmat for EMS,* St Louis, 1995, Mosby (videotape and guidebook).

DOT: *1996 North American emergency response guidebook,* Office of Hazardous Materials Transportation, Research and Special Programs Administration, Washington, DC, 1996, US Department of Transportation.

Guidelines for public sector hazardous materials training. 1998 ed, HMEP Curriculum Guidelines, Emmitsburg, Md, 1998, National Emergency Training Center.

Hazardous materials response training program, New Jersey/New York, 1988, Hazardous Materials Worker/Training Program.

National Fire Protection Association: *NFPA 471, Recommended practice for responding to hazardous materials incidents,* Quincy, Mass, 1992, The Association.

Noll GG, Hildebrand MS, Yvorra JG: *Hazardous materials: managing the incident,* ed 2, Stillwater, Okla, 1995, Fire Protection Publications.

Ricks RC, Leonard RB: *Hospital emergency department of radiation accidents,* Washington, DC, 1984, Emergency Management Institute, National Emergency Training Center.

Tokle G, editor: *Hazardous materials response handbook,* ed 2, Quincy, Mass, 1993, National Fire Protection Association.

Varela J, editor: *Hazardous materials handbook for emergency responders,* New York, 1996, Van Nostrand Reinhold.

4

Chemistry Overview

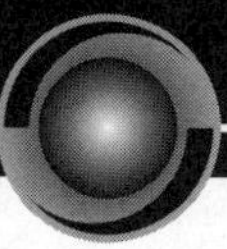

Phil Currance

CHAPTER OBJECTIVES

At the conclusion of this chapter the student will be able to:

- Discuss the importance of determining the state of matter involved in the incident.
- Given physical properties of a specific chemical, identify the state of matter, and describe the probable movement pattern.
- Discuss how water solubility and vapor pressure relate to a patient's chemical exposure.
- Define BLEVE, and describe the hazard potential involved.
- Identify five types of chemical hazard potential.
- Determine the fire potential of a hazardous chemical.
- Determine the corrosive potential of a hazardous chemical.
- Determine the reactive potential of a hazardous chemical.
- Explain the difference between organic and inorganic chemicals.
- Identify common types of radiation exposure, and discuss how they relate to patient management.
- Discuss protection measures to guard against radiation exposure.

CASE STUDY

Fire and Emergency Medical Services (EMS) responders are called to a water treatment plant for a chlorine release in which three employees were injured. On arrival they find a ton cylinder releasing a large vapor cloud of chlorine with one employee apparently unconscious and lying within the vapor cloud (Fig. 4-1). Two employees who had been briefly exposed at the edge of the vapor cloud are complaining of eye irritation and shortness of breath.

- What types of injuries can be expected?
- How large will the chlorine cloud get?
- Will the vapor stay on the ground or rise in the air?
- Is the population located downwind in danger?

Medical responders at a hazardous materials incident must have a basic understanding of chemistry. A knowledge of where the chemical will go and what it will do is essential. EMS responders need this information to predict exposure patterns/levels and anticipate the injuries that may occur with specific products. Probably the most important issue for EMS responders is the ability to predict chemical movement, which will allow them to stage equipment in a safe area and also to predict the pattern of exposure.

State of Matter

The state of matter of the chemical will directly affect victim exposure. Chemicals can be found in either solid, liquid, or gas/vapor form. Solids have a high molecular attraction for each other and will not usually move farther than their volume allows (Fig. 4-2). Physical means, such

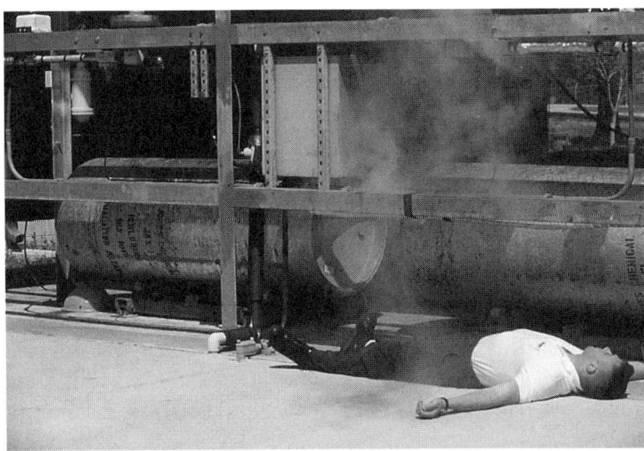

FIG. 4-1 One patient is unconscious in the chlorine cloud.

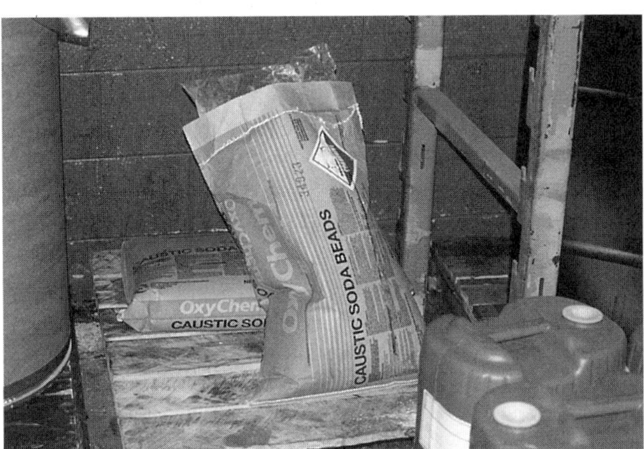

FIG. 4-2 A bag of solid chemical.

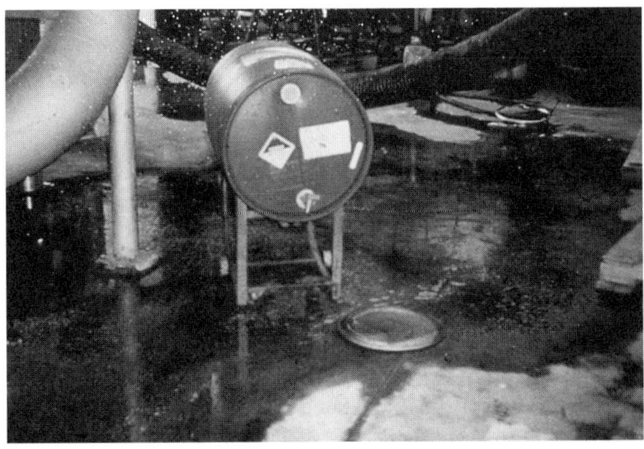

FIG. 4-3 Liquid chemicals are affected by gravity and will flow downhill.

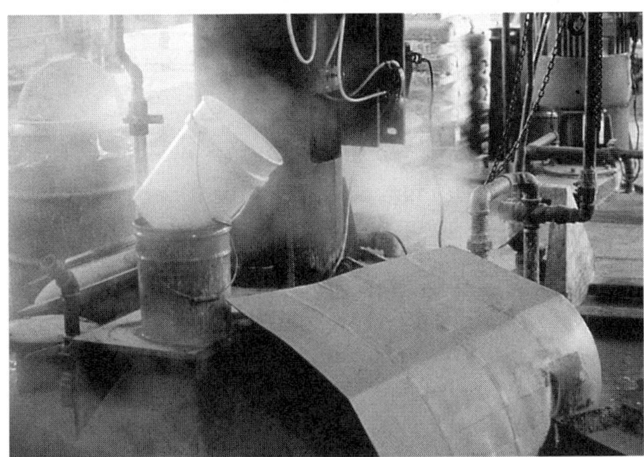

FIG. 4-4 Vapors can move with air currents, expanding as they go.

as wind, ventilation systems, and people, can cause the product to move. Solids, when mobile, can present an inhalation, ingestion, or skin contact hazard.

Liquids are more mobile than solids (Fig. 4-3). They will conform to the shape of their container as much as their volume allows. They are affected by gravity and will flow downhill. Liquids also can evaporate, creating a greater problem. Liquids can present an inhalation, ingestion, skin contact, and skin absorption hazard.

Gases and vapors present the greatest hazard (Fig. 4-4). They will always conform to the shape of their container. When released, their new container is the atmosphere. They will move with air currents, diluting and expanding as they go, possibly resulting in a wide exposure pattern. Exposure to gases usually results in inhalation, skin contact, and possibly a skin absorption hazard.

A common hazardous materials response tactic is to control chemical movement by changing the state of matter. For example, spraying water on a chlorine cloud will control the cloud's movement by turning it into a hydrochloric acid solution on the ground. EMS responders must be aware that changing the state of matter will not eliminate the hazard potential of the chemical. This manipulation of the state of matter also explains many of the injury patterns associated with exposure to hazardous materials. For example, chlorine gas, on contact with the moisture in the respiratory tract, will become soluble and cause irritation and corrosive damage.

The state of matter can be determined by assessing the melting and boiling points of the chemical. These properties may be found in the chemical's Material Safety Data Sheet (MSDS) and other resources. At the melting point a solid turns to a liquid, and at the boiling point a liquid chemical produces maximum vapor (vapor pressure equals atmospheric pressure). By assessing these properties and the ambient temperature, the responder can predict the state of matter of a known material that will be released. The temperature of the product also will directly affect injuries. For example, as temperature increases, so does the evaporation rate of a liquid, resulting in an increase of vapors and, consequently, inhalation exposures. The temperature of the product may present its own hazards. Cryogenics is an excellent example. Cryogenic materials are gases that have been liquified by supercooling. They have temperatures of less than −130° F (−90° C).

State of matter: Matter may exist as either a solid, liquid, or gas. States are separated by the melting and boiling points.

Melting point: The temperature at which a solid changes to a liquid. Ice melts at 32° F (0° C). Sodium hydroxide solids melt at 605° F (318° C).

Boiling point: The temperature at which the vapor pressure of the material being heated equals atmospheric pressure (760 mm Hg). Water boils at 212° F (100° C). Acetone boils at 133° F (56° C). Ethylene glycol boils at 387° F (197° C).

Solution: A homogeneous mixture in which all of the ingredients are completely dissolved. Solid pesticides often are dissolved in a hydrocarbon, such as xylene, to form a solution that can be sprayed.

Slurry: A pourable mixture of a solid and a liquid.

Chemical Movement

Once the state of matter has been identified, movement of the chemical can be predicted by assessing physical and chemical properties. Movement of liquid in water can be predicted by considering the chemical's specific gravity and water solubility. How quickly the chemical will evaporate and present an inhalation hazard can be assessed by considering the chemical's vapor pressure and sublimation ability.

Specific gravity: The ratio of a liquid's weight compared with an equal volume of water (Fig. 4-5). Water is given a constant value of 1.0. Materials with a specific gravity of less than 1.0 will float on water, and materials with a specific gravity greater than 1.0 will sink.

Water solubility: The degree to which a material or its vapors are soluble in water. Materials that are completely soluble in water are called *miscible,* or *polar,* solvents. Nonsoluble materials are called *immiscible,* or *nonpolar,* solvents.

Viscosity: A measure of the thickness of a liquid. It will determine how quickly a substance flows. Liquids with high viscosity are not very fluid and do not flow or absorb easily. Liquids with low viscosity will spread easily, thereby increasing the size of the endangered area. Low-viscosity liquids also present a greater chance of skin absorption.

Volatility: A measure of how quickly a material will pass into the vapor, or gas, state. The greater the volatility, the greater its rate of evaporation. Vapor pressure is a measure of volatility.

Vapor pressure: The pressure exerted by a vapor against the sides of a closed container. It is temperature-dependent; that is, as the temperature increases, so does vapor pressure. Thus, more liquid evaporates or vaporizes. Values for vapor pressure most often are given as millimeters of mercury (mm Hg) at a specific temperature. Vapor pressure is used to indicate how quickly a liquid will evaporate. Water has a vapor pressure of approximately 20 mm Hg at 70° F and will evaporate slowly at room temperature. If a chemical has a higher vapor pressure, it will evaporate faster and present an increased inhalation hazard. Sometimes a chemical's vapor pressure is listed in atmospheres. One atmosphere is equal to 760 mm Hg. Chemicals with vapor pressures in excess of 1 atm will turn to vapor almost immediately after being released from their container.

Sublimation: Most substances pass from solid to liquid to gas states. In sublimation, certain substances can pass from the solid to the gas state without first becoming a liquid. As temperature increases, so does the rate of sublimation. Dry ice turning directly into carbon dioxide is an example of sublimation.

The properties of water solubility and vapor pressure are of special importance to EMS responders. Inhaled

Specific Gravity

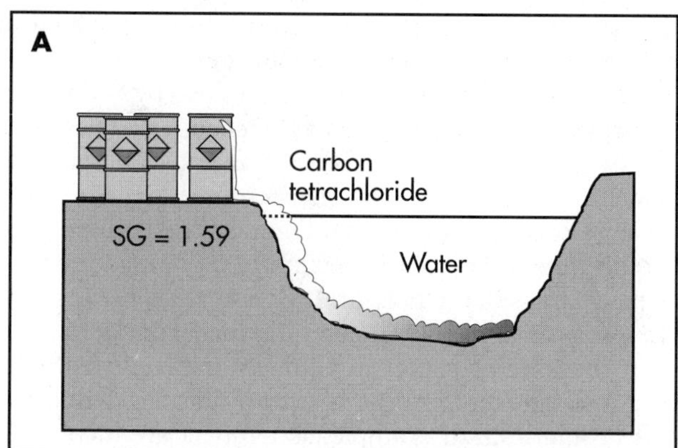

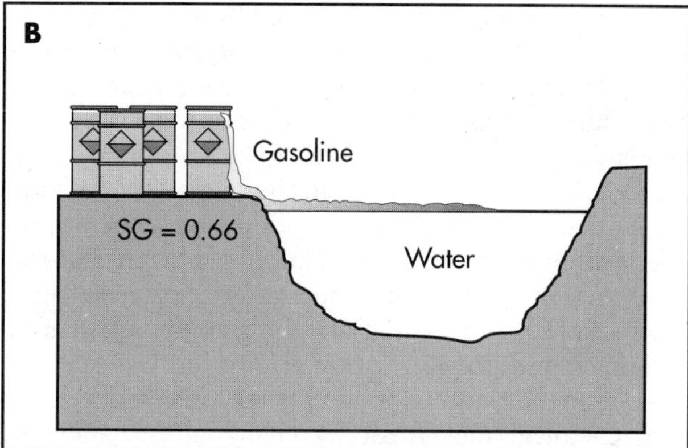

FIG. 4-5 Some liquids will float on water; others may sink.

chemicals that are highly water soluble will result in upper airway symptoms, and chemicals with lower solubility tend to result in lower airway symptoms. Chemicals with high vapor pressures will evaporate very quickly, resulting in an increased inhalation risk.

Boiling point and vapor pressure are closely related. Vapor pressure will control the product's boiling point. This is the reason that liquified gases, such as liquified petroleum gas (LPG), can be kept in a liquid state inside a container even though the temperature is well above its boiling point. Liquified gases usually have an extremely high expansion ratio. The expansion ratio will determine how much vapor will result when liquids evaporate. For example, 1 cubic foot of liquid expands to 100 cubic feet of pure gas (an expansion ratio of 100 to 1). LPG expands 270 to 1, chlorine 450 to 1, and anhydrous ammonia 840 to 1. Once a liquified gas is released from its container, it will form an extremely large vapor cloud. When containers of liquids and liquified gases under pressure suddenly are breached, the product may rapidly boil and expand. If the product is flammable, a large fireball may result. This is known as a *boiling liquid expanding vapor explosion (BLEVE)* (Fig. 4-6).

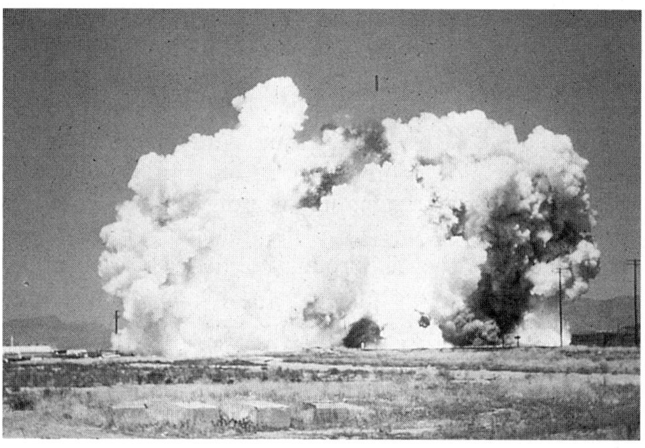

FIG. 4-6 Large BLEVE.

Even nonflammable products can present a BLEVE hazard. The increase in pressure can cause the container to violently rupture, resulting in a large vapor release. The container or projectiles may travel great distances. In most cases, BLEVEs are caused by thermal stress. A fire on the outside of the container will heat the product inside, causing an increase in vapor pressure. If the container is equipped with a pressure relief valve, it usually will reduce the pressure and therefore the risk of a BLEVE. However if the pressure exceeds the ability of the relief valve to adequately reduce the pressure, or if the strength of the container is reduced by heat, a BLEVE can result. Besides thermal stress, other factors, such as mechanical damage to the container or chemical reaction inside the container, may also result in a BLEVE.

Physical properties can also be used to predict the movement of gases and vapors. The property of vapor density is similar to specific gravity. With vapor density, the chemical is compared with air. Assessing a chemical's vapor density will determine if it will float or sink compared with air. With this information the EMS responder can better predict dispersion patterns and exposure risk.

Vapor density: The weight of a volume of pure gas compared with the weight of an equal volume of pure, dry air (Fig. 4-7). Air is given a constant value of 1.0. Materials with a vapor density less than 1.0 are lighter than air. Materials with a vapor density greater than 1.0 are heavier than air. Most vapors have densities greater than 1.0. Heavier air vapors can flow and settle in low areas, presenting a greater risk of exposure and fire should they reach an ignition source.

Hazard Potential

To properly prepare for injuries at hazardous materials incidents, EMS responders must be able to predict the type of damage a chemical can do. Standard chemical

Vapor Density

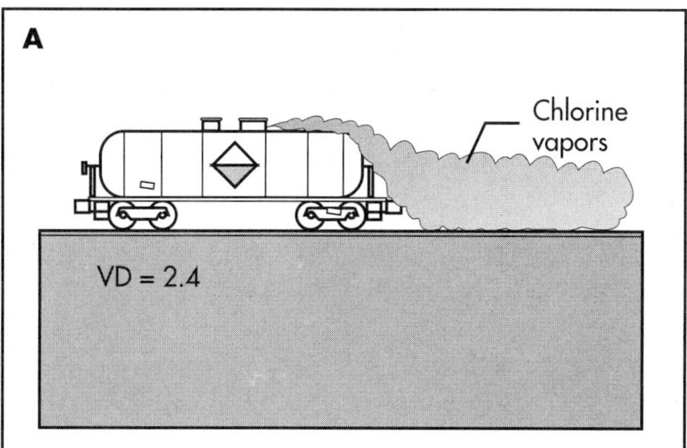

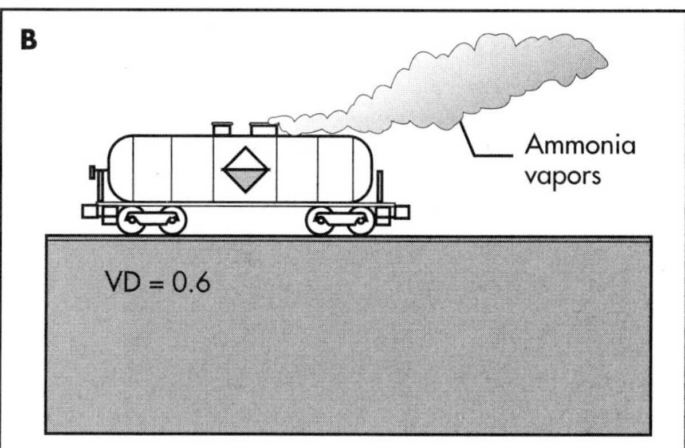

FIG. 4-7 Some gases are heavier than air.

identification methods (placards, labels, NFPA 704) may not accurately identify all of the expected hazards. Responders should always assess the hazard potential of a chemical by checking the chemical properties, not by placards/labels alone. Responders should assess the flammability, corrosivity, reactivity, radioactivity, and toxicity of chemicals. This section will address flammability, corrosivity, reactivity, and radioactivity concerns. Toxicity will be addressed in Chapter 5.

Flammability

A large percentage of chemicals used in industry are flammable (Fig. 4-8). A chemical's flammability can be assessed by knowing its flash point, fire point, autoignition temperature, lower flammable limit (LFL), and upper flammable limit (UFL).

Flash point: The minimum temperature at which a substance evaporates fast enough to form an ignitable mixture with air near the surface of the substance.

Fire point: The temperature at which a liquid gives off sufficient vapor such that the air-vapor mixture contains enough fuel to continue burning after ignition.

Autoignition point: The temperature at which a material will ignite and burn without an ignition source.

Lower flammable limit (LFL) or lower explosive limit (LEL): The minimum concentration of fuel in the air that will ignite. Below this point there is too much oxygen and not enough fuel to burn (too lean).

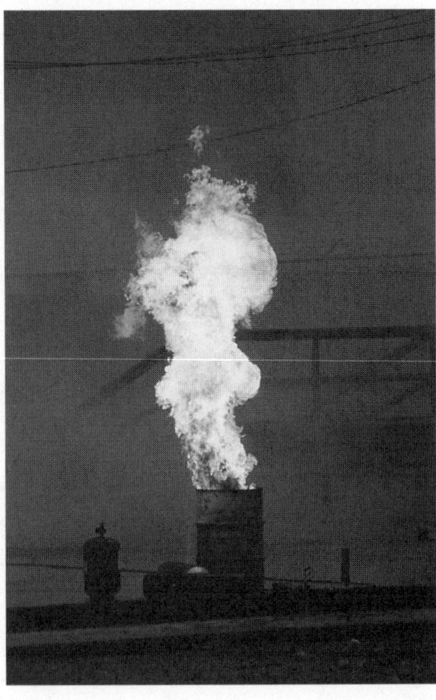

FIG. 4-8 Many industrial chemicals are flammable, including this liquid.

Upper flammable limit (UFL) or upper explosive limit (UEL): The concentration of fuel in the air above which the vapors cannot be ignited. Above this point there is too much fuel and not enough oxygen to burn (too rich).

Chemicals often are classified by their flash point. Many people use terms such as flammable, combustible, and noncombustible without understanding their true definition. By definition, the difference between a flammable, a combustible, and a noncombustible liquid is the chemical's flash point. It is not the liquid that burns but rather the vapors that come off the liquid that present a flammability risk. At a chemical's flash point, enough vapors exist to create a fire hazard. Flammable chemicals have a flash point below 141° F (60.5° C). Combustible products have a flash point between 141° F (60.5° C) and 200° F (93° C). Noncombustible products have a flash point in excess of 200° F (93° C). If a noncombustible product is spilled onto a surface that has been heated to above its flash point and an ignition source is present, it will burn.

At its autoignition temperature, a chemical will burn without an ignition source. Some chemicals have autoignition temperatures below room temperature. The chemical's flammable range also is an indication of its inherent flammability (Fig. 4-9). The flammable range is the concentration of vapors that exists between the LFL or LEL and the UFL or UEL, and contains enough oxygen and fuel for combustion if an ignition source is present. The wider the flammable range, the easier it is to find an ignition source and a flammable mixture. At the point of release the mixture may be too rich to burn, but as vapors disperse and mix with air, the flammable range may be found at a distance from the point of release.

The flammability of a chemical must be assessed by evaluating the chemical properties, not just by looking at the label. The flammability of anhydrous ammonia is a

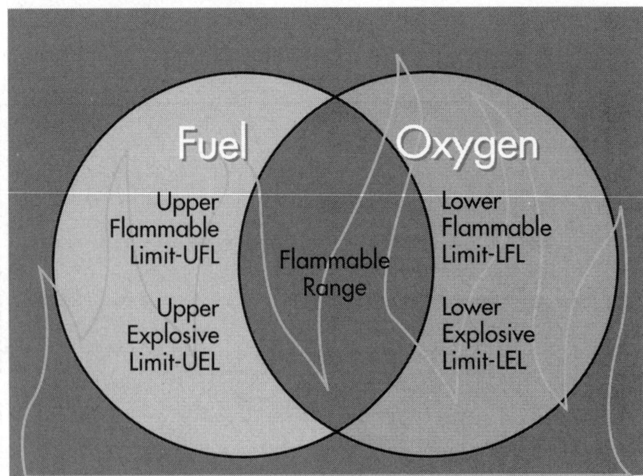

FIG. 4-9 The flammable range is partially determined by the concentration of vapors between the lower and upper flammable limit.

good example. The Department of Transportation (DOT) defines a flammable gas as any material that is a gas at 68° F or less, is ignitable at 14.7 psi (atmospheric pressure) when in a mixture of 13% or less by volume with air, or has a flammable range at 14.7 psi with air of at least 12% regardless of the LEL. According to DOT information, anhydrous ammonia has an LEL of 15.5% and a UEL of 27%. Because the LEL is above 13% and the flammable range is only 11.5%, anhydrous ammonia does not meet the specifications of a flammable gas, and therefore the DOT considers it to be a nonflammable gas. This means that at concentrations in the flammable range of anhydrous ammonia, it will burn and has been the cause of some serious fires in the past, but it is transported with a nonflammable placard. Do not be lulled into a false sense of security. Always check the data to be sure.

Corrosivity

Another injury hazard is corrosivity. The DOT defines a corrosive product as one that damages human tissue or has a severe corrosion rate on steel (Fig. 4-10).

A more in-depth assessment of a corrosive can be accomplished by determining the chemical's pH. The pH scale is used to define corrosivity and determine if the product is an acid or base (Fig. 4-11).

Acids: Materials with a pH value less than 7. Examples include hydrochloric acid and sulfuric acid.

Bases or caustics: Materials with a pH value greater than 7. Examples include sodium hydroxide and potassium hydroxide.

Understanding how the pH scale works will allow EMS responders to assess the potential hazards associated with the chemical. The pH scale is an inverse, logarithmic representation of the amount of hydrogen ions that are available. This is an important factor in assessing a corrosive chemical's strength. On the pH scale, 7 is neutral. Because the pH scale is inverse, or opposite, the lower the number, the greater the amount of hydrogen and the stronger the acid. The higher numbers on the scale represent decreasing amounts of hydrogen ions but increasing amounts of hydroxide ions. The more hydroxide ions, the more alkaline, or base, the substance is. The Environmental Protection Agency (EPA) defines an extremely corrosive product as one with a pH value of 2 or less, or a pH value of 12.5 or greater. Both strong acids and strong alkalis will cause extensive tissue damage. Because the pH scale is a logarithmic scale, for each number change, up or down from 7, the strength increases by 10 times (e.g., a 6 is 10 times stronger than a 7, a 5 is 100 times stronger).

Strength: Term used to describe the corrosiveness of a solution. It refers to the amount of hydrogen or hydroxide ions that are available to go into solution in water.

Concentration: A comparison of the amount of corrosive to the amount of water that is present in a solution. Concentration is not the same as strength. It is possible to have a high concentration of a weak acid or a low concentration of a strong acid.

It is important to remember that both sides of the scale are corrosive. Strong alkalis usually result in deeper burns because of their ability to penetrate tissue. When assessing the hazards of a corrosive chemical, vapor pressure also should be assessed. Chemicals with high vapor pressure will evaporate, and the corrosive vapors will cause an inhalation exposure and tissue damage.

Hazardous materials (HAZMAT) response teams frequently neutralize corrosive chemicals. Although this is an effective way to deal with the released chemical on the ground, corrosive chemicals on skin should *never* be neu-

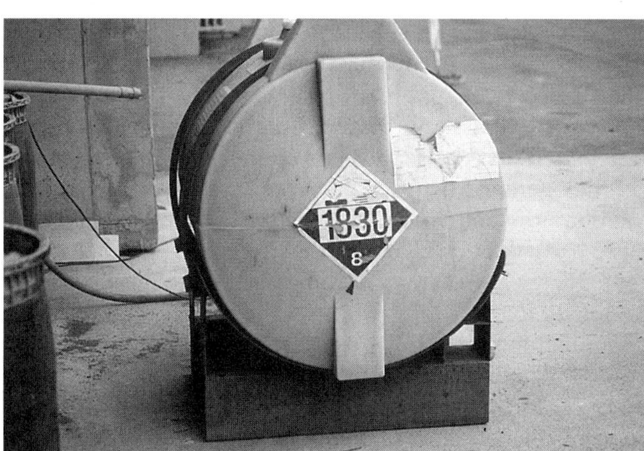

FIG. 4-10 Corrosive liquids can damage human tissue or have a severe corrosion rate on steel.

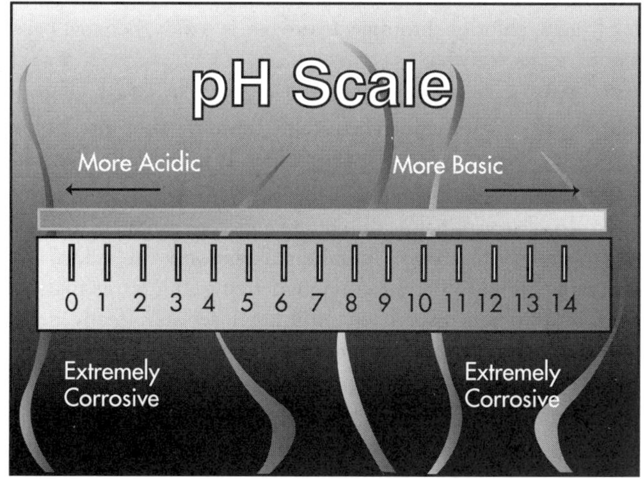

FIG. 4-11 Acids have a pH value of less than 7. Bases have a value greater than 7.

tralized. Neutralization causes an exothermic (heat-releasing) reaction that generates a tremendous amount of heat, increasing the amount of tissue damage. Immediate flushing with copious amounts of water is the treatment of choice.

Neutralization reaction: The process of counteracting an acid or base to form a salt and water. This reaction can produce a tremendous amount of heat.

Reactivity

Chemicals also should be assessed for their reactivity hazard. Chemicals may interact to produce heat or increased corrosivity, causing container failure or increased toxicity when mixed with other chemicals. Some chemicals may ignite and burn when exposed to air or water. Others are able to give off oxygen. Chemical compounds can break down into component parts with a tremendous release of energy. Chemicals also frequently become more toxic when they decompose under fire or heat conditions (toxic products of combustion). Commonly used terms related to chemical reactivity include:

Water-reactive materials: Will violently decompose and/or burn vigorously when they come in contact with moisture. Sodium reacts with water to form sodium hydroxide and hydrogen. Sulfuric acid reacts violently with water because of the heat of solution generated. This can form vapor clouds of steam and sulfuric acid.

Air-reactive materials: React with atmospheric moisture and rapidly decompose. White phosphorous will react and burn in air at temperatures above 85° F. Chlorosulfonic acid reacts violently with moisture in the air, creating heat and a vapor cloud to form hydrochloric acid and sulfuric acid.

Pyrophorics: Substances that form self-ignitable, flammable vapors when in contact with air.

Oxidation ability: The ability of a substance to release oxygen readily to stimulate combustion. Many chemicals (e.g., nitric acid, chlorine, bromine, hydrogen peroxide, benzoyl peroxide) act as oxidizers.

Polymerization: A chemical reaction in which two or more smaller molecules chemically combine to form larger molecules. The reaction often is violent. If it takes place inside a closed container, the container will usually fail.

Inhibitor: Chemicals that are added to products to control chemical reactions. Inhibitors commonly are added to monomers to keep them from polymerizing. Inhibitors may be time or heat sensitive. If an inhibitor loses its effectiveness, polymerization may occur, resulting in container failure.

Catalyst: Products that are used to control the rate of a chemical reaction. Catalysts can either speed up or slow down a chemical reaction. If chemical reaction speed is increased, pressure may build up, causing container failure.

Unstable materials: Materials that in the pure state will vigorously polymerize, decompose, condense, or become self reactive, and undergo other violent chemical changes. For example, ether will decompose to form peroxides, which are shock sensitive. Benzoyl peroxide will decompose explosively at 176° F (80° C).

With the many chemicals available, predicting reactivity can be a major problem. Labeling systems do not always accurately relate reactivity hazards. The yellow section on the NFPA marking indicates reactivity but uses strict criteria. The NFPA reactive criteria include reaction with water and the ability to explode. It may not reflect reactivity when multiple chemicals are mixed. Some reactivity can be assessed by understanding the chemical structure. Organic materials are derived from living or once living materials. Organic compounds are formed by covalent bonding. In covalent bonding the elements combine into compounds by sharing of electrons. This type of bonding can produce very complicated chemical compounds.

Hydrocarbons are organic compounds that contain chains of carbon atoms and hydrogen. Saturated, unsaturated, and aromatic all are types of hydrocarbons. In many cases their reactivity will differ. Saturated hydrocarbons (alkanes) are straight chain or branched hydrocarbons with only single covalent bonds. In other words, all of the carbons are "saturated" with hydrogen. This saturation generally makes the chemical relatively stable. Hydrocarbons that end in "ane" (i.e., methane, pentane, butane) are examples of saturated hydrocarbons.

With unsaturated hydrocarbons (alkenes and alkynes) double or triple bonds exist between some of the carbon atoms in the molecule. In other words, not all of the carbon molecules are saturated with hydrogen. These double or triple bonds generally are weaker than single bonds and make the chemical more reactive than saturated hydrocarbons. Hydrocarbons that end in "ene" (i.e., pentene, butene) and "yne" (i.e., ethyne) are examples of unsaturated hydrocarbons.

Aromatic hydrocarbons contain a benzene ring structure. Examples of aromatic hydrocarbons include benzene, toluene, and xylene. They are relatively nonreactive solvents but, in the case of benzene, can be toxic. Another term that you may hear is *halogenated hydrocarbon*. In a halogenated hydrocarbon, an element known as a *halogen* (chlorine, bromine, fluorine, iodine) has been attached in place of a hydrogen atom. Many solvents contain halogenated hydrocarbons (i.e., carbon tetrachloride, trichloroethylene, trichloroethane). They usually are more toxic than nonhalogenated hydrocarbons. Most organic materials react with oxidizers and are flammable or combustible.

Inorganic compounds usually do not contain carbon. Some may contain carbon atoms but lack carbon chains. Inorganic compounds form by ionic bonding. In ionic bonding, elements form compounds by giving off or taking on an electron. This type of bonding limits the size of the chemical structure. Inorganic compounds range from extremely stable (i.e., water) to some that are extremely reactive with water (i.e., sulfuric acid, lithium hydride) and with air (i.e., phosphine, silane).

Radioactivity

Responders also may come into contact with radioactive substances (Fig. 4-12). Radioactivity is the spontaneous disintegration of unstable nuclei accompanied by the emission of nuclear radiation.

Ionizing radiation is either particles or pure energy that produces changes in matter by creating ion pairs. Responders or patients exposed to electromagnetic radiation sources emitting gamma rays will be irradiated. They are not contaminated and pose no risk of secondary contamination. Conversely, exposure to particle radiation sources (alpha and beta particles, neutrons, protons, and positrons) in the form of dusts, liquids, or gases will result in contamination and present a secondary contamination risk. The most common types of radioactive sources encountered are as follows:

Alpha particles: The largest of the radioactive particles. They are the same size as the nucleus of the helium atom, can travel less than 10 inches, and can be stopped by a sheet of paper.

Beta particles: The same size as an electron. They can travel approximately 10 feet and be stopped by a 1-mm–thick piece of aluminum.

Gamma rays: These are weightless forms of pure energy, which can travel great distances and are stopped by heavy shielding such as lead.

Half-life is a measure of the rate of decay of a radioactive material. It indicates the time needed for half of a given amount of a radioactive material to change to another nuclear form or element.

Time, distance, and shielding are means of protection against ionizing radioactive materials. The exact length of time, distance, and thickness of shielding needed for protection will depend on the type and amount of radioactive source present. Radiation experts, using special detection equipment, can assist with these decisions. In all cases, the shorter the exposure time, the farther the distance from the source, and/or the greater the shielding, the lower the dosage. For radioactive particulate exposure, proper protective equipment and decontamination must be added.

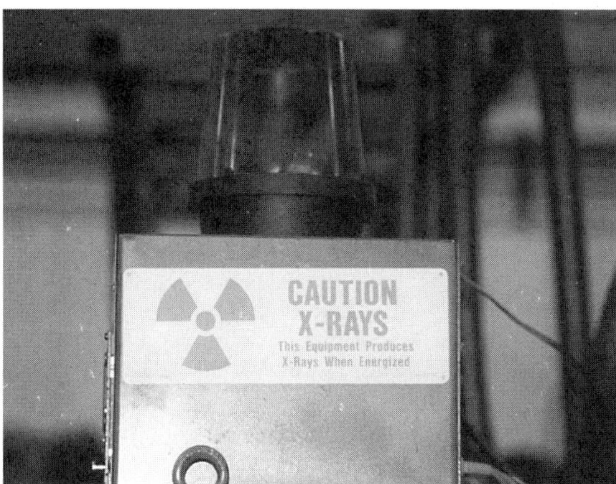

FIG. 4-12 Radioactive warning.

Summary

Although not every EMS responder must be a chemist, an understanding of chemical movement and what type of harm chemicals present is vital to safe response and patient management. By assessing the chemical and physical properties, responders will have a better idea of what they are facing during a hazardous materials emergency. Physical properties, such as boiling and melting points, specific gravity, vapor pressure, and vapor density, can help responders predict the movement of hazardous chemicals and injury patterns. Chemical properties will assist responders in identifying the harm that a chemical can do. Flash point, fire point, autoignition temperature, and upper/lower explosive limits can identify flammability risk. To assess a chemical's corrosive potential, pH should be assessed. Chemical structure can help to determine a chemical's reactive potential. Radioactivity threat can be assessed by identifying the type of radiation threat present.

CHAPTER REVIEW QUESTIONS

1. Which physical properties can be used to determine a chemical's state of matter?
2. Define cryogenic gas.
3. Which physical properties can be used to predict the movement of liquid chemicals?
4. Which physical properties can be used to predict the movement of gases or vapors?
5. Explain the relationship between vapor pressure and boiling point.
6. Which chemical properties can be used to determine the flammability hazard of a chemical?
7. Which chemical properties can be used to determine the corrosive hazard of a chemical?
8. How can a chemical's reactivity be assessed?
9. Explain the difference between a saturated and an unsaturated hydrocarbon.
10. Name the three most common types of radioactivity encountered, and discuss how their identification relates to patient management.

BIBLIOGRAPHY

Andrews LP, editor: *Emergency responder training manual for the hazardous materials technician,* New York, 1992, Van Nostrand Reinhold.

Bowen JE: *Emergency management of hazardous materials incidents,* Quincy, Mass, 1995, National Fire Protection Association.

Bronstein AC, Currance PL: *Emergency care for hazardous materials exposure,* ed 2, 1994, St Louis, Mosby.

Coleman RJ, Williams KH: *Hazardous materials dictionary,* Lancaster, Pa, 1988, Technomic Publishing.

EPA: *EPA standard safety operating guidelines,* Washington, DC, 1984, US Government Printing Office.

Guidelines for public sector hazardous materials training. 1998 ed, HMEP Curriculum Guidelines, Emmitsburg, Md, 1998, National Emergency Training Center.

Hazardous materials response training program, New Jersey/New York, 1988, Hazardous Materials Worker/Training Program.

National Fire Protection Association: *NFPA 471, Recommended practice for responding to hazardous materials incidents,* Quincy, Mass, 1992, The Association.

Noll GG, Hildebrand MS, Yvorra JG: *Hazardous materials: managing the incident,* ed 2, Stillwater, Okla, 1995, Fire Protection Publications.

Strong CB, Irvin TR: *Emergency response and hazardous chemical management: principles and practices,* Delray Beach, Fla, 1996, St. Lucie Press.

Sullivan JB, Kreiger GR, editors: *Hazardous material toxicology, clinical principles of environmental health,* Baltimore, 1992, Williams & Wilkins.

Tokle G, editor: *Hazardous materials response handbook,* ed 2, Quincy, Mass, 1993, National Fire Protection Association.

Varela J, editor: *Hazardous materials handbook for emergency responders,* New York, 1996, Van Nostrand Reinhold.

5

Basic Principles of Hazardous Materials Toxicology

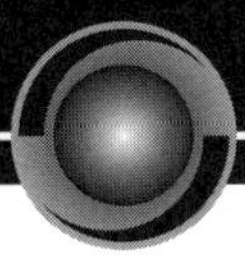

Alvin C. Bronstein, M.D., FACEP

CHAPTER OBJECTIVES

At the conclusion of this chapter the student will be able to:

- Define the specialty of medical toxicology.
- Define a poison.
- Describe four ways a poison may enter the body.
- Understand the concept of workplace exposure limits.
- Describe a poison's toxicity in terms of its route and duration of exposure.

CASE STUDY

Toluene ($C_6H_5CH_3$), or methylbenzene, is an aromatic hydrocarbon solvent. It is used in various chemical manufacturing processes. Toluene is sold as a solvent and chemical reagent. It also is a component in many paints, glues, solvent mixtures, and gasoline.

For several days, three employees of a company that manufactures model airplane cement experience increasing lightheadedness and fatigue, which they describe as a drunklike feeling. On the third day, the employees contact the plant health and safety officer. She instructs them to leave the area and report to the occupational health nurse. The safety officer mobilizes the plant hazardous materials (HAZMAT) team to survey the area. Their detection equipment finds low air levels of volatile organic compounds. No evidence of a chemical spill is found. Subsequent industrial hygiene monitoring reveals toluene air concentrations of 60 ppm, which is below the OSHA PEL of 100 ppm but above the ACGIH-TLV of 50 ppm.

- Are these employees' symptoms consistent with toluene exposure?
- Why was the plant HAZMAT team mobilized to inspect the scene?
- What is a PEL?
- What is a TLV?
- How are PELs and TLVs used to decide if a work environment is safe?
- How should the employees and workplace be evaluated to identify the cause of the health complaints?

Across the United States, workers may be exposed to hundreds of chemicals in varying amounts. Many of these are newly made compounds that do not exist in nature. Thousands of new chemicals are synthesized every year. These agents are transported throughout the country by truck, rail, and air. Collectively these agents are known as *hazardous materials.* Hundreds of local, state, and federal regulations have been established to control the transport and use of hazardous materials. Workplace chemical exposure limits, such as TLVs and PELs, have been established to keep the work environment safe. These and other exposure-limited systems are a major part of hazardous materials toxicology. This chapter discusses basic hazardous materials toxicology principles and their practical application. We will begin by looking at some of the ways hazardous materials are classified.

Definition of Hazardous Materials

The United States Occupational Safety and Health Administration (OSHA) has defined a hazardous material as a substance that on exposure results, or may result, in adverse effects on the health and safety of humans. Several systems exist to classify hazardous materials. All of these systems have limitations. One system widely used to classify hazardous materials is known as the *International Hazard Class System (IHCS)* (Box 5-1). The IHCS format separates hazardous materials into nine classes.

Substances in each class are assigned a four-digit identification number (e.g., 1075 = liquified petroleum gas). Each class also has an associated hazard symbol. This system is used in the *North American Emergency Response Guide.* The IHCS is of limited use in predicting a substance's health hazard potential and human exposure effect. Chemicals are assigned by their most dangerous physical characteristic (e.g., explosion risk or flammability). Other potential dangers, such as an agent's ability to cause cancer or birth defects, are not considered. This system provides even less insight into treating poisoning symptoms from hazardous materials exposure. To estimate human exposure effects, it is more valuable to examine the physical properties of a chemical. For example, it is useful to know the state of matter in which a particular chemical typically exists. Is the chemical a solid, liquid, or gas at room temperature? Other physical properties, such as vapor pressure, may influence the chemical's human toxicological effects. Specific facts, such as whether the chemical is a carcinogen, must also be known. Knowledge about these factors can help the EMS responder predict the health effects of a potential chemical poison.

BOX 5-1

INTERNATIONAL HAZARD CLASS SYSTEM

Explosives
Gases
Flammable liquids
Flammable solids
Oxidizers
Poisons
Radioactives
Corrosives
Miscellaneous hazardous materials

Any of the chemicals in the hazard classes just described can be toxic. The ability of a chemical or hazardous material to poison humans is of special importance in toxicology, the science of poisons. Medical toxicologists are physicians specially trained in the diagnosis and treatment of human poisoning. Some medical toxicologists may specialize in the health effects of hazardous materials. The Emergency Medical Services (EMS) and HAZMAT responder also must be aware of the general health effects of chemicals on humans. To do so the EMS responder must be familiar with basic occupational and environmental toxicological concepts as they apply to hazardous materials toxicology. These principles have been designed specifically to apply to occupational and hazardous materials exposure. In assessing the potential toxic effects of a chemical, the EMS responder must consider the chemical characteristics and potential toxicity of the product, and the duration and route of exposure.

Poisons

What is a poison? This seemingly simple question is crucial because in the right dose, almost any chemical can be considered a poison. Over the centuries, scientists have struggled to adequately define a poison. The first to address this issue was Philippus Theophrastus Bombastus von Hohenheim, a sixteenth-century Swiss alchemist and early toxicologist. He is known to medical toxicology as Paracelsus, and his *Third Defense* usually is regarded as the first scientific discussion to address the theory of the dose/response relationship. Paracelsus wrote: "All substances are poisons; there is none which is not a poison. The right dose differentiates a poison from a remedy."

Dose/Response Relationship

In the simplest sense, it is the dose that separates a poison from a remedy. Paracelsus's idea led to the modern concept of the dose/response relationship. This idea plays a central role in our understanding, categorization, and definition of a poison. Not only did Paracelsus give us the concept of the dose/response relationship, but also he emphasized the need for the application of scientific methodology to toxicology. He emphasized the need to study and document a chemical's actions to describe its therapeutic and toxic properties.

The toxicity of a particular hazardous material usually may be described in terms of a dose/response relationship. In general, the larger the dose, the greater the toxicological response. Conversely, the smaller the dose, the less likely the person is to be harmed. This relationship applies to most hazardous materials exposures except for compounds thought to be carcinogens (e.g., asbestos, benzene, benzidine). In cases of exposure to these agents, even relatively small amounts have the potential to cause damage. For agents such as these, no safe exposure dose has been universally recognized. Although no definition of a poison is perfect, the dose/response relationship as described offers a practical system for the HAZMAT responder.

Development of Occupational Exposure Limits

During the latter part of the twentieth century, medical toxicologists, industry, and occupational health specialists have become increasingly aware of the need to reduce workplace chemical exposures. Understanding that a zero-tolerance occupational exposure level is not practical, industrial hygienists and other health professionals have struggled with concern over acceptable vs. safe exposure standards. Current thought emphasizes proper workplace environmental and work practice controls to minimize worker exposure. This method of limiting exposure is preferred to placing the employee in cumbersome personal protective equipment (PPE), which may be difficult to use and maintain. Overall, emphasis is placed on preventing the exposure rather than treating the poisoning.

Because it is almost impossible to ensure a zero chance of workplace exposure, various industry, governmental, and private groups have developed safe occupational exposure limits for workers to identify potentially dangerous levels of exposures. These limits have been developed with the healthy, adult worker in mind. Workplace exposure limits usually assume a 40-hour (i.e., 8 hours a day for 5 days) work week. Acceptable exposure levels have been established by industry, other nongovernmental, and governmental agencies for many workplace hazardous chemical exposures. Exposure limits for the same chemical may vary among groups and agencies. It is important to review all relevant documentation for a specific substance to determine the most appropriate exposure limit for the work area in question. In the United States, occupational exposure standards are published by the American Conference of Governmental and Industrial Hygienists (ACGIH), a private agency; the National Institute of Occupational Safety and Health (NIOSH), an agency of the Centers for Disease Control (CDC); and OSHA, of the United States Department of Labor. Each group publishes various documents listing their respective exposure limits. Sometimes, if a chemical compound has an extremely specialized, limited use, the company using the chemical may determine its own exposure limits. Although most material safety data sheets (MSDS) list the chemical's exposure limits, it is a good practice to also check the source documentation from the aforementioned agencies.

One of the most important concerns of medical toxicologists, occupational medicine physicians, and industry and governmental agencies has been to develop a system to designate safe workplace exposure limits for individuals who may be exposed daily to hazardous materials. As previously discussed, the preferred occupational method is to implement engineering and work practice controls rather than use cumbersome PPE. Eliminating all potential sources of exposure may not be a practical solution in selected situations. Proactive industries often will adopt a lower exposure limit than the OSHA or ACGIH exposure limits. Obviously, in cases of hazardous materials emergencies, work practice or engineering controls are not easily achieved, and responders must rely more on PPE to ensure their safety.

In the United States, five basic systems are used to describe safe workplace exposure limits for potentially hazardous environments. They are as follows:

- Threshold Limit Values (TLVs)
- Permissible Exposure Limits (PELs)
- Recommended Exposure Limits (RELs)
- Immediately Dangerous to Life and Health (IDLH)
- Lethal Dose 50 (LD_{50})
- Lethal Concentration 50 (LC_{50})

Threshold Limit Values

ACGIH, a private consortium of governmental, university, and industrial members, has developed a system called *threshold limit values (TLVs)* for chemical substances and physical agents. The ACGIH defines TLVs as the airborne concentrations of substances and representative conditions under which it is believed that nearly all workers may be repeatedly exposed day after day without adverse health effects. It also is recognized that individual susceptibility varies widely, and certain individuals may become ill even if their exposure is below the TLV limit. Sometimes this situation occurs because of aggravation of a preexisting condition or synergy with other agents such as tobacco smoking, which may enhance the toxic effects of chemicals or impair the body's defense mechanisms. Some individuals also may be hypersusceptible to substances in the workplace because of age, genetic factors, medications, or personal habits. Individuals with a history of prior exposure to a particular toxin may be more susceptible to chemical injury. These individuals require additional medical toxicology or occupational medicine consultation to determine if additional protective precautions or medical monitoring are necessary.

TLVs usually refer to airborne exposure concentrations. Some substances, such as toluene, benzidine (a recognized bladder carcinogen), and diethylamine, have a special "skin" notation regarding the importance of cutaneous absorption, including mucous membranes and eyes, in addition to the inhalation potential in assessing workplace exposure. The ACGIH also classifies chemicals with respect to their carcinogenicity potential based on available human and animal data. That classification system is as follows:

- A1: Confirmed human carcinogen
- A2: Suspected human carcinogen
- A3: Animal carcinogen

- A4: Not classifiable as a human carcinogen
- A5: Not suspected as a human carcinogen

No carcinogenicity designation is given to a specific chemical if no data are reported on its carcinogenic potential.

Remember also that TLVs were designed for adults, not children. TLVs, for example, do not apply to situations, such as home environments, where people spend many more hours than at work.

TLVs are based on animal research, experimental human studies, and industrial experience. Although it probably is best to base TLV determination on data from all three areas, because of limited data for some chemicals, not all TLVs are based on data from all three areas. Therefore, the ACGIH states that TLVs should be considered guidelines. These limits should not be considered exact lines between safety and toxicity. Because of the many ambiguities and potential pitfalls in interpretation, application of TLVs should be done by individuals specially trained in their use and interpretations.

TLVs usually are expressed in units of parts per million (ppm) (parts of vapor or gas per million parts of air by volume at 25° C and 760 mm Hg barometric pressure). One ppm can be visualized as 1 drop of water in a swimming pool. TLVs also may be expressed in units of mg/m^3 (milligrams of a substance per cubic meter of air). TLVs expressed as ppm may be converted to mg/m^3 using the following formula:

TLV in ppm = (TLV in mg/m^3) × (24.45)/(gram molecular weight of substance)

Rearranging the equation, TLVs in mg/m^3 can be converted to ppm as follows:

TLV in mg/m^3 = (TLV in ppm) × (gram molecular weight of substance)/24.45

These conversion formulas are based on a barometric pressure of 760 mm Hg and a temperature of 25° C (77° F), and where 24.45 equals molar volume in liters. Resulting values are rounded to two significant figures below 100 and three significant figures above 100. This is done not to give any converted value a greater precision than that of the original TLV, but to avoid increasing or decreasing the TLV significantly merely by the conversion of units. For example, the TLV for toluene is 50 ppm. Toluene's molecular weight is 92.13. Therefore, to convert the TLV in ppm to mg/m^3, calculate as follows:

TLV (mg/m^3) = (50) × (92.13)/24.45

TLV (mg/m^3) = 188

The ACGIH has devised three types of TLVs. These types are as follows:

- Threshold Limit Value–Timed Weighted Average (TLV–TWA)
- Threshold Limit Value–Short Term Exposure Limit (TLV–STEL)
- Threshold Limit Value–Ceiling (TLV–C)

The *TLV–TWA* refers to a time-weighted average air concentration of a substance for a normal 8-hour workday and a 40-hour work week, to which nearly all workers may be repeatedly exposed, day after day, without adverse effect. The *TWA–STEL* was developed in response to the fact that conditions may exist in which a worker must be unavoidably exposed to higher air concentrations than the TLV–TWA value. The TWA–STEL usually applies to chemicals that are thought to exhibit primarily chronic health effects but that may have acute, high-level health effects. The TLV–STEL is a 15-minute TWA exposure, which should not be exceeded at any time during the workday, even if the 8-hour TWA is within the TLV–TWA. Exposures above the TLV–TWA and up to the STEL should not exceed 15 minutes and should not occur more than four times a day. A period of at least 60 minutes should elapse between exposures. No irritation, chronic or irreversible tissue damage; or narcosis of sufficient degree to increase the likelihood of accidental injury, impair self-rescue, or materially reduce work efficiency should occur provided that the daily TLV–TWA is not exceeded. This level usually is higher than the TWA for a given substance.

The *TLV–C* refers to the concentration that should not be exceeded during any part of the working exposure. This value has been established as the maximum level to be used in computing the TWA and STEL limits. The ceiling value is under the IDLH limit for a given substance (see the discussion of the IDLH system later in this chapter). As previously stated, TLVs are recommendations and are not legally enforceable. Most of these different limits are for airborne exposures occurring in occupational settings. These values are expected to provide appropriate protection for 90% to 95% of the worker population. Because the conditions for which these values were established differ from those at an uncontrolled spill site, it is difficult to interpret exactly how these values should be used by emergency medical personnel dealing with a hazardous materials incident. It should also be remembered that TLVs were developed to control workplace exposures. Therefore, the TLV system does not apply to home living environments or emergency response activities. These values are reviewed annually by the Physical Agents TLV Committee of the ACGIH. This information is published annually in the ACGIH booklet *Threshold Limit Values for Chemical Substances and Physical Agents and Biological Exposure Indices.*

NIOSH Recommended Exposure Limits

NIOSH also has established its own system of safe workplace limits. Because NIOSH is primarily a research institution with no governmental regulatory ability, these exposure guidelines are called *recommended exposure limits*

(RELs). NIOSH values may differ from both the TLV and the OSHA PEL (see the discussion of OSHA exposure limits later in this chapter) for a specific chemical. NIOSH has established three main types of RELs. These types are as follows:

- Recommended Exposure Limit–Timed Weighted Average (REL–TWA)
- Recommended Exposure Limit–Short Term Exposure Limit (REL–STEL)
- Recommended Exposure Limit–Ceiling (REL–C)

The TWA exposure recommendation is based on a 40-hour work week. The STEL is based on a time-weighted average for 15 minutes, no more than four times a day, with at least 60 minutes of rest between each exposure and no demonstrable health effects (specifically, central nervous system [CNS] or cardiorespiratory depression). A ceiling air concentration also has been established. The *REL–C* is a maximum exposure air concentration that should never be exceeded.

The REL is defined as a TWA for up to a 10-hour day during a 40-hour work week, to which nearly all workers may be repeatedly exposed without adverse effects. These levels are not legally enforceable. NIOSH designates potential carcinogenic agents with a "Ca" notation.

OSHA Exposure Limits

Through OSHA the federal government has developed similar exposure limits to TLVs and RELs; these are called *permissible exposure limits (PELs)* and are the allowable air concentration of a substance in the workplace 8 hours a day, 40 hours a week. As enforced by OSHA (Box 5-2), PELs are governmental standards to which industry must adhere to provide safe workplace environments. PELs are developed from the REL and TLV data and are legally enforceable. The PEL–TWAs and PEL–Cs carry the same definition as RELs, except that PELs refer to an 8-hour workday, 5 days a week.

The original federal legislation establishing OSHA was enacted in 1970. Because the law was written before its 1970 passage, it adopted the 1968 ACGIH TLVs in effect to establish the original OSHA PELs. Since then the PELs may have remained the same or changed according to updates in OSHA regulations. Many times, PELs are the same as the corresponding TLVs (which may or not change annually); but, depending on the chemical in question, they may be higher or lower than the current ACGIH TLV. OSHA also designates carcinogens with a "Ca" notation. Through a regulatory process, OSHA may adopt RELs as PELs or change the PEL value based on current information.

IDLH System

Firefighters, EMS, and HAZMAT team members encounter various hazardous materials conditions in their work. To define absolute safe entry environments for emergency situations, a limits system termed *Immediately Dangerous to Life and Health (IDLH)* has been developed by the Environmental Protection Agency (EPA) and NIOSH. Developed in the 1970s, these originally were developed for respirator selection. IDLH values define air concentrations that can cause unconsciousness, incapacitation, or intolerable irritation during an exposure time of 30 minutes. The IDLH is the maximum environmental air concentration of a substance from which a person could escape within 30 minutes without symptoms of impairment or irreversible health effects. Because the IDLH system was devised for acute emergency exposure potentially causing death, the 30-minute window is arbitrary and does not take into account chemicals that may be carcinogens. Therefore, the idea of immediate evacuation must be emphasized.

Table 5-1 lists the differences in TLVs for toluene using the four systems just discussed. As can be seen, the quoted TLVs for this chemical differ considerably. These differences are representative for most chemicals with exposure limits designated by multiple groups.

BOX 5-2

OSHA PELs

Permissible Exposure Limit–Time Weighted Average (PEL–TWA)
Permissible Exposure Limit–Short Term Exposure Limit (PEL–STEL)
Permissible Exposure Limit–Ceiling (PEL–Ceiling)

TABLE 5-1

TLV COMPARISON

1998 TOLUENE	ACGIH TLV	NIOSH REL	OSHA PEL
TWA ppm =	50,A4	100	200
TWA mg/m3 =	188,A4	375	
STEL/CEIL (C) ppm =		150	C 300 500, 10-minute peak per 8-hr shift
STEL/CEIL (C) mg/m3 =		560	
Skin notation	Yes	No	No
IDLH VALUE = 500 ppm			

Because of the inadequacies of PELs and TLVs in assessing exposures in the general population and home environments, special exposure limits have been established. Emergency Response Planning Guidelines (ERPGs), Short-term Public Emergency Guidance Levels (SPEGLs), and the Level of Concern all are designed to aid the emergency responder in making decisions regarding non-workplace exposures.

- Emergency Response Planning Guidelines (ERPGs)—published by the American Industrial Hygiene Association, these exposure limits are designed for emergency planning. There are three levels of ERPGs: ERPG-3 is the level to which individuals could be exposed for 1 hour without experiencing or developing life-threatening effects; ERPG-2 is the level for a 1-hour exposure that should not cause irreversible adverse or other serious health effects or symptoms that could impair an individual's ability to take protective action; ERPG-1 is the level for a 1-hour exposure that should not result in health effects more severe than sensory perception or mild irritation. Only a small number of ERPGs are established.
- Short-term Public Emergency Guidance Levels (SPEGLs)—established by the National Research Council, these are concentrations considered acceptable for public exposures during emergencies. Only a small number of SPEGLs are established.
- Level of Concern (LOC)—established by the Environmental Protection Agency (EPA) for public exposures to chemicals that have IDLH limits. This level is set at one tenth the level of the IDLH. This was developed as an interim level until more appropriate exposure limits are developed to protect the public during short-term exposures.

Lethal Dose System

A lethal dose system of chemical lethality has been developed based on animal research studies for oral, dermal, and inhaled exposures. The values associated with this system are the so-called Lethal Dose 50% (LD_{50}) or Lethal Concentration 50% (LC_{50}) measurements. The LD_{50} value for a particular chemical is determined from animal experiments. This number identifies the oral dose of a substance that will kill 50% of an exposed animal population (e.g., rats, mice, or rabbits). The animals are exposed to the chemical either dermally or orally. LC_{50} refers to the air concentration of a substance that will kill half of the research animal population in a particular study. This number denotes the product of the concentration (C) and the length of exposure time (t) it takes to achieve a 50% animal kill.

Although the lethal dose system may have some limited usefulness in the particular animal species tested and in comparing the relative toxicity of chemicals in the same chemical family, the concept is of limited medical usefulness. This system has serious deficiencies when used to rate the risk for human hazardous materials exposure. The animal model lethal dose cannot be extrapolated across species lines to humans to predict exposure signs and symptoms. Remember, the LD or LC number is based on lethal dose and not harmful effects. Table 5-2 lists the most poisonous human nerve agents, ranked according to descending order of toxicity, and their LD_{50} and LC_{50} values.

The toxicity ranking is the same for the two routes of exposure, but the differences are much greater in skin exposure. This difference mainly is attributable to the more volatile nerve agents evaporating from naked skin. If evaporation is prevented (e.g., by tightly fitting clothing), the difference will be less. Therefore, the LD_{50}/LC_{50} system has some usefulness in ranking chemicals in the same class. However, in this case, the military airborne exposure Limit (AEL [similar to a TLV]) for these agents is 0.0001 mg/m^3 because even 1 drop on the skin of any of these agents can be lethal, making the LD_{50} or LC_{50} values of these agents of academic interest only. In summary, the lethal dose system has some usefulness to the medical toxicologist in estimating risk but does not establish harmful effect levels for humans.

All of the hazardous materials exposure parameters described in this chapter usually are listed in the chemical's MSDS or other standard toxicological references. At best, these exposure levels can be used as a benchmark for determining a hazardous material's relative toxicity, and perhaps for assistance in selecting appropriate protective equipment. If a HAZMAT team equipped with appropriate air monitoring devices is on scene, the team members may provide responders with more accurate estimates of a material's toxic potential. It must be remembered that these limits are generic in nature. They do not take into account extremes of age, individual sensitivity, or preexisting medical conditions. Some people will experience adverse effects at or below the established exposure limits. Special considerations exist for mixtures of hazardous materials. Standard protocols exist to combine TLVs for mixtures. These may be found in ACGIH

TABLE 5-2
NERVE AGENT TOXICITY

AGENT	LC_{50} (Inhalation) mg/min/m^3	LD_{50} (Skin) mg/individual
Tabun (GA)	200	4000
Sarin (GB)	100	1700
Soman (GD)	100	300
VX	50	10

and OSHA documentation and standard industrial hygiene reference texts.

The exposure systems described in this chapter are used in the United States. Other countries have their own systems. Although some countries refer to the ACGIH TLVs, Germany has its own system, referred to as the *Federal Republic of Germany Maximum Concentration Values in the Workplace,* or *MAK,* system. Carcinogenic properties for various agents are reviewed by the International Agency for Research on Cancer (IARC). IARC monographs on the carcinogenic properties of various hazardous materials are available.

When selecting the most appropriate exposure limit, one should consult several standard references. Review the various exposure limits for the substance(s) in question. Once this process has been completed, follow this simple rule for choosing the safest exposure limit for a particular chemical: *select the lowest practical exposure limit.*

Routes of Exposure

Poisons generally enter the body by four different, but not mutually exclusive, routes. They are as follows:

- Lung inhalation
- Oral ingestion
- Skin/eye absorption
- Intravenous, intramuscular, or subcutaneous injection

Determining the route by which a chemical enters the body is important. Poisons may enter the body in numerous ways. Damage may be either localized to the exposed area, or systemic, or both. Local injury refers to damage that is present at the point of chemical contact. Many absorbed products can cause systemic, or remote, damage as well.

Inhalation is the quickest and most frequently encountered route of exposure for occupational and hazardous materials-related poisonings. Products that are small enough to reach the alveoli may quickly enter the bloodstream. Even if the product is not absorbable through the respiratory tract, extensive damage can be done by irritant or corrosive effects, leading to lung damage and pulmonary edema.

Skin

The skin is the body's largest organ. Intact skin provides a barrier to toxins. Once this barrier is breached, systemic absorption may occur. With skin contact, substances damage the skin and may be absorbed into the systemic circulation. Certain substances easily pass through the skin and cause systemic poisoning. Skin absorption is increased in cases of skin damage or hot weather. Certain areas of the body are more susceptible to chemical absorption than others. For instance, the groin area will absorb chemicals many times faster than the hand or foot. Most solvents and pesticides are examples of chemicals that are highly skin absorbable.

Ingestion

Toxins also can enter the body by ingestion. Although ingestion typically does not happen often in cases of hazardous materials poisoning, it may occur because of accidental poisoning, suicide attempts, smoking, failure to properly decontaminate one's hands before eating, or breathing in particulate matter that then is swallowed. After chemicals are absorbed across a body surface membrane (e.g., lungs, intestine, skin), they are distributed throughout the body. The hazardous material is either metabolized or stored in various organs or adipose (fat) tissue. Substances may be stored first and then slowly or never metabolized, or metabolized and then stored. Poisons may be metabolized to a more toxic product than the parent compound (lethal synthesis, e.g., methanol, ethylene glycol) or excreted unchanged (e.g., nitrogen gas). Metabolism usually takes place in the liver. Excretion occurs by the lungs, kidneys, skin, or gastrointestinal system. For most substances, no specific measures exist to prevent metabolism once they are absorbed. Therefore, prevention of hazardous materials exposure and absorption is vital.

Inhalation

As just discussed, occupational or environmental hazardous materials exposures usually occur through inhalation (Fig. 5-1). Hazardous materials are found in various states of matter or configurations that allow for inhalation exposure. Gases and vapors are the two main terms used to describe respirable agents. *Gases* refer to substances that are in a gaseous state at room temperature and standard pressure. The term *vapor* refers to the gaseous state of a chemical that usually is in a solid or liquid state at room temperature and pressure.

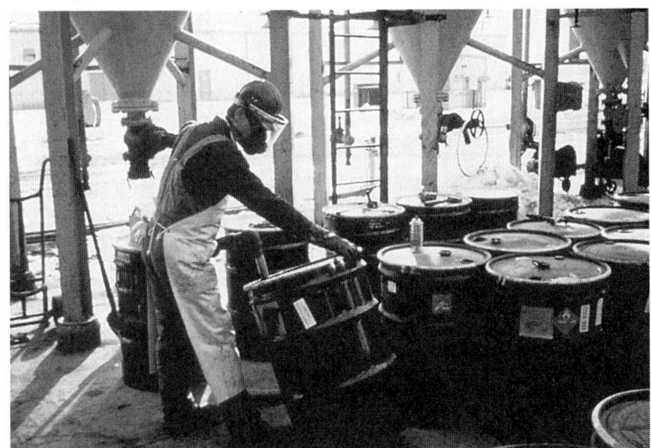

FIG. 5-1 Inhalation is the most common route of workplace exposure.

Vapor pressure (VP) is a useful concept to determine if a solid or liquid will release enough of itself in the gaseous form to be a respiratory threat. VP describes the atmospheric pressure force produced by the vapors given off from the chemical in question. Knowledge of a substance's VP is useful in estimating the inhalation risk from the chemical agent off-gassing. Knowledge of the VP helps the health care provider or hazardous materials responder estimate the inhalation risk for a particular chemical exposure. The lower the VP, the less likely that the chemical will volatilize (i.e., produce respirable gas). Conversely, the higher a chemical's VP, the more likely it will exist as a vapor at room temperature. Thus a chemical with a high VP presents a greater risk for inhalation exposure than does a chemical with a lower VP. Standard reference texts list vapor pressure for various commonly encountered chemical compounds. For example, water has a VP of approximately 20 mm Hg at 70° F. The VP of acetone is generally listed at 250 mm Hg. Therefore, acetone vaporizes much faster than does water and presents a higher inhalation exposure risk (Fig. 5-2).

Besides gases and vapors, several other terms are used to describe the physical properties of inhaled agents. Solid particulate matter is called *dust.* These particles usually vary in size. The term *aerosol* refers to a suspension of liquids or solids (particles) in air. Condensation of liquid droplets on particles produces *mists,* or *fogs.* Combustion of vapors creates *mists.* The water solubility of gases and liquids generally determines how far into the respiratory tract the substance will reach. For particulates, the location of pulmonary system deposition depends on the size of the particle.

To better understand these issues, a review of the respiratory tract anatomy is needed. The respiratory system is divided into the upper and lower respiratory tract. The upper respiratory tract comprises the nasal cavity, oral cavity, pharynx, larynx, and trachea. The trachea terminates and divides into the right and left mainstem bronchi. The lower respiratory tract consists of the air passages (bronchial tubes) and alveoli.

The passages continue to subdivide into secondary bronchi, terminal bronchioles, respiratory bronchioles, and alveolar ducts, terminating in alveolar sacs composed of individual alveoli. This system acts as an increasingly fine sieve, with the smallest particles being deposited in the lowest levels of the respiratory tree. This sieve is the most important factor in determining the location of particle deposition. Generally, particles ranging from 5 to 30 μm are deposited in the nose, oral pharynx, and larynx. Particles in the 3- to 5-μm range make it to the trachea and mainstem bronchi. Particles must be 1 μm or less to be deposited in the alveoli. Other factors that play a role in pulmonary toxicity are the toxicity of the agent; the ability of respiratory cells, such as the respiratory tract macrophages, to interact with the toxic substances; the anatomy of the respiratory tract; and the patient's breathing rate (Fig. 5-3).

For gases and liquids, the water solubility of the compound is the major factor determining the deposition site. Chemicals with high water solubility are more likely to react on contact with water in the upper respiratory tract and cause upper respiratory symptoms such as irritation and bronchitis. Lower water-soluble compounds

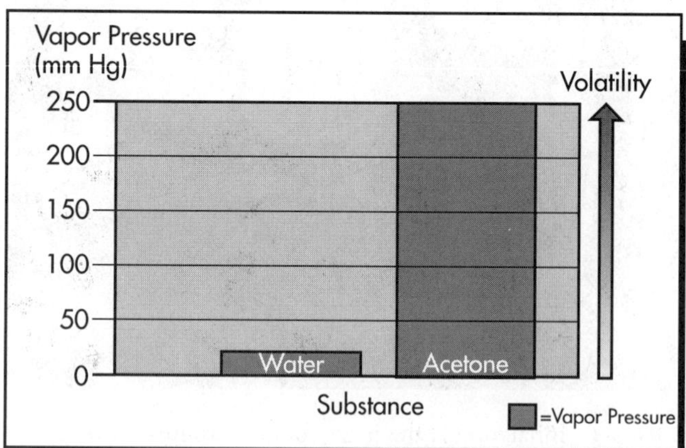

FIG. 5-2 Acetone has a higher vapor pressure than water.

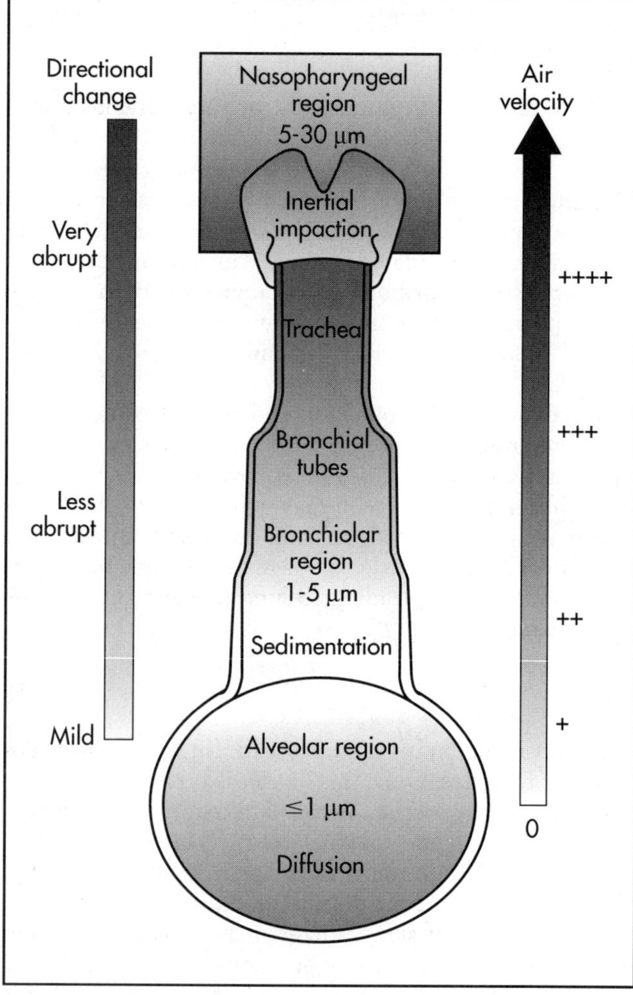

FIG. 5-3 Particles can be deposited throughout the respiratory tract.

tend to reach the lower respiratory tract and cause reactions such as pulmonary edema.

Another important factor in pulmonary toxicology is the enormous pulmonary surface area available for chemical absorption. The total lung surface area in the average adult available for chemical absorption measures between 140 and 150 m^2, resulting in a surface approximately 3 feet wide and 1½ times the length of a football field. On the other hand, the average adult skin surface area is approximately 1.7 m^2. Although dermal absorption is the second most common route of exposure, the lungs have more than 70 times more surface area than does skin available for chemical absorption. Therefore, most occupational exposure guideline standards have been developed for respiratory exposures.

Water solubility in large part determines the time of onset for many respiratory exposures. When a chemical is inhaled, depending on the particle size, it will contact the respiratory tract at different levels along the respiratory tree, where it will combine with water found along the tract. Agents that are highly water soluble react with water rapidly, usually causing immediate symptoms. Less water-soluble chemicals are slower to react and cause delayed symptoms. Highly water-soluble chemicals usually cause early respiratory tract irritation with immediate upper respiratory tract symptoms of coughing and congestion. Lower water-soluble chemicals may penetrate lower into the respiratory tract, eliciting delayed onset with fewer symptoms of acute exposure. Low water-soluble compounds are more likely to cause direct lung damage, leading to pulmonary edema, which may be delayed 6 to 12 hours. The following are examples of highly soluble, corrosive vapors/gases with immediate symptom onset:

- Acetaldehyde (CH_3CHO)
- Acrolein (CH_2CHCHO)
- Ammonia (NH_3)
- Hydrogen chloride (HCl)
- Sulfur dioxide (SO_2)
- Chlorine (Cl_2)

The following low-soluble, corrosive vapors/gases have a relatively delayed symptom onset:

- Nitric acid (HNO_3)
- Nitrogen oxides (NO_x)
- Ozone (O_3)
- Phosgene (CCl_2O)

Examples of corrosive liquids are hydrochloric acid (HCl) and sulfuric acid (H_2SO_4). Other chemicals, such as hydrocarbon solvents (e.g., toluene or hydrofluoric acid [HF]), may exhibit delayed symptom onset because of their systemic toxicity mechanisms.

Asphyxiants

Asphyxiants are chemicals that impair the body's ability to either get or utilize oxygen. Asphyxiants are divided into two classes: simple and chemical. Simple asphyxiants are inert gases or vapors that displace oxygen (O_2) in inspired air. A number of gases and vapors, when present in high concentrations in air, act primarily as simple asphyxiants without other significant physiological effects. By OSHA rule, the minimal O_2 content in inspired air should be at least 19.5% by volume under normal atmospheric pressure (equivalent to a partial pressure [PO_2] of 135 mm Hg). Atmospheres deficient in O_2 because of displacement by simple asphyxiants do not provide adequate warning properties. Remember also that most simple asphyxiants are odorless. Several simple asphyxiants (e.g., hydrogen) also present an explosion hazard. Simple asphyxiants include argon, ethane, ethylene, helium, hydrogen, methane, neon, nitrogen, and propane.

Chemical asphyxiants are substances that either prevent O_2 delivery or utilization for energy production in the cell. The most common example of a substance that prevents hemoglobin from transporting O_2 to tissues is carbon monoxide (CO). Hydrogen sulfide (H_2S) and cyanide (CN) act primarily by blocking the metabolism of O_2 in the mitochondria for the generation of adenosine triphosphotase.

Duration of Exposure

The duration of exposure also is an important index of toxicity. Obviously the shorter the exposure time, the lower the absorbed dose and presumably the lower the response. Exposure time frames have been described as acute or chronic. An acute exposure usually refers to a high-dose, single exposure occurring over less than 24 hours. Usually, acute exposures may be observed after a hazardous materials spill or release has occurred. EMS personnel are at risk for these exposures while working at a hazardous materials incident site. Chronic exposures are thought of as low-dose exposures occurring over a longer period, usually a month or more. These exposures commonly occur daily in the workplace. Symptom onset from these exposures may be confusing. A common misconception is that an acute exposure should result in immediate onset of symptoms. However, this is not always the case. Acute exposures may result in immediate symptom onset, delayed onset that may occur hours to days later, or long-term exposure, with symptoms that can be delayed for years. Examples of chemicals with long-term symptom onset are as follows:

- Carcinogens: Vinyl chloride, benzene
- Reproductive toxins (mutagens, teratogens): Lead, mercury
- Pulmonary toxins: Asbestos
- Allergens/sensitizers: Phthalates, glutaraldehyde, latex
- Heavy metals poisoning: Lead, cadmium, mercury, arsenic

The concepts just discussed are important for hazardous materials responders. Knowledge of a chemical's toxicological properties (exposure limits, chemical reactions), physical state, and vapor pressure are critical in gauging the severity of a potential exposure. This information, coupled with a material's solubility and particle size, can be used to predict the site of and rapidity of action. Characterizing the exposure as acute or chronic helps predict the timeline of the exposure. Systematically applying these principles will aid responders in their duties and protect them from harm by helping to choose the most optimal personal protective equipment plan.

Summary

A basic knowledge of hazardous materials toxicology is necessary to be able to respond to hazardous materials accidents. Developing a focused, logical approach to assessment of the toxicological dangers is mandatory. Hazardous materials toxicology is constantly evolving. The basic principles that have been discussed in this chapter provide a foundation for further study.

CHAPTER REVIEW QUESTIONS

1. What is a poison?
2. Name four ways a poison can enter the body.
3. Define vapor pressure.
4. How big is 1 part per million (ppm)?
5. What is the ACGIH?
6. Define the three types of workplace exposure limits.
7. Compare and contrast PELs and TLVs.
8. Describe the mechanism by which an LD_{50} is determined.
9. Give two examples of simple asphyxiants.
10. Why is the water solubility of an inhaled chemical useful in determining its possible toxic effects?

BIBLIOGRAPHY

American Conference of Governmental and Industrial Hygienists: TLVs and other occupational exposure values, 1997. Cincinnati, Ohio, ACGIH, 1997 CD ROM.

American Conference of Governmental and Industrial Hygienists: *1998 TLVs and BEIs. Threshold limit values for chemical substances and physical agents: biological exposure indices.* Cincinnati, Ohio, ACGIH, 1998.

Ballantyne B, Sullivan JB: Basic principles of toxicology. In Sullivan JB, Krieger GR, editors: *Hazardous material toxicology,* Baltimore, 1991, Williams & Wilkins.

Bronstein AC, Currance PL: *Emergency care for hazardous materials exposure,* ed 2, St. Louis, 1994, Mosby.

Cohen KS: Hazardous material information resources, *Occup Health Saf* 52:15-17, 1983.

Greenberg MI, Cone DC, Roberts JR: Material safety data sheet: a useful resource for the emergency physician. *Ann Emerg Med* 27:347-352, 1996.

IARC: Monographs on the evaluation of carcinogenic risk of chemicals to man. Overall evaluations of carcinogenicity to humans as evaluated in IARC monographs, vol 1-71 (a total of 834 agents, mixtures, and exposures). Last updated March 5, 1998 (cited July 10, 1998). Available from URL: http://193.51.164.11/monoeval/crthall.html.

Lerman SE, Kipen HM: Material safety data sheets. Caveat emptor, *Arch Intern Med* 150:981-984, 1990.

Marsick DJ, Byrd DM: Resources for material safety data sheet (MSDS) preparation. *Fundam Appl Toxicol* 15:1-5, 1990.

Solomon CJ: Understanding and using the MSDS: material safety data sheets. *OHN J* 36:376-379, 1988.

6

Emergency Response Information Sources

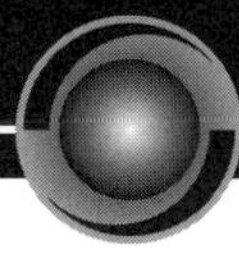

Phil Currance

CHAPTER OBJECTIVES

At the conclusion of this chapter the student will be able to:

- Identify the information that can be found in the *North American Emergency Response Guidebook* and cite its limitations.
- Identify other written reference sources that may be useful for Emergency Medical Services (EMS) responders.
- Identify telephone reference sources that may be useful for EMS responders.
- Identify computer references that may be useful for EMS responders.

CASE STUDY

Numerous individuals were exposed to methyl ethyl ketone during an industrial accident. One patient is experiencing seizure activity, while the other patients are alert and oriented. Fire department personnel are seeking information on the extent of decontamination needed, and EMS responders need information on medical management and personal protective equipment (PPE) needs.

- What information can be accessed from the *North American Emergency Response Guidebook?*
- Where can detailed information regarding chemical and physical properties be found?
- Where can detailed medical management information be found?

It is impossible to memorize chemical data on all of the many chemicals with which EMS responders may come into contact. Likewise a see this–do this, or "cookbook," approach to hazardous materials emergency response is too general and will not work. Successful hazardous materials management and treatment of the resultant injuries depend on specific information. Each chemical and situation must be evaluated on its own merits. By researching the physical and chemical properties of the hazardous material, decisions can be made on its exposure potential and ability to cause harm. Chemicals may have the potential to cause harm by flammability, corrosivity, reactivity, radioactivity, or any combination of these. By assessing the chemical data, responders can make informed decisions on exposure potential, harmful effects, protective equipment needs, decontamination needs, and treatment modalities.

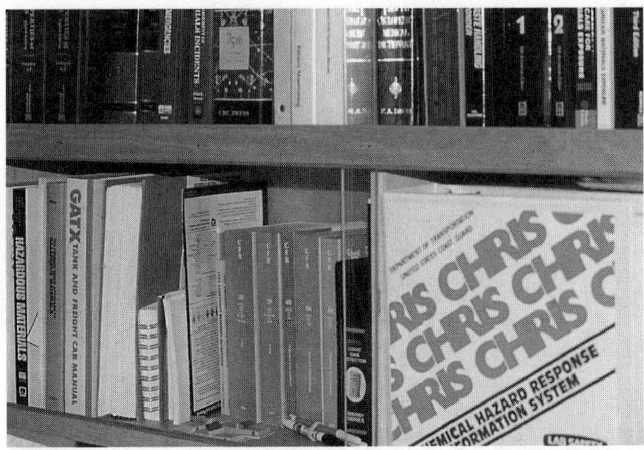

FIG. 6-1 Resource library in hazardous materials response vehicle.

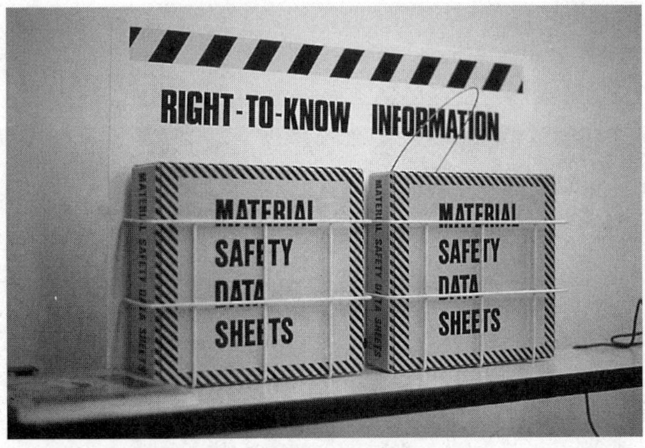

FIG. 6-2 Industrial MSDS station.

Resources that allow responders to assess chemical threats and guide treatment should be readily available. This chapter will discuss popular references (written, telephone, and computer) that may be available to the EMS responder. Written references are the most cost effective and readily available to emergency response personnel (Fig. 6-1).

Written Resources

The North American Emergency Response Guidebook

The *North American Emergency Response Guidebook (NAERG)* is probably the reference most familiar to responders. It has been available for many years in the United States as the *DOT Emergency Response Guidebook.* In Canada a similar reference was available as the CANUTEC *Dangerous Goods Initial Emergency Response Guide.* In 1996 these two references, as well as information from Mexico, was combined into the NAERG. This reference, which is available from the U.S. Government Printing Office Bookstore or numerous private sources, is a quick-response guide written for first responders to use at a hazardous materials emergency. A chemical can be referenced by placard, chemical name, or a four-digit ID number (see Chapter 3). Information can be found in guidelines that have been developed for chemicals with similar hazards and management needs. This information includes:

- Fire and explosion hazards
- Health hazards
- Public safety information
- Protective clothing needs
- Evacuation concerns
- Fire response
- Spill/leak response
- Basic first aid information
- Protective distances

Material Safety Data Sheets

Under the Occupational Safety and Health Administration's (OSHA) Hazard Communication Standard (also known as the *Worker Right to Know*), employers must provide chemical information to their employees by ensuring that containers are labeled and a Material Safety Data Sheet (MSDS) is readily available for each chemical with which workers may come into contact. MSDSs are supplied by the chemical manufacturer (Fig. 6-2). This valuable resource usually can be found in industrial settings. Although OSHA does not mandate the exact format that the MSDS must follow or the depth of information that it must contain, it does require that basic information be included. Responders may find MSDSs with very detailed information or MSDSs with very limited information. The American National Standards Institute (ANSI) is working on a voluntary format to standardize MSDSs, but this may not be available for some time. Information that is required on the MSDS includes:

- Chemical name
- Physical data
- Chemical ingredients
- Fire and explosion hazard data
- Health hazard data
- Reactive data
- Spill or leak procedures
- Special protection information
- Special precautions

The National Institute of Occupational Safety and Health *Pocket Guide to Chemical Hazards*

A reference that has been available for some time is the National Institute of Occupational Safety and Health (NIOSH) *Pocket Guide to Chemical Hazards.* This cost-effective reference is available from the U.S. Government Printing Office Bookstore. This easy-to-use guide indexes chemicals in alphabetical order and provides chemical identification, properties, PPE needs, and basic medical information. Information in this guide includes:

- Synonym, trade names
- Exposure limits (REL, PEL, IDLH)
- Physical hazards
- Chemical and physical properties
- Incompatibilities and reactives
- Personal protection
- Respirator selection
- Health hazards (routes of exposure, symptoms, first aid, target organs)

The Chemical Hazardous Response Information System Manual

The *Chemical Hazardous Response Information System (CHRIS)* Manual, which is developed by the U.S. Coast Guard, is available from the U.S. Government Printing Office Bookstore. This four-volume document is designed to provide information to the Coast Guard Hazardous Materials Strike Teams. The second volume, *Hazardous Chemicals Data,* is the most useful to EMS responders. This volume comprises a large document that fills three 3 inch binders. It provides chemical identification information, chemical and physical data, and emergency response information, including the following:

- Chemical identification
- Emergency information
- Response to discharge
- Health and fire hazards
- Reactivity hazards
- Physical and chemical properties

Threshold Limit Values for Chemical Substances and Physical Agents and Biological Exposure Indices

This reference, published annually by the ACGIH, provides the most up-to-date chemical exposure levels (TLVs), information on medical surveillance, and other industrial health and safety concerns. Contents include:

- Latest TLV levels
- Biological exposure indices
- Heat exposure information
- Cold exposure information
- Hand and arm vibration exposure information
- Noise exposure information
- Laser exposure information

Emergency Care For Hazardous Materials Exposure

The references discussed so far contain emergency response information and chemical data. First aid information is included in some of these texts, but it is very basic. *Emergency Care For Hazardous Materials Exposure,* available from Mosby, is designed for EMS responders, nurses, physicians, and health and safety officers. Although it does not provide data on chemical and physical properties, it does provide field recognition and management guidelines for hazardous materials exposure and associated medical emergencies. More than 3000 chemicals are indexed. Similar in format to the NAERG, chemicals can be referenced by placard/label, four-digit ID number, chemical name, or chemical family. A total of 109 guidelines are given, with information that includes the following:

- Substance identification
- Routes of exposure
- Target organs
- Life threat
- Signs and symptoms by body system
- Symptom onset for acute exposure
- Co-exposure concerns
- Medical conditions possibly aggravated by exposure
- Decontamination
- Immediate first aid
- Basic and advanced medical treatment
- Initial emergency department considerations
- Treatment protocols
- Drug protocols
- EMS/HM operating procedures
- References

Clinical Toxicology of Commercial Products, available from Williams & Wilkins, was written to assist physicians in managing acute chemical poisonings resulting from misuse of consumer products. This text was not written to be used as a quick field guide, but it can be useful when detailed information is needed. This text is divided into seven sections. Sections II and III are the most useful for EMS responders. Section II ("Ingredients Index") lists 1646 chemicals and gives a brief description and toxicity information. Many chemicals are referenced to "reference congeners" in Section III. Section III ("Therapeutics Index") summarizes clinical and experimental data on 85 compounds or classes of compounds (reference congeners.) Each entry in Section III typifies toxicology for a group of related substances. Section III focuses on toxic signs and symptoms (symptomatology) and recommended treatment. Each entry spans numerous pages but concludes with a summary for symptomatology and treatment. Sections are as follows:

- Section I—"First Aid and General Emergency Treatment"
- Section II—"Ingredients Index"
- Section III—"Therapeutics Index"
- Section IV—"Supportive Treatment"
- Section V—"Trade Name Index"
- Section VI—"General Formulations"
- Section VII—"Manufacturers' Names and Addresses"

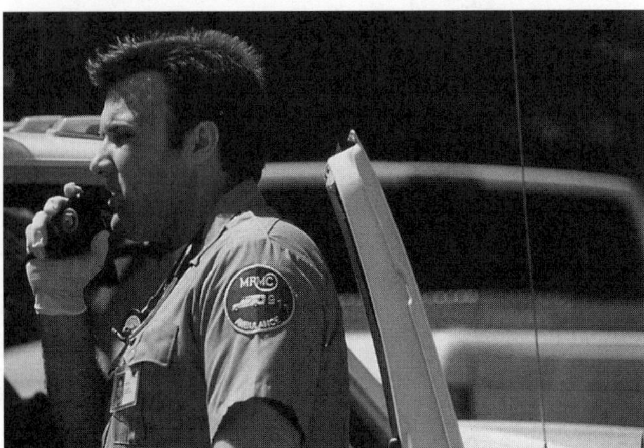

FIG. 6-3 An EMS responder should be able to use the 24-hour contact number in an emergency.

FOR PRODUCT EMERGENCY
Spill, Leak, Fire, Exposure or Accident
CALL CHEMTREC-DAY OR NIGHT
800-424-9300
OUTSIDE THE UNITED STATES CALL COLLECT 202-483-7616

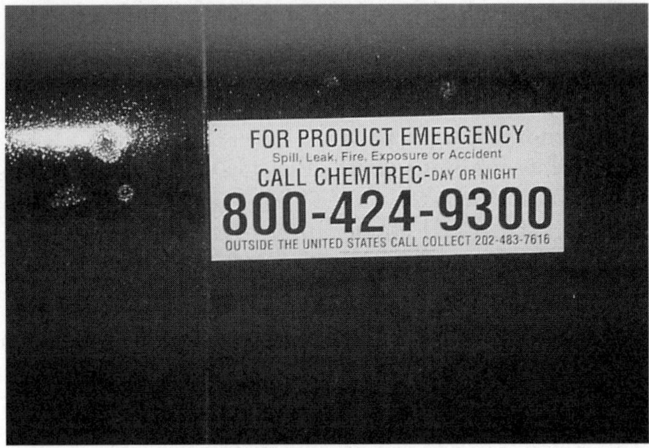

FIG. 6-4 Immediate response information is available through several organizations, one of which is CHEMTREC.

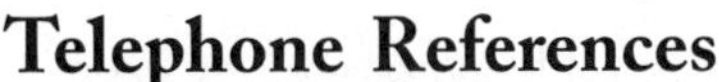

Telephone References

Telephone references can be extremely valuable to responders who do not have the room to carry multiple written texts or the budget to purchase a laptop and all the necessary software. One of the drawbacks of telephone references is the mistakes that can occur when transcribing information. The availability of a fax or cellular fax will minimize this problem.

New Department of Transportation (DOT) regulations require that shipping papers for hazardous materials transport contain an emergency contact telephone number that is accessible 24 hours a day (Fig. 6-3).

The Chemical Manufacturers Association

The Chemical Manufacturers Association (CMA) CHEMTREC and MEDTREC programs are telephone contact resources sponsored by the CMA and designed to provide emergency responders with immediate response information and to make contacts with manufacturers, shippers, and product experts when more detailed information is necessary. Under the MEDTREC program, medical responders can access medical information from the San Francisco Poison Center by calling the CHEMTREC number (Fig. 6-4), which follows:

- CHEMTREC: (800) 424-9300

The Agency of Toxic Substances and Disease Registry

The Agency of Toxic Substances and Disease Registry (ATSDR), a department of the U.S. Public Health Service, provides this 24-hour emergency telephone number, which can provide the emergency responder with chemical identification, detailed toxicological support, and decontamination information. That number is as follows:

- ATSDR: (404) 639-0616

The Centers for Disease Control

Another department of the U.S. Public Health Service is the Centers for Disease Control and Prevention (CDC). The CDC is available for assistance in handling infectious-disease–related incidents. The telephone number is as follows:

- CDC: (404) 633-5313

The Regional Poison Center

A valuable resource for EMS responders needing immediate toxicological information is the regional poison center. Regional poison centers are staffed by specially trained medical personnel, including toxicologists. Know the telephone number for the poison center in your area.

Computer References

Many EMS, fire, and hazardous materials (HAZMAT) response agencies are managing information using computers. An advantage of computers is they are a way to access numerous sources of information without having to tote a lot of weight. A laptop loaded with the most current software will provide emergency responders with a wealth of information (Fig. 6-5).

Probably the most detailed computer program is the *TOMES Plus* system available from Micromedex. This program, on CD-ROM, is actually a compilation of 14 databases designed for medical, environmental, and safety professionals. The Meditext database provides detailed medical management information, and the Hazardtext database provides in-depth hazardous materials response information. In addition to these two databases, the program contains 12 other databases. They are as follows:

- *NAERG—North American Emergency Response Guidebook*

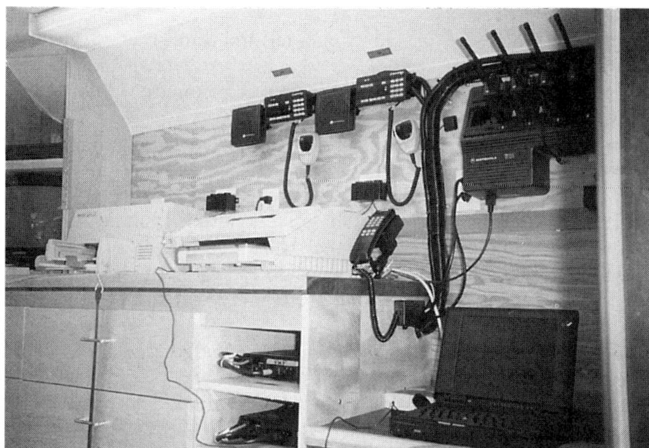

FIG. 6-5 Hazardous materials response vehicle incident command post supplied with radios, computers, fax, and printer/copier.

- RTECS—Registry of Toxic Effects of Chemical Substances
- New Jersey Hazardous Substance Fact Sheets
- HSDB—Hazardous Substance Data Bank
- *CHRIS—Chemical Hazard Response Information System*
- OHM/TADS—Oil and Hazardous Materials/Technical Assistance Data System
- IRIS—Integrated Risk Information System
- Reprotext System
- TERIS—Teratogen Information System
- Shepard's Catalog of Teratogenic Agents
- NIOSH Pocket Guide of Hazardous Substances
- Reprotox System

CCINFO

A detailed database program is *CCINFO,* from the Canadian Centre for Occupational Health and Safety. Three CD-ROMs are available. The red and yellow disks are the most useful for emergency responders. The red disk contains approximately 80,000 individual MSDSs and a compilation of emergency information called *CHEMINFO.* The yellow disk contains detailed chemical databases, including the following programs:

- Chemical Evaluation Search and Retrieval System (CESARS)
- CHEMINFO
- Chemical Hazard Response Information System (CHRIS)
- New Jersey Hazardous Substance Fact Sheets
- PRIS: Insecticide Information Systems

Computer-Aided Management of Emergency Operations

The *Computer-Aided Management of Emergency Operations (CAMEO)* is a computer database that was developed by the National Oceanographic and Atmospheric Administration (NOAA). It is now available from the National Safety Council. It was originally designed to manage the Superfund Amendment and Reauthorization Act (SARA) Title III information and assist emergency planners. Its chemical database has been updated recently to contain more than 3000 chemicals and more than 14,000 synonyms and trade names. The complete program will allow responders to track inventory, show building plans, list resource locations, locate special population areas that may require evacuation, show transportation routes, predict vapor plume dispersion, create incident reports, and conduct training. The chemical database will assist in the identification of chemicals and provide an MSDS-type printout with detailed emergency response information. Database information includes:

- General description
- Chemical/physical properties
- Health hazards
- First aid
- Fire hazards
- Firefighting information
- Protective clothing suggestions
- Nonfire response

Automated Resource for Chemical Hazard Incident Evaluation

A free program, called the *Automated Resource For Chemical Hazard Incident Evaluation (ARCHIE),* is available from the Federal Emergency Management Agency (FEMA). This program was not designed for use during an emergency response but rather to test emergency plans to see if they are realistic. It allows responders and planners to predict the damage that can occur when a chemical is released from its container. The program allows responders to:

- Estimate the discharge rate of a liquid or gas
- Estimate the area of the liquid pool
- Estimate the vaporization rate of the liquid pool
- Evaluate a toxic vapor dispersion hazard
- Evaluate a pool fire radiation hazard
- Evaluate a fireball radiation hazard
- Evaluate a flame jet hazard
- Evaluate a vapor cloud/plume fire hazard
- Evaluate a vapor cloud explosion hazard
- Evaluate a tank overpressurization rupture hazard
- Evaluate solid/liquid explosion hazards

Summary

We have discussed only a few of the quality references available to the emergency responder. Many other excellent written, telephone, and computer references are available. Responders must find a mix of references that provides assistance in identification, chemical/physical data, emergency response information, and medical management information. No single reference can supply responders with all the information that is necessary. The rule of thumb in using references is to consult a minimum of three sources and take the worst-case data into consideration. Numerous available forms allow this information to be copied in a user-friendly manner. This process can be carried out on high-hazard chemicals in the area as a preplanning measure that will speed information gathering.

CHAPTER REVIEW QUESTIONS

1. What types of information can be obtained from the NAERG?
2. Where can MSDSs be found?
3. List at least two other common written hazardous materials references.
4. List at least two written hazardous materials references that focus on medical management.
5. Identify at least three telephone references that can supply medical management information.
6. What are the advantages and limitations of computer references?
7. List at least three computer hazardous materials references.
8. Why is a mix of different reference sources necessary?
9. The reference source rule of thumb states how many references should be used?

BIBLIOGRAPHY

American Conference of Governmental and Industrial Hygienists: *1997-1998 threshold limit values for chemical substances and physical agents and biological exposure indices,* Cincinnati, Ohio, 1997, ACGIH.

Bronstein AC, Currance PL: *Emergency care for hazardous materials exposure,* ed 2, St Louis, 1994, Mosby.

CAMEO: Chicago, National Safety Council.

CCINFO (Canadian OSH database): Hamilton, Ontario, Canada, Canadian Centre for Occupational Health and Safety.

DOT: *CHRIS hazardous chemical data,* US Department of Transportation/US Coast Guard, Washington, DC, 1984, US Department of Transportation.

DOT: *1996 North American emergency response guidebook,* Office of Hazardous Materials Transportation, Research and Special Programs Administration, Washington, DC, 1996, US Department of Transportation.

Gosselin RE, Smith RP, Hodge HC: Clinical toxicology of commercial products, ed 5, Baltimore, 1994, Williams & Wilkins.

Lewis RJ: Hazardous chemical desk reference, New York, 1993, Van Nostrand Reinhold.

NIOSH: *NIOSH pocket guide to chemical hazards,* Washington, DC, 1994, DHHS (NIOSH) Publication No. 94-116, US Government Printing Office.

Olson KR, editor: Poisoning and drug overdose, ed 2, East Norwalk, Conn, 1994, Appleton & Lange.

Tomes Plus, Lakewood, Colo, Micromedex.

7

Medical Surveillance

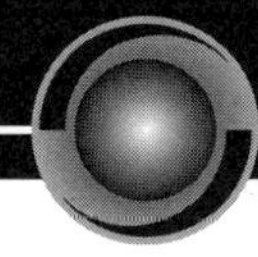

Alvin C. Bronstein, M.D., FACEP

CHAPTER OBJECTIVES

At the conclusion of this chapter the student will be able to:

- Describe the purpose of a medical surveillance program.
- Discuss the definition of a HAZMAT team.
- Define a health hazard as described by OSHA.
- Discuss the four basic types of evaluations that compose a medical surveillance plan.
- Discuss the components of the medical surveillance examination.

CASE STUDY

You are the chief of a newly designated fire department hazardous materials (HAZMAT) team located in a coastal city. As part of your job duties, a medical surveillance program must be established for the team. Not having expertise in this area, you contact your family physician. The physician agrees to meet with you to discuss the issues. At the meeting it becomes clear that setting up a medical surveillance program is complex. Your physician tells you that he has never set up such a program and recommends that you contact the regional poison center or an occupational medicine physician.

- How can a primary care physician assist in setting up a medical surveillance program?
- Describe the goals of a medical surveillance program.
- What are the necessary components for a quality surveillance program?
- What is the role of a constant in the medical surveillance program?
- What resources are available from the regional poison center?

HAZMAT team responders must be ready to respond to various environmental emergencies. Because of the myriad of potential health threats, many of which are unknown, a comprehensive medical surveillance program is required to ensure the health and safety of the responders. The goal of the medical monitoring or screening program is to promote (1) early diagnosis of hazardous-materials–related occupational disease, (2) early intervention and treatment, (3) effective management of an occupational disease process, and (4) illness prevention. The medical program requires comprehensive planning by medical personnel knowledgeable in the team's response duties and the health effects of hazardous materials exposure.

HAZMAT Teams

According to Occupational Safety and Health Administration (OSHA) standard 1910.120, a "hazardous materials (HAZMAT) response team" is defined as an organized group of employees, designated by their employer, who are expected to perform work to handle and control actual or potential leaks or spills of hazardous substances requiring possible close approach to the substance. Team members respond to releases or potential releases of hazardous substances to control or stabilize the incident. A HAZMAT team is not a fire brigade, nor is a typical fire brigade a HAZMAT team. A HAZMAT team, however, may be a separate component of a fire brigade or fire department. Their work requires them to participate in a medical monitoring program. This lengthy definition can be applied to many HAZMAT team configurations, from industrial response teams to fire department HAZMAT teams.

Hazardous materials responders may be involved in various activities, ranging from emergency response operations with uncontrolled and unknown hazards to site cleanup operations in which the specific health hazards may be known. Emergency response may consist of entering areas of known chemical or pathological agents, with the added danger of chemical reaction or combustion product exposure. Cleanup activities present additional potential exposure problems, ranging from containing and removing products to product neutralization reactions to product incineration. Because of these various exposure scenarios, a HAZMAT team's health care program must be customized to the team's usual type of hazardous materials response, as well as to anticipation of theoretical health threats. Development of a comprehensive medical surveillance program requires the participation of a medical toxicologist or occupational medicine physician knowledgeable in the team's activities and potential exposure threats.

The HAZMAT team faces many potential health hazards. OSHA (29 CFR 1910.120) defines a health hazard as a chemical, mixture of chemicals, or a pathogen for which there is statistically significant evidence based on at least one study conducted in accordance with established scientific principles that acute or chronic health effects may occur in exposed employees. The term *health hazard* includes chemicals defined as carcinogens, toxic or highly toxic agents, reproductive toxins, irritants, corrosives, sensitizers, heptaotoxins, nephrotoxins, neurotoxins, agents that act on the hematopoietic system, and/or agents that damage the lungs, skin, eyes, or mucous membranes (Box 7-1). It also includes physiological stress caused by temperature extremes.

BOX 7-1

HAZMAT Team Health Hazards

Carcinogens
Highly toxic agents
Reproductive toxins
Irritants
Corrosives
Sensitizers
Heptaotoxins
Nephrotoxins
Neurotoxins
Blood poisons
Pulmonary poisons
Skin and eye poisons
Temperature extremes

OSHA also mandates that employers shall develop and implement a written safety and health program for their employees who are involved in hazardous waste operations. The program shall be designed to identify, evaluate, and control safety and health hazards, and provide for emergency response for hazardous waste operations. This plan has two major parts: (1) identification of the operations that have been identified by the employer to be part of the hazardous materials response and (2) the design and operation of a medical surveillance program. The program should be responsive to the hazards potentially encountered by the team.

The law requires the employer to identify potential hazards. This is accomplished using a two-step process: preliminary and detailed surveys. All suspected conditions that may pose inhalation or skin absorption hazards that are immediately dangerous to life or health, or other conditions that may cause death or serious harm, shall be identified during the preliminary survey and comprehensively evaluated during the detailed survey. Examples of such hazards include, but are not limited to, confined space entry, potentially explosive or flammable situations, visible vapor clouds, or areas in which biological indicators, such as dead animals or vegetation, are located. Additionally, HAZMAT team members must be provided with any information describing the hazards they may encounter. Any information concerning the chemical, physical, and toxicological properties of each substance known or expected to be present on site that is available to the employer and relevant to the duties an employee is expected to perform shall be made available to the affected employees before beginning their work activities. The employer may use information developed for the hazard communication standard for this purpose. Obviously, this complicated procedure is most applicable to industry-based teams working in a permanent facility. Fire department and other emergency response teams do not always have the luxury of preidentifying potential team health hazards. Therefore, the medical surveillance program must cover the most likely exposure scenario and be as comprehensive as possible, given fiscal constraints (Box 7-2).

BOX 7-2

Individuals for Whom Medical Surveillance Is Required

All employees at hazardous waste sites who are exposed to chemicals above the permissible exposure limit
All employees who wear a respirator more than 30 days a year
All employees who become ill or injured from exposure to hazardous materials
Members of a hazardous materials response team

OSHA further requires a medical surveillance program for the following workers:

1. All employees at hazardous waste sites who are, or may be, exposed to hazardous substances or health hazards at or above the permissible exposure limit (PEL) or, if there is no PEL, above the published exposure levels for these substances, without regard to the use of respirators, for 30 days or more a year
2. All employees who wear a respirator for 30 days or more a year or as required by OSHA 1910.134
3. All employees who are injured, become ill, or develop signs or symptoms caused by possible overexposure involving hazardous substances or health hazards from an emergency response or hazardous waste operation.

Planning the Medical Surveillance Program

Types of Medical Surveillance Examinations

Four basic types of evaluations make up the medical surveillance plan. They are as follows:

- Baseline
- Annual or periodic
- Job termination or exit
- Exposure-specific and medical follow-up examinations

The frequency of medical examinations and consultations also is specified by OSHA. Medical examinations and consultations are conducted according to the following schedule:

1. Baseline: Before assignment on the HAZMAT team
2. Annual or periodic: At least once every 12 months for each employee covered unless the attending physician believes a longer interval (not greater than every 2 years) is appropriate
3. Exit: At termination of employment or reassignment to an area where the employee would not be covered, if the employee has not had an examination within the past 6 months
4. Exposure Specific: As soon as possible on notification by an employee that the employee has developed signs or symptoms indicating possible overexposure to hazardous substances or health hazards, or that the employee has been injured or exposed above the PELs or published exposure levels in an emergency situation

Additional medical follow-up examinations may be required at more frequent times, if the examining physician determines there is a medical necessity (e.g., for employees who may have been injured or suffered health impairment because of a hazardous materials response). Included would be individuals with signs or symptoms that may have resulted from exposure to hazardous substances resulting from an emergency incident, or during an emergency incident to hazardous substances at concentrations above the PELs or the published exposure levels without the necessary personal protective equipment (PPE) being used.

Physician Involvement

OSHA requires that all medical examinations and procedures be performed by or under the supervision of a licensed physician (Fig. 7-1). Preferably, this is a physician who is knowledgeable in toxicology, occupational medicine, and hazardous materials exposure. The employer is required by OSHA to provide the physician with a copy of the OSHA standard and its appendices. For each employee, the employer should furnish:

1. A description of the employee's duties as they relate to the employee's exposures
2. The employee's exposure levels or anticipated exposure levels
3. A description of PPE used or to be used
4. Information from previous medical examinations of the employee that is not readily available to the examining physician

At the examination, the physician obtains a comprehensive health history from the patient. This usually is done using a questionnaire. The health history includes a detailed occupational and exposure history, with emphasis on symptoms related to the handling of hazardous substances and other health hazards. The team members' ability to wear required PPE under conditions such as temperature extremes also is assessed. Based on the HAZMAT team member's responses to the history, cer-

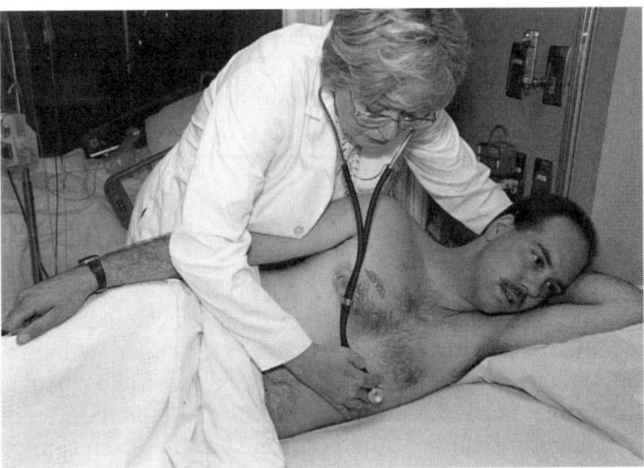

FIG. 7-1 Medical examinations should be performed by or under the supervision of a licensed physician.

tain areas of the physical examination may require more emphasis than others. The medical toxicologist or occupational physician considers whether special risk factors for the team member exist. These may include immunological competence, use of steroid medication such as prednisone, chemotherapy, pregnancy, or cigarette smoking.

Physical examination

Following the comprehensive health history-taking, a complete physical examination is done, including near and far vision testing. Pertinent positive findings are noted. Forms should be developed so that physical findings are easy to track from year to year.

Laboratory testing

Baseline laboratory tests are obtained as part of the screening process. A detailed matrix of appropriate laboratory examinations or biochemical profiles should be developed. Depending on specific HAZMAT team needs, this list will vary with team and region. The biochemical profile usually includes tests of serum electrolytes, blood glucose, and kidney and liver function. The following is an example of the laboratory components of a comprehensive medical surveillance examination:

- Complete blood count (CBC)
- Blood tests of kidney and liver function
- Glucose
- Blood urea nitrogen (BUN)
- Creatinine
- Sodium
- Potassium
- Chloride
- Magnesium
- Calcium
- Phosphorous, inorganic
- Protein, total
- Albumin
- Globulin
- Bilirubin, total
- Alkaline phosphatase (Alk Phos)
- Lactate dehydrogenase (LDH)
- Gamma glutamyl transpeptidase (GGTP)
- Aspartate aminotransferase (AST)
- Alanine aminotransferase (ALT)
- Uric acid
- Urine tests, including urinalysis and urine drug screen for drugs of abuse

Additional biochemical tests or specific toxicological examinations, such as plasma and/or red blood cell cholinesterase, may be required depending on the particular hazardous materials exposure likely to be encountered. These additional tests are performed at the discretion of the medical director. Because few chemicals have specific blood markers for easily and economically available screening programs, most physicians must rely on assessment of general health status to determine the presence of possible hazardous materials health exposure effects.

Other tests include a baseline resting electrocardiogram (ECG). Hearing testing consists of a hearing questionnaire and audiogram. Hearing conservation counseling should be done in conjunction with the audiometric testing. Further testing includes pulmonary function tests (PFTs), chest radiographs, and tuberculosis skin testing (PPD). PFTs must include evaluation of forced expiratory volume at 1 second (FEV_1), forced vital capacity (FVC), and FEV_1/FVC ratio and use accepted normative data for comparison.

Because being a member of a HAZMAT team requires strenuous physical work at extremes of temperature and humidity, physical fitness, cardiac stress testing, and strength and agility testing may be added to the examination regimen.

Medical surveillance programs usually are customized to the potential toxins involved. For example, an asbestos monitoring program focuses on the cardiovascular and respiratory systems and the individual's ability to wear a respirator.

Annual medical examination

The annual medical examination repeats all of the baseline testing except for the chest radiograph. An interval medical history is obtained. The annual screening examination updates the medical and occupational history in the team member's medical file. Any exposures during the previous year are reviewed. If a specific exposure has occurred, then more specific testing may be required.

Termination or exit examination

At team exit, job transfer, or termination, a comprehensive history and physical examination is conducted. All baseline laboratory tests are repeated. An interval medical history is obtained. The exit examination updates the medical and occupational history in the team member's medical file. Any exposures since the last examination are reviewed. If a specific exposure occurred, then more specific testing may be required.

Exposure-specific examination

If a HAZMAT team member is exposed, regardless of the presence of symptoms, then an exposure-specific examination is conducted. This includes a physical examination and laboratory tests geared toward evaluating the exposure and potential short- or long-term problems.

Reports and recordkeeping

SUMMARY REPORT FOR EMPLOYEE (BASELINE, ANNUAL, EXIT). Once the history, physical, and laboratory examinations are completed, the physician prepares a summary report. This report is supplied to the employee and must contain the following information:

1. Medical condition(s) that would place the employee at increased risk of medical impairment from con-

tinued work on a HAZMAT team or from respirator use
2. Fitness for duty status, with any recommended work restrictions
3. Disclosure to the employee of the results of the medical examination and tests
4. A statement that the employee has been informed by the physician of the results of the medical examination and of any medical conditions that require further examination or treatment

Summary Report for Employer (Baseline, Annual, Exit). The written opinion obtained by the employer should not reveal specific findings or diagnoses unrelated to occupational exposures. This report usually includes the following:

1. Fitness-for-duty statement, including whether the HAZMAT team member is medically fit to wear a respirator
2. Report stating whether the employee has any medical problem that would preclude him or her from being on the HAZMAT team

Exposure-Specific Examination Summary Report for Employee. The exposure-specific examination physician report should include the following:

1. A description of the signs and symptoms of exposure that the employee is experiencing, if any
2. Recommendation for further medical follow-up
3. Results of the medical examination and any associated tests
4. Any medical condition that was found, which might place the employee at increased risk as a result of the exposure to a hazardous chemical found in the workplace

Exposure-Specific Examination Summary Report for Employer. This report should include the following:

1. A statement that the employee has been informed by the physician of the results of the medical examination
2. Any medical condition that requires further examination or treatment
3. Fitness for duty and ability to wear a respirator

The written physician opinion should not reveal specific findings of diagnoses unrelated to occupational exposure.

Medical surveillance generally is defined as the systematic collection, analysis, and evaluation of health data in a defined population to identify patterns or trends suggesting an adverse health effect or the need for further investigation or remedial action. Some examples of medical surveillance are serial examination of liver function tests over time because of specific exposures, periodic monitoring of pulmonary function and chest radiograph data for asbestos exposure, and periodic monitoring of heavy-metal exposure. An accurate record of the medical surveillance examinations must be retained for the duration of employment plus 30 years.

Summary

Comprehensive medical surveillance programs protect the health of the HAZMAT team responder. These programs require careful planning. Proper implementation ensures accurate results. For these programs to achieve their goal, the health care provider must work closely with the team to ensure reliability and quality. Implementation of a medical monitoring program requires the involvement of physicians with specialized knowledge of hazardous materials and their potential health effects. This individual usually will be a medical toxicologist or occupational medicine physician. If no one is available in your area, then consultation with the regional poison control center should be arranged.

CHAPTER REVIEW QUESTIONS

1. List the four goals of a medical surveillance program.
2. Name three types of HAZMAT team health hazards.
3. What are the four types of hazardous materials medical surveillance examinations?
4. Describe the parts of a hazardous materials surveillance medical examination.
5. Who needs to be in a medical monitoring program?
6. What governmental agency specifies the frequency of medical surveillance examinations?
7. When should an exposure-specific examination be conducted?
8. Before the medical examination, what information should the employer furnish to the physician?
9. List three laboratory tests that may be done as part of the medical surveillance examination.
10. How long must medical surveillance records be kept on file?

BIBLIOGRAPHY

American Conference of Governmental and Industrial Hygienists: *TLVs and other occupational exposure values, 1997.* Cincinnati, Ohio, ACGIH, 1997 (CD-ROM).

American Conference of Governmental and Industrial Hygienists: *1998 TLVs and BEIs. Threshold limit values for chemical substances and physical agents: biological exposure indices.* Cincinnati, Ohio, ACGIH, 1998.

Bronstein AC, Currance PL: *Emergency care for hazardous materials exposure,* ed 2, 1994, St. Louis, Mosby.

Code of Federal Regulations: 29 CFR 1910.120, Washington, DC, US Government Printing Office, 1997.

Cohen KS: Hazardous material information resources. *Occup Health Saf* 52:15-17, 1983.

IARC: Monographs on the evaluation of carcinogenic risk of chemicals to man. Overall evaluations of carcinogenicity to humans as evaluated in IARC monographs, vol 1-71 (a total of 834 agents, mixtures, and exposures). Last updated March 5, 1998 (cited July 10, 1998). Available from URL: http://193.51.164.11/monoeval/crthall.html.

Krieger GR, Balge M: Principles of medical surveillance and human exposure standards. In Sullivan JB, Krieger GR, editors: *Hazardous material toxicology,* Baltimore, 1991, Williams & Wilkins.

Mullan RJ, Murthy LI: Occupational sentinel health events: an updated list for physician recognition and public health surveillance, *Am J Ind Med* 19:775-799, 1991.

SECTION TWO

Emergency Medical Services/Hazardous Materials Field Operations

8

Personal Protective Equipment

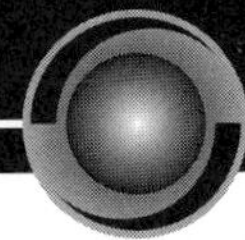

Phil Currance

CHAPTER OBJECTIVES

At the conclusion of this chapter the student will be able to:

- Discuss the role that preplanning plays in selecting personal protective equipment.
- Explain the use and limitations of standard and specialized EMS protective equipment in hazardous materials incidents.
- Identify adverse effects that can be caused by the use of personal protective equipment.
- Identify mitigation techniques that should be used in conjunction with personal protective equipment.
- Identify three types of respiratory-protective equipment, and discuss their limitations.
- Given chemical identification and concentrations, select the proper level of respiratory-protective equipment.
- Describe respiratory-protective equipment fit test procedures.
- Discuss the difference between vapor- and splash-protective clothing.
- List the four EPA-designated levels of protection, and discuss the use and limitations of each.
- Describe the three ways that chemical-protective clothing may fail.
- Discuss the process for selecting proper levels of personal protective equipment.
- Describe donning and doffing procedures for personal protective equipment.
- Discuss maintenance and inspection procedures for personal protective equipment.

CASE STUDY

A railcar of hydrochloric acid is leaking at a local switching yard. Four railroad employees who tried to repair the leak have been injured, and two employees are unconscious in the hot zone. The fire department hazardous materials (HAZMAT) team is donning Level A protective equipment to rescue the downed patients and perform containment operations on the leaking tankcar. Emergency Medical Services/hazardous materials (EMS/HM) Level 2 responders are on scene and have been asked to assist with medical management of the patients during decontamination.

- ◆ What level of respiratory protection is appropriate for the EMS/HM Level 2 responders?
- ◆ What level of skin protection is appropriate for the EMS/HM Level 2 responders?
- ◆ What type of protective clothing fabric will provide the best protection against hydrochloric acid?
- ◆ To what risks are the HAZMAT team responders wearing Level A suits exposed?

Responders at hazardous materials incidents must be adequately protected from potential exposure and injury. The purpose of personal protective equipment (PPE) is to shield or isolate individuals from the chemical, physical, and biological hazards that exist when responding to hazardous materials incidents (Box 8-1). Protective equipment concerns must be addressed before any response activity. Protective equipment decisions must be based on responder involvement. Activities in clean, safe areas, such as management of decontaminated patients, can be safely carried out in PPE commonly used for body substance isolation (Fig. 8-1). This will include gloves, mask, eye protection, and a suit to keep liquids from contacting the responder's uniform. This type of PPE is not adequate for use in the contaminated area or for use during primary decontamination activities. In these areas, chemical protective equipment is needed (Fig. 8-2). Equipment that is chemical protective includes chemical-resistant clothing and gloves that are specifically compatible with the chemical, and either an air-purifying respirator (APR) or a self-contained breathing apparatus (SCBA). The use of this equipment requires special training and selection by a knowledgeable, experienced person.

Responders should not attempt to utilize PPE without proper preplanning, training, medical examinations, and fit testing as required. Selection of equipment by an informed and knowledgeable individual using appropriate reference sources is essential. Having equipment is not enough. The equipment must be compatible with the chemical. Another problem is that chemical-protective equipment usually does not provide protection against fire or heat. Initial hands-on training and repeated practice with all the protective equipment is essential for safe and effective use.

In addition to EMS responders' protection, knowledge of protective equipment concerns is vital for the support of the HAZMAT response team. The use of PPE can itself create significant worker hazards such as heat stress; physical and psychological stress; and impaired vision, mobility, and communication. In general, greater levels of PPE protection can cause the associated risks to increase. For any given situation, equipment and clothing should be selected that provide an adequate level of protection. Gross overprotection, as well as underprotection, can be hazardous and should be avoided.

No single combination of PPE and clothing is capable of protecting against all hazards. Thus PPE should be used in conjunction with other protective methods. All potential hazards should be identified. Once identified, as many hazards as possible should be mitigated. Examples of hazard mitigation include:

- Ventilation of structures/confined spaces
- Use of foam to suppress vapors
- Use of nonsparking tools
- Control of ignition sources
- Avoidance of contact with hazardous substances as much as possible
- Adequate decontamination before removal of PPE

BOX 8-1

PPE Needs for EMS/HM Response

STANDARD PROTECTIVE EQUIPMENT

Body substance isolation equipment for cold-zone operations
Eye protection
Mask
Gloves (latex under gloves and chemical-resistant outer gloves)
Fluid-resistant gowns
Fluid-resistant shoe covers
Rain gear

SPECIALIZED PROTECTIVE EQUIPMENT

For warm- or hot-zone operations
Self-contained breathing apparatus
Air-purifying respirators
Chemical-resistant gloves (with latex under gloves)
Chemical-resistant suits
Boots or shoe covers

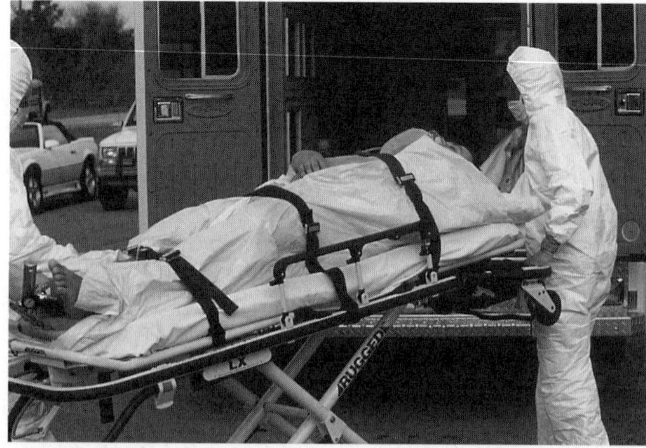

FIG. 8-1 EMS responder in body substance isolation PPE.

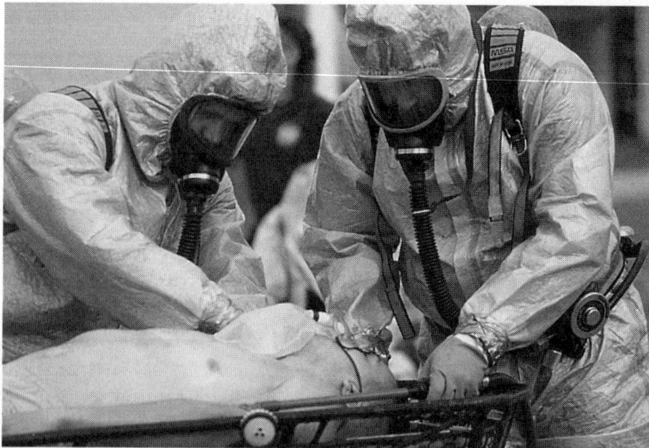

FIG. 8-2 EMS responder in chemical-protective PPE.

Respiratory Protection

The most vulnerable route of exposure is inhalation. Responders must have adequate respiratory protection. Respiratory protection can be provided by APRs (Fig. 8-3), positive-pressure SCBA (Fig. 8-4), or positive-pressure, supplied-air respirators (SAR, or air lines).

Occupational Safety and Health Administration (OSHA) standards mandate specific requirements for respirator use. These include mandates for a written program, proper selection of respirators, medical monitoring, fit tests, user training, and storage/inspection. Proper use procedures, such as restrictions on facial hair, also are included in the standards. The selection of the proper respirator is based on several factors:

- ◆ Oxygen concentration in the area
- ◆ Identity of the substance
- ◆ Concentration of the substance
- ◆ Chemical and physical properties of the substance
- ◆ Warning properties of the substance
- ◆ Area in which responders must operate
- ◆ Specific tasks to be completed

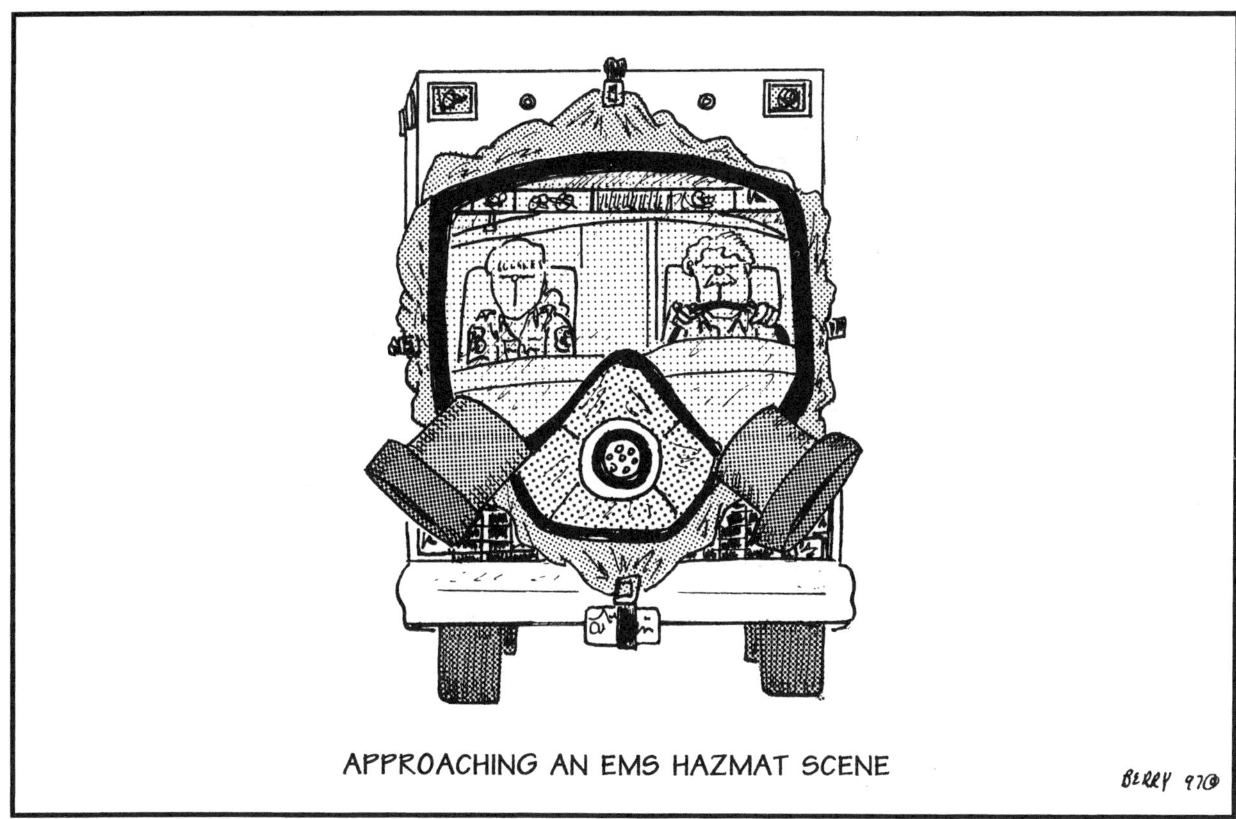

Reprinted with permission from Steve Berry's *I'm Not an Ambulance Driver* cartoon book series.

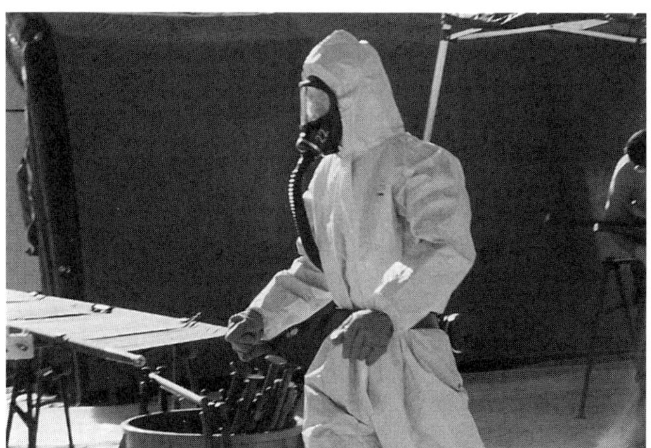

FIG. 8-3 EMS responder wearing a powered air-purifying respirator.

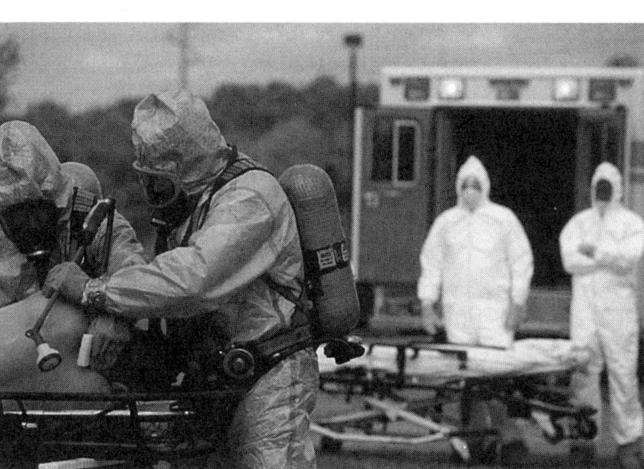

FIG. 8-4 EMS responders wearing SCBAs.

BOX 8-2

PROTECTION FACTORS (PF) FOR VARIOUS RESPIRATORS

Half-face APR	10
Full-face APR	50
Powered air-purifying respirator (PAPR)	50
Positive-pressure SCBA	10,000+
Positive-pressure air line with escape bottle	10,000+

MAXIMUM USE CONCENTRATION FORMULA:

PEL × PF = MUC

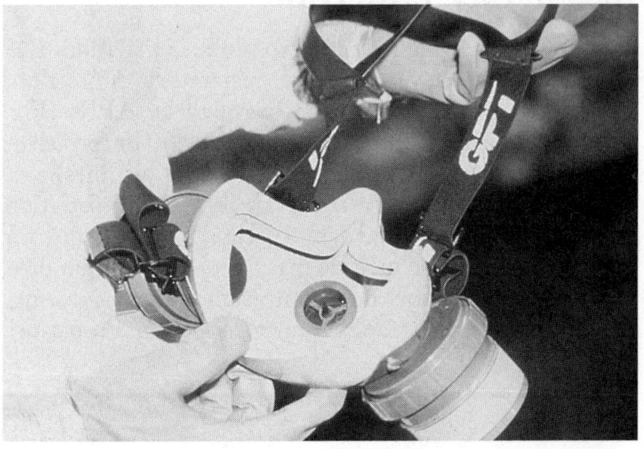

FIG. 8-5 Half-face air-purifying respirator.

The level of protection that can be provided by a respirator is indicated by the respirator's protection factor (PF). This number, which is determined experimentally by measuring face piece seal and exhalation valve leakage, indicates the relative difference in concentrations of substances outside and inside the face piece that can be maintained by the respirator. The PF is multiplied by the chemical's exposure limit (permissible exposure limit [PEL]–time weighted average [TWA] or threshold limit value [TLV]–TWA) to determine the maximum use concentration (MUC) of the respirator (Box 8-2). APRs should never be used at concentrations above either the chemical's Immediately Dangerous to Life and Health (IDLH) value or MUC (PF × PEL–TWA = MUC). Above these levels, SCBAs or SARs are required.

Several factors can affect the proper fit of a respirator and reduce the PF. These factors are as follows:

- Facial hair that contacts the sealing surface
- Facial deformities
- Extreme heat or cold
- Eyeglasses with temple bars or straps

Air-Purifying Respirators

Air-purifying respirators (APRs) use filters or sorbent materials to remove harmful substances from the air. They range from simple disposable masks to sophisticated, powered air-purifying respirators (PAPRs) (Fig. 8-5).

APRs consist of a face piece and an air-purifying device, which is either a removable component on the face piece or an air-purifying apparatus worn on a body harness and attached to the face piece by a corrugated breathing tube. APRs selectively remove airborne contaminants by filtration, absorption, adsorption, or chemical reactions. They are approved for use in atmospheres containing specific chemicals up to designated concentrations. The use of APRs is limited, especially for emergency response operations, and is only appropriate when:

- Atmospheric oxygen is above 19.5%.
- The chemical substance is known.
- The chemical substance can be filtered, absorbed, or neutralized.
- The chemical substance has an adequate warning property (odor, irritation, or taste detectable below the PEL and consistent to above the IDLH).
- The airborne concentration of the chemical substance is known.
- The airborne concentration of a chemical substance does not exceed 1000 ppm, the calculated MUC or the established IDLH.
- There is a NIOSH-approved cartridge.
- No firefighting activities are involved.
- Users have been properly trained, fit-tested, and under gone medical monitoring.

WARNING: Some contaminants cannot be removed by APRs. These respirators are *not* used in oxygen-deficient or IDLH situations, or when the contaminants are unknown.

During emergency response operations, initial entry into the contaminated area must be considered as an IDLH situation and atmosphere-supplying respirators used. Once the substance has been identified and quantified, and all criteria are met, APRs may be of limited use. In these circumstances they may be used during decontamination or in low-risk cleanup activities.

Air-purifying cartridges and canisters are designed for specific materials at specific concentrations. The respirators that are being used by EMS personnel to protect against tuberculosis are high efficiency particulate air (HEPA) cartridges. These respirators may provide protection against asbestos and other particulates, but will allow gases and vapors to pass through.

To aid the user, manufacturers have color-coded the cartridges and canisters to indicate the chemical or class of chemicals against which the device is effective (Fig. 8-6). The National Institute of Occupational Safety and Health (NIOSH) recommends that the use of a cartridge not exceed one work shift. However, if breakthrough of the

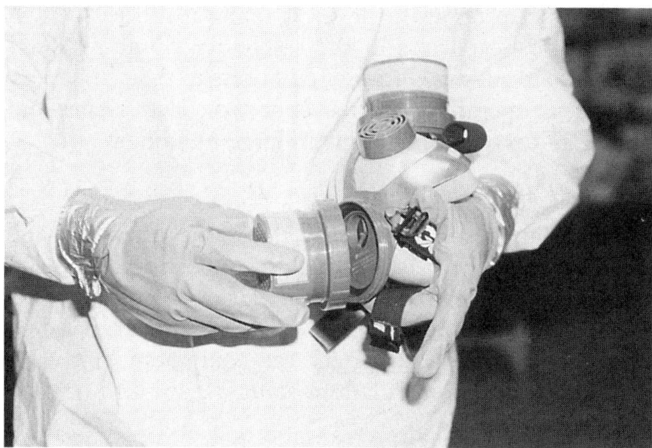

FIG. 8-6 APR and combination cartridge (HEPA and organic vapor/acid gas).

contaminant or difficulty breathing occurs first, then the cartridge or canister must be replaced immediately.

Atmosphere-Supplying Respirators

Atmosphere-supplying respirators are designed to provide breathable air from a clean air source other than the surrounding contaminated atmosphere (Fig. 8-7).

Atmosphere-supplying respirators supply certified breathing air to the face piece. These respirators must be operated in a positive-pressure or pressure-demand mode. Pressure-demand respirators maintain a positive pressure in the face piece during both inhalation and exhalation. In these respirators, a pressure regulator and an exhalation valve on the mask maintain the mask's positive pressure. If a leak develops in a pressure-demand respirator, the regulator sends a continuous flow of clean air into the face piece, preventing penetration by contaminated ambient air. This is in contrast to negative-pressure respirators such as APRs. In a negative-pressure system the user inhales, creating a negative pressure inside the mask and allowing air to move through the filter medium to the inside of the mask. If there are any facial fit leaks, contaminated air will be drawn into the mask. Atmosphere-supplying respirators come in three types:

- ◆ SCBA
- ◆ SARs, or air lines
- ◆ Escape-only respirators

Self-contained breathing apparatus

Self-contained breathing apparatuses (SCBAs) are the most common respiratory protection device used by emergency responders. SCBA respirators can be purchased as open- or closed-circuit design. An open-circuit SCBA exhausts exhaled air directly into the environment (Fig. 8-8). Air is supplied by either a single-stage (conventional) or a two-stage National Aeronautic and Space Administration (NASA) regulator. Single-stage regulators reduce the air pressure from the air cylinder only once before reaching the wearer. This type of SCBA usually is characterized by a corrugated low-pressure tube connecting the face piece to the regulator. Two-stage regulators are characterized by an initial reduction of cylinder air pressure immediately exiting the air cylinder. A second regulator then is placed at the face piece.

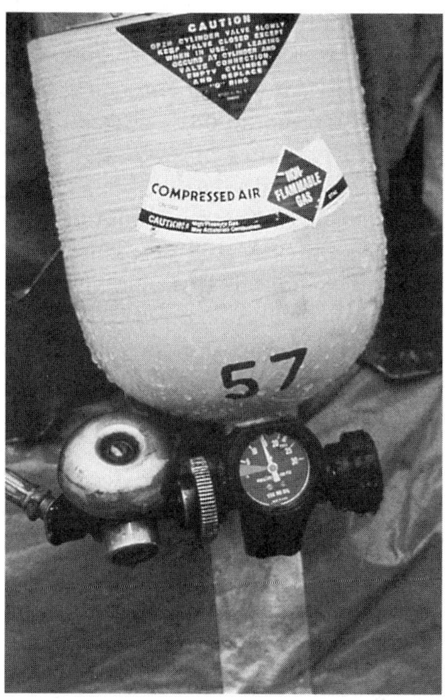

FIG. 8-7 Atmosphere-supplying respirator (SCBA).

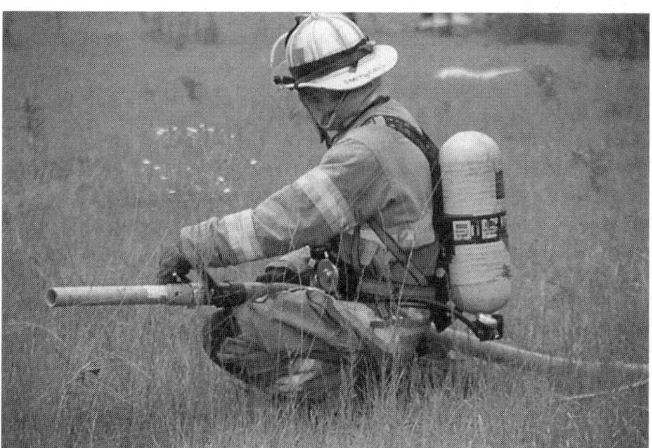

FIG. 8-8 Responder wearing open-circuit SCBA.

Open-circuit SCBAs provide respiratory protection from most types and levels of airborne contaminants. However, the air supply is a limiting factor. The duration of the air supply is limited by the amount carried in the tank (tank pressure pounds per square inch [psi]), the rate of consumption, and the type of work being done. The size, physical condition, breathing rate, and lung volume (tidal volume) of the responder using the equipment will determine the rate of consumption. Open-circuit SCBAs typically are described as high- or low-pressure systems.

Low-pressure systems with standard-size bottles, commonly referred to as *30-minute units,* have service pressures of 2216 psi, while high-pressure systems with standard-size bottles, commonly referred to as *1-hour units,* have service pressures of 4500 psi. High-pressure units also are available with smaller bottles that are rated at 30 or 45 minutes. Most users will not get the 30-, 45-, or 60-minute use time. A common rule of thumb is 1 minute for each 100 pounds in a standard-size cylinder.

An alarm (e.g., bell, whistle, or vibrator) is set to function when 25% of the service pressure (approximately 500 psi for low-pressure bottles) is reached. During hazardous materials emergencies, the alarm should not be depended on as a signal to withdraw from the contaminated area. Personnel will have to be decontaminated before removing the respirator face piece. Time must be allocated for exit from the contaminated area and decontamination.

Other negative aspects of open-circuit SCBAs are bulk and weight. Responders wearing SCBAs may be unable to operate in tight spaces. These units will provide EMS personnel with the highest level of protection during patient decontamination, but the weight and bulk will limit the responders' ability to carry out some patient care activities. The weight of the SCBA will contribute to the physical and heat stress of the wearer. An increased risk of back injuries exists and is a result of a change in the wearer's center of gravity when wearing SCBA.

A closed-circuit breathing apparatus recycles the wearer's exhaled air (Fig. 8-9). Closed-circuit units consist of a carbon dioxide (CO_2) scrubber unit and a bottle of compressed oxygen. These units have a tube that carries air to the mask and a second tube that carries exhaled air back to the unit. The CO_2 is chemically removed, and fresh oxygen is introduced.

This type of breathing apparatus is commonly referred to as a *rebreather.* Advantages of a closed-circuit unit are lighter weight and longer service duration (up to 6 hours in some units). Disadvantages include higher prices, higher operating costs, and heat build-up caused by the exothermic reaction in the CO_2 removal process, which can add to heat stress in the responder. Some response agencies are adding closed-circuit units to their inventory for special operations such as confined space rescues and search and rescue operations in large buildings.

Supplied-air respirators

Supplied-air respirators (SARs), or air lines, provide clean air to a face mask through a connecting hose from a large tank of certified breathing air or a certified compressor located in a safe, clean area (Fig. 8-10). A safety escape bottle must be part of the equipment in IDLH conditions. OSHA regulations state that the air line cannot exceed 300 feet.

Advantages of air-line systems include an increased work time and reduced weight and bulk. Disadvantages include the close proximity of the air source to the contaminated area and the vulnerability of the air line. The air line may be damaged by chemicals or cut by sharp edges or debris, or may kink, cutting off the air supply. In addition, responders have limited mobility. They must retrace their steps to exit the area. Additional responders must be assigned to manage the air source and air lines.

Air lines are extremely useful for responders carrying out decontamination activities or rescue in confined spaces. Air lines also can be combined with open-circuit SCBAs. This combination can provide for mobility and increased work time in isolated areas or increased time for decontamination.

Escape-only respirators

Escape-only respirators provide continuous air flow from a small bottle to a plastic hood that goes over the head. Escape bottles typically are 5- or 10-minute duration. They supply direct, continuous-flow air but are not pressure-demand units. They are used by otherwise nonprotected personnel to escape from hostile areas. Another use for escape bottles is the rescue of patients from contaminated areas or confined spaces (Fig. 8-11).

The escape-bottle hood is placed over the head of the

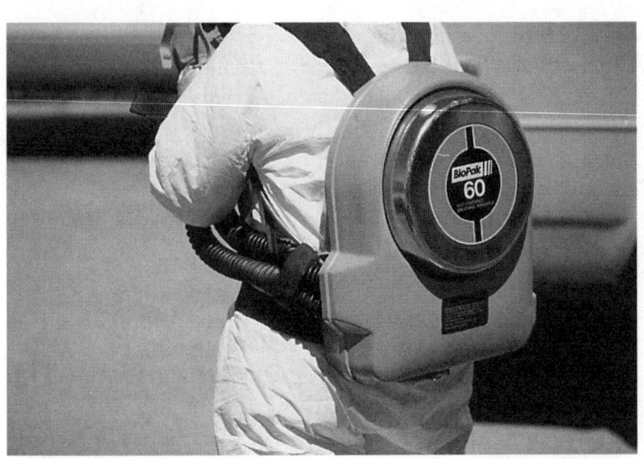

FIG. 8-9 Responder wearing closed-circuit SCBA.

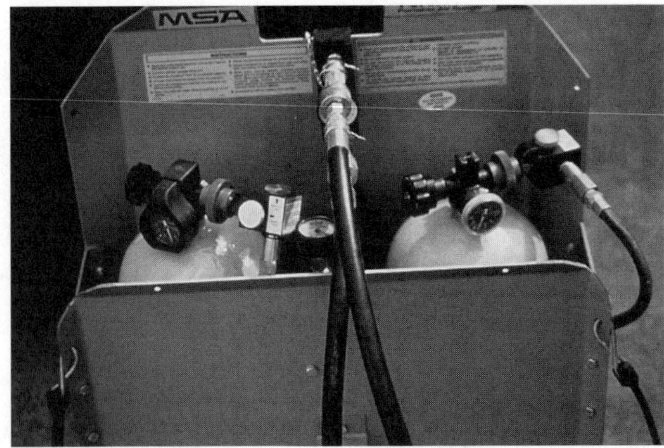

FIG. 8-10 An air-line system.

spontaneously breathing patient, giving the patient 5 or 10 minutes of clean air during the rescue. Most of these units have hoods that are tightened by using a drawstring around the neck. Spinal immobilization can be maintained while donning the hood by a responder stabilizing the head and neck from the front. A second responder slides the hood over the patient's head and the first responder's hands. Once the hood is in place the second responder takes over immobilization, and the first responder removes his hands and tightens the drawstring.

Respirator Fit Testing

All users of respirators (especially negative-pressure–type respiratory-protective devices) must be fit-tested to ensure proper face piece-to-face seal of the respirator. The fit test should be accomplished using standard OSHA methods. Fit testing can be conducted by qualitative or quantitative testing, depending on the respirator type. In qualitative testing the wearer is exposed to isoamyl acetate vapors (banana oil), irritant smoke, or saccharin (Fig. 8-12). During the test the wearer reads out loud and conducts simple exercises. A failure occurs if the wearer can detect the test agent.

In quantitative testing a computerized device attached to the mask is used to detect facial leaks. Quantitative testing is more accurate. Personnel should be tested into a specific brand, model, and size of respirator. Fit testing should be done annually. Fit testing also is required if the user gains or loses 20 lbs or more, has facial/dental surgery that would interfere with the facial fit, or changes to a different brand or model of respirator.

In addition to the annual fit test, a fit check should be performed every time a respirator is donned. The purpose of this check is (1) to ensure that a proper fit is possible and (2) to check the patency of the exhalation valve of the mask. This is accomplished by means of a positive-negative fit check. To conduct a positive fit check, gently exhale while covering the exhalation valve to ensure that a positive pressure can be built up. Failure to build a positive pressure indicates a poor fit. To conduct a negative-pressure check, close the inlet part with the palm of the hand or squeeze the breathing tube so it does not pass air, and gently inhale for about 10 seconds (Fig. 8-13). Any inward rushing of air indicates a poor fit or failure of the exhalation valve.

Respirator Maintenance

Respirators should be inspected before and after each use. Respirators that are not used routinely should be inspected at least monthly. Inspections should include a check of the tightness of the connections; a check of the face piece, valves, connecting tube, and filters (in APRs);

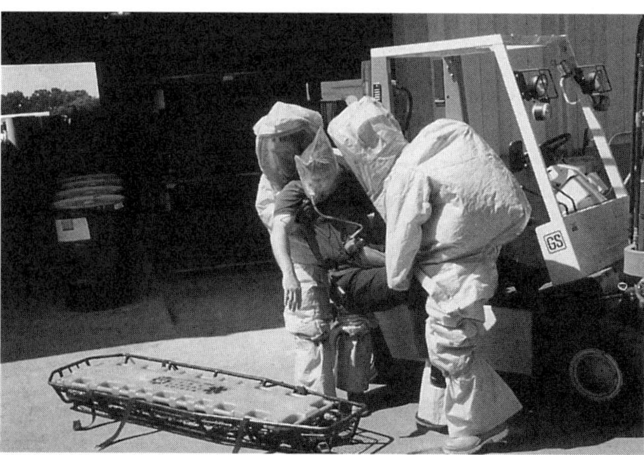

FIG. 8-11 Responders performing a rescue using an escape-only respirator for the patient.

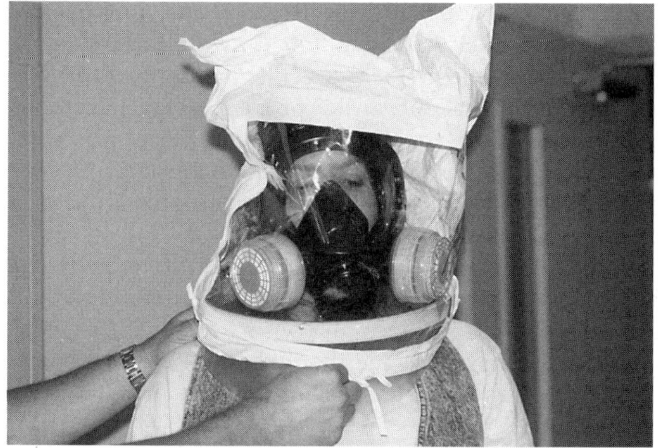

FIG. 8-12 In a qualitative fit test, a failure occurs if the wearer can detect a test agent.

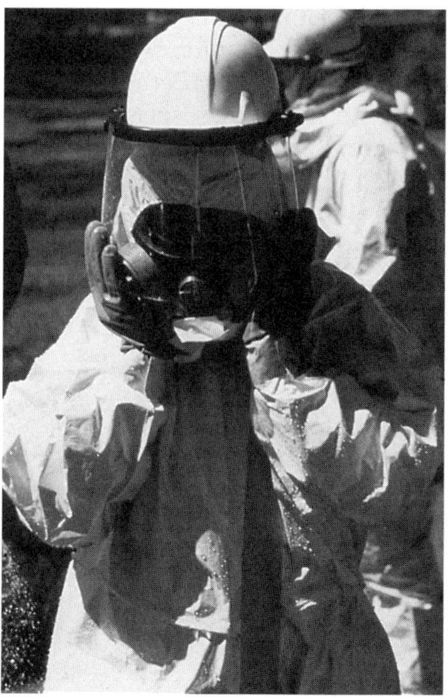

FIG. 8-13 In a negative fit check, an inward rushing of air indicates a poor fit.

and a check of the regulator and warning devices on SCBAs for proper functioning.

Respirators should be cleaned and disinfected after each use. Maintenance should be performed by factory-trained personnel, or the respirator returned to the factory for service. APRs can be stored in sealed plastic bags. Filters or cartridges should not be stored with the respirator, but should be unsealed and installed just before use. SCBAs can be stored in quick-don racks or in their factory cases.

Protective Clothing

When activities are conducted at sites in which chemical contamination is known or suspected to exist, chemical-protective clothing (CPC) must be worn. Street clothing or uniforms will offer little or no protection from chemical exposure. Even structural fire gear will offer little protection against most chemicals. The predominant physical and chemical or toxic properties of hazardous materials will dictate the type and degree of chemical protection that is required. The maximum level of protection can only be determined when complete identification of a hazard has been made.

Vapor-protective clothing is designed to provide the highest level of protection against skin-destructive and skin-absorbable substances. It consists of a fully encapsulating, vapor-tight suit and the highest degree of respiratory protection (pressure-demand SCBA or SAR with escape bottle).

Chemical-splash protective clothing is designed to provide protection against liquid splash or particulates. It does not provide protection against vapors. Tape often is used with splash-protective clothing to seal openings, gloves, and boots. Sealing splash-protective suits with tape will not make them vapor protective. A key component with splash-protective clothing is the type of respiratory protection used. In most cases, splash-protective equipment and an atmosphere-supplying respirator are adequate for patient management during decontamination.

EPA Protective Clothing and Respiratory Protection Levels

The Environmental Protection Agency (EPA) has divided protective clothing and respiratory protection into four categories according to the degree of protection afforded.

Level A

Level A protection should be worn when the highest level of respiratory, skin, eye, and mucous membrane protection is needed (Fig. 8-14). This level usually is used for protection against skin-toxic or corrosive vapors. It also is needed when gross liquid contact is possible, such as when working on overhead pipes, and for extremely hazardous materials. PPE for this level includes the following:

- Positive-pressure (pressure-demand) SCBA (approved by the Mine Safety and Health Administration [MSHA] and NIOSH)
- Fully encapsulating, vapor-tight, chemical-resistant suit, inner gloves, chemical-resistant outer gloves, chemical-resistant boots with steel toe and shank
- Underwear, cotton, long-john type*
- Hard hat (under suit)*
- Cooling vest*
- Coveralls (under suit)*
- Two-way radio communicators (that are intrinsically safe)*

Even if Level A protection is used, responders should try to keep any contact with the substance to an absolute minimum.

Level B

Level B protection should be selected when the situation requires the highest level of respiratory protection, but a lesser level of skin and eye protection (Fig. 8-15). This

*Optional.

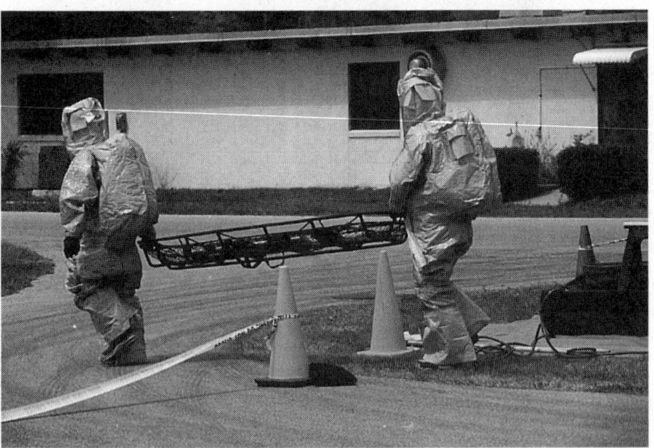

FIG. 8-14 Level A suits are worn when the highest level of protection is needed.

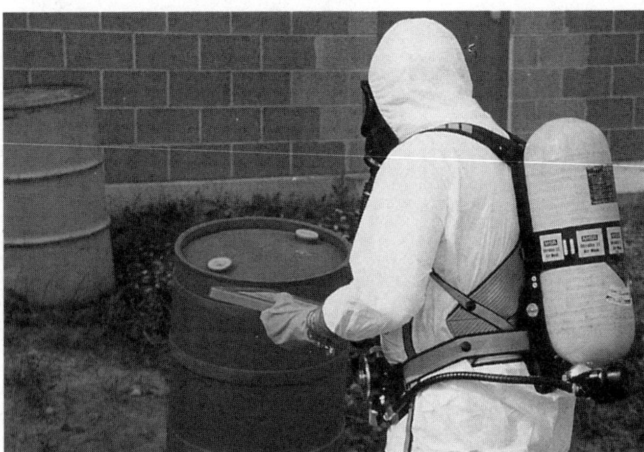

FIG. 8-15 Level B protective equipment should be selected when the highest level of respiratory protection, but a lesser level of skin and eye protection, is needed.

level usually is used for protection against inadvertent liquid splash or particulates. A relatively new style of splash-protective suits is a fully encapsulating, nonvapor-tight suit that offer a higher degree of skin protection and protect the SCBA. PPE for this level includes the following:

- Positive-pressure (pressure-demand) SCBA (approved by the MSHA and NIOSH)
- Chemical-resistant clothing (overalls and long-sleeved jacket; coveralls; hooded, two-piece, chemical-splash suit; disposable, chemical-resistant coveralls; or fully encapsulated, nonvapor-tight suit)
- Coveralls (under splash suit)*
- Inner gloves
- Chemical-resistant outer gloves, taped to suit
- Chemical-resistant boots with steel toe and shank
- Cooling vest*
- Two-way radio communicators (that are intrinsically safe)*
- Hard hat*

Level C

Level C protection should be selected when the type of airborne substance is known, its concentration has been measured, the criteria for using APRs have been met, and skin exposure is unlikely (Fig. 8-16). Periodic monitoring of the air must be performed when this level of protection is used.

PPE for this level includes the following:

- Full-face APR (MSHA/NIOSH approved)
- Chemical-resistant clothing (one-piece coverall; hooded, two-piece chemical-splash suit; disposable, chemical-resistant overalls)
- Inner gloves
- Chemical-resistant outer gloves, taped to suit

*Optional.

- Chemical-resistant boots, with steel toe and shank
- Coveralls (under splash suit)*
- Two-way radio communicators (that are intrinsically safe)*
- Cooling vest*
- Hard hat*
- Escape mask*

Level D

Level D protection is primarily a work uniform. It should not be worn on any site where respiratory or skin hazards exist (Fig. 8-17).

In many cases the initial survey of a hazardous materials incident should be done in a minimum of Level B protection. If skin-toxic chemicals are present or suspected, Level A protection should be used. The level of protection is then upgraded or downgraded accordingly as information becomes available. The type of equipment used and the overall level of protection should be constantly reevaluated as additional information about the incident is obtained, and as responders are required to perform different tasks.

Reasons to upgrade protection levels include:

- Known or suspected presence of chemicals that can cause skin damage
- Occurrence or likely occurrence of gas or vapor emission
- Change in work task that will increase contact or potential contact with hazardous materials

Reasons to downgrade protection levels include:

- New information indicating that the situation is less hazardous than was originally thought
- Change in site conditions that decreases the hazard
- Change in work task that will reduce contact with hazardous materials

*Optional.

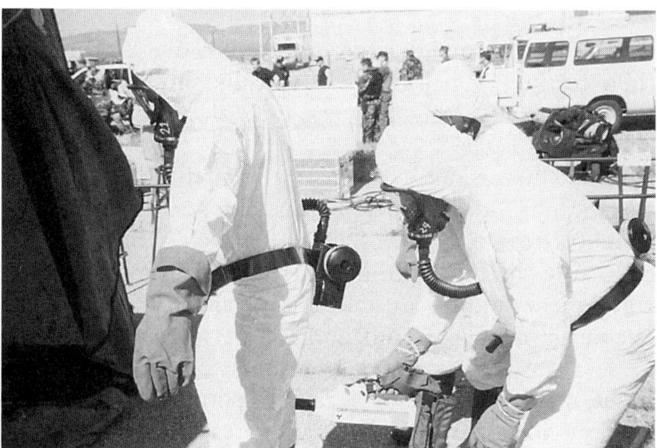

FIG. 8-16 Responders in Level C protective equipment.

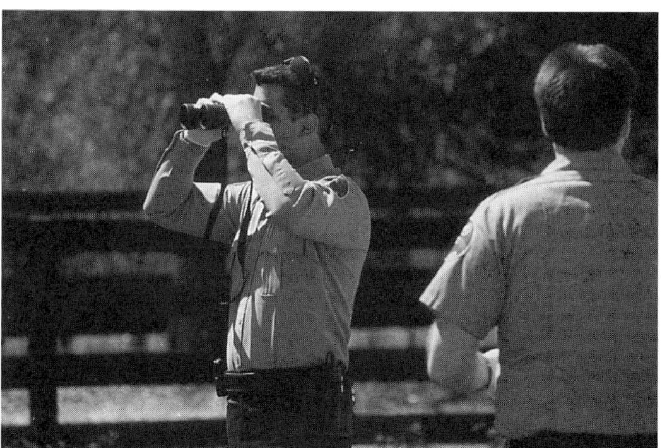

FIG. 8-17 Level D protective equipment is primarily a work uniform.

National Fire Protection Association Standards

A weakness with the EPA levels of protection is that they only provide a design specification instead of a performance specification. An EPA-designated Level A suit may be used, but users have little idea if it meets their protection need. The National Fire Protection Association (NFPA) has developed standards for chemical-protective suits. The standards cover certification, documentation requirements, design and performance requirements, and test methods. NFPA 1991 applies to vapor-protective suits used for chemical protection in the hot zone. NFPA 1992 applies to liquid-splash–protective suits used in the hot zone. NFPA 1993 applies to garments worn by personnel outside the hot zone who are in support functions such as decontamination or remedial cleanup. These standards will assist responders in the understanding and selection of protective clothing.

CPC Materials

Selecting the correct fabric is just as important as selecting the level of protection. CPC materials are those that by their physical and chemical makeup are able to resist the physical and chemical hazards that are inherent in various hazardous substances. These products have excellent-to-fair resistance to selected chemicals. *No material has total resistance to all chemical exposures.* Very often chemical resistance is extremely limited.

Chemical resistance

Chemical resistance is the ability of a material to physically resist degradation, permeation, and penetration by a contaminant (Fig. 8-18).

- *Degradation* is the loss in physical properties caused by an exposure to a chemical. Damage to the material may be so slight that it may not be visible to the naked eye.
- *Permeation* is the process by which a chemical moves through a material on a molecular level, or diffusion. Permeation typically is measured by the time it takes to pass from the outer side of a material (once exposed) and be measured on the inside. This is referred to as *permeation time. Permeation rate* is the rate or amount at which the chemical passes through.
- *Penetration* is the flow of a substance or material through openings such as zippers, seams, stitches, holes, or tears in the garment.

The degree of resistance is measured by testing a particular material or substance against a specific product or chemical. To assist users of specialized protective clothing, manufacturers of materials submit their product or fabric sample to a research laboratory or agency for testing.

Chemical resistance is represented by charts or tables distributed by manufacturers of protective clothing or their testing agencies. They typically show their resistance or relative effectiveness against specific classes of chemicals (Table 8-1).

Many hazardous chemicals are mixtures, for which specific data with which to make a good selection of chemical-resistant fabrics are not available. Because of a lack of testing, only limited permeation data for multi-component liquids are currently available. Mixtures of chemicals can be significantly more aggressive toward CPC materials than can any single component alone. Even small amounts of a rapidly permeating chemical may provide a pathway that accelerates the permeation of other chemicals. NIOSH currently is developing methods for evaluating CPC materials against mixtures of

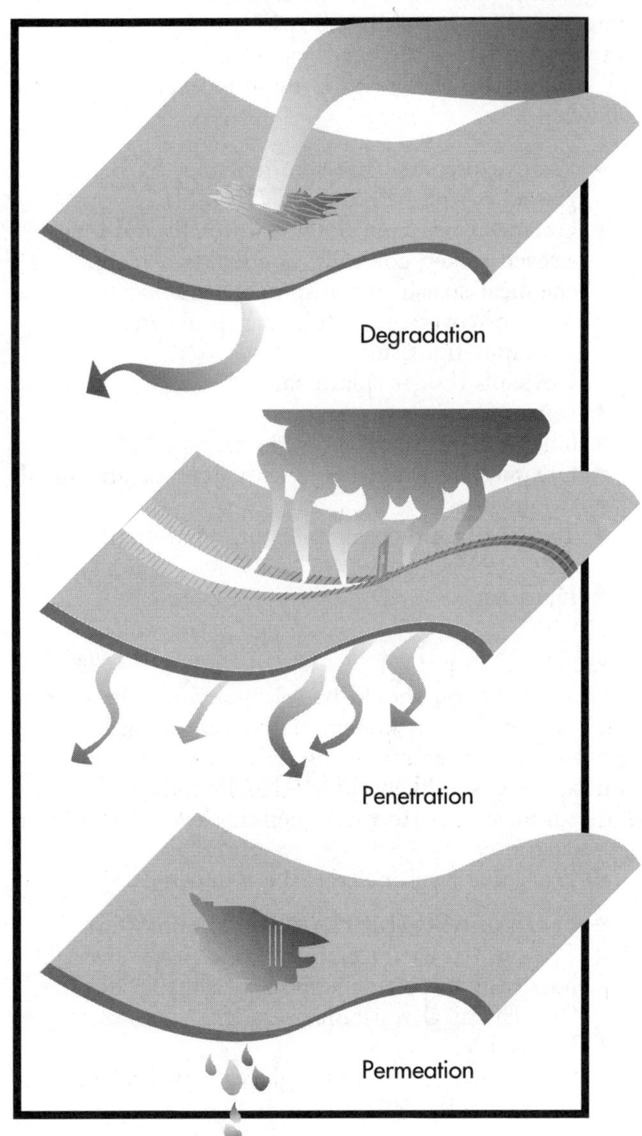

FIG. 8-18 Degradation, penetration, and permeation.

chemicals and unknowns in the field. For emergency response operations, CPC should be selected that offers the widest range of protection against the chemicals expected at the incident. Vendors are now providing CPC material composed of two or even three different materials laminated together. These multilaminate fabrics are able to provide the best features of each material.

EMS responders should not expect their protective clothing and gloves to provide protection against all chemicals. A selection of fabrics should be stocked and compatibility with the chemical checked before use.

Heat transfer characteristics

The heat transfer characteristics of CPC may be an important selection factor. Because most CPC is virtually impermeable to moisture, evaporative cooling is limited. The *clo value (thermal insulation value)* of CPC is a scientific measure of the capacity of CPC to dissipate heat loss through means other than evaporation. The larger the clo value, the greater the insulating properties of the garment and, consequently, the lower the heat transfer. A clo value of 1 is equal to the heat loss capacity of a three-piece business suit. Given other equivalent protective properties, protective clothing with the lowest clo value should be selected in hot environments or for high-work rates. Unfortunately, clo values currently are available for only a few CPC ensembles.

Responders using Level A or Level B PPE must be monitored for the effects of heat stress and fatigue. EMS responders should anticipate that heat stress injuries will occur. Procedures to limit heat stress should be in place. These procedures include monitoring for heat stress, the use of ice vests, having responders take frequent breaks, and frequent oral hydration to replace lost body fluids.

Other factors

In addition to chemical resistance and heat transfer, several other factors must be considered during clothing selection. These factors affect not only chemical resistance, but also the responder's ability to perform the required task. Included among these factors are the following:

- Durability
- Flexibility
- Temperature effects
- Ease of decontamination
- Compatibility with other equipment
- Duration of use

Fire, explosion, heat, and radiation are considered special conditions that require special protective equipment. Aluminized "flash suits" are available for many brands of chemical-protective suits. These garments offer limited protection against flash fires but do not offer the protection necessary for wear in proximity to high temperatures or for firefighting operations. Additional fire protection may be offered with the use of coveralls, gloves, and hoods made from a fire-resistant fabric such as Nomex or PBI.

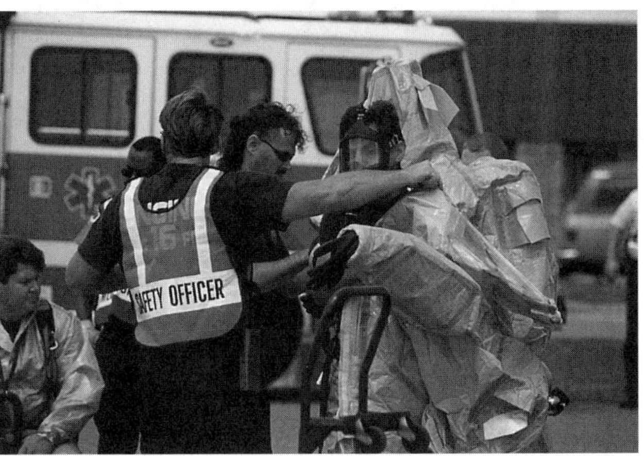

FIG. 8-19 Responders should assist in donning chemical-protective equipment to decrease the probability of suit damage.

Donning and Doffing PPE

A routine should be established and practiced periodically for donning PPE. Assistance should be provided for donning and doffing because these operations are difficult to perform alone, and solo efforts may increase the possibility of suit damage (Fig. 8-19).

Once the equipment has been donned, its fit should be evaluated. If the clothing is too small, it will restrict movement, thereby increasing the likelihood of tearing the suit material and accelerating responder fatigue and heat stress. If the clothing is too large, the possibility of snagging the material is increased, and the dexterity and coordination of the responder may be compromised.

While wearing PPE, responders should immediately exit the hot zone and report any perceived problems or difficulties. Problems include, but are not limited to, the following:

- Visible damage to the suit
- Degradation of the suit
- Respirator malfunction
- Perception of odors
- Skin irritation
- Physical discomfort
- Interference with vision or communication
- Restriction of movement
- Personal responses such as rapid pulse, nausea, and dizziness

Exact procedures for removing fully encapsulating suit/SCBA ensembles must be established and followed to prevent contaminant migration from the hot zone and contaminant transfer to the wearer and other responders. Doffing procedures should be performed only after de-

TABLE 8-1
PERMEATION DATA TABLE

Class	Subclass	Chemical	Physical Phase	TYVEK QC Breakthrough Time Normalized (min)	TYVEK QC Perm Rate (μg/cm²/min)	TYCHEM SL Breakthrough Time Normalized (min)	TYCHEM SL Perm Rate (μg/cm²/min)
Hydroxylic compounds	**316** Aromatic phenols	Cresol (mixed isomers)	L	112	0.43	480	0.17
		Dinitro-o-cresol (sat. sol. in methanol)	L	nt	nt	nt	nt
		Pentachlorophenol (sat. sol. in methanol)	L	nt	nt	nt	nt
		Phenol, 85%	L	immed.	0.4	>480*	<0.28
		Phenol (45° C)	L	nt	nt	nt	nt
Elements	**330** Elements	Bromine	L	immed.	high	nt	nt
		Chlorine (20 ppm)	G	>480*	nm	>480*	nm
		Chlorine gas	G	immed.	>50	>480	<0.7
		Chlorine liquid (−70° C)	L	nt	nt	nt	nt
		Iodine	S	440*	30	>480*	<70
		Mercury	L	nt	nt	>480	<0.00046
Inorganic salts (solutions)	**340** Inorganic salts (solutions)	Mercuric chloride, sat.	L	nt	nt	>480*	<0.28
		Potassium acetate, sat.	L	nt	nt	>480*	<0.51
		Potassium chromate, sat.	L	nt	nt	>480*	<0.51
		Sodium fluoride, sat.	L	nt	nt	>480*	<0.28
		Sodium hypochlorite, 5.25%	L	>480*	nm	>480*	nm
	345 Inorganic cyano compounds	Hydrogen cyanide liquid	L	60*	110	nt	nt
		Potassium cyanide, 10%	L	>480	<0.1	nt	nt
		Sodium cyanide, 95%	L	nt	nt	>480*	<0.28
Inorganic gases and vapors	**350** Inorganic gases and vapors	Ammonia gas	G	immed.	3.1	32	0.15
		Ammonia liquid (−60° C)	L	nt	nt	>480	<0.1
		Ammonia liquid (−70° C)	L	nt	nt	nt	nt
		Carbon monoxide	G	nt	nt	nt	nt
		Chlorine (20 ppm)	G	>480*	nm	>480*	nm
		Chlorine gas	G	immed.	>50	>480	<0.7
		Chlorine liquid (−70° C)	L	nt	nt	nt	nt
		Chlorine trifluoride	G	nt	nt	nt	nt
		Hydrogen bromide	G	nt	nt	nt	nt
		Hydrogen chloride	G	immed.	9.3	>480	<0.1
		Hydrogen fluoride gas	G	immed.*	6	20*	3
		Hydrogen fluoride liquid (0° C)	L	nt	nt	nt	nt
		Hydrogen sulfide	G	nt	nt	nt	nt
		Nitrogen dioxide	G	nt	nt	>480*	<0.00004
		Nitrogen tetroxide	G	nt	nt	nt	nt
		Nitrogen tetroxide (0° C)	L	nt	nt	nt	nt
		Phosgene	G	nt	nt	nt	nt
		Sulfur dioxide	G	immed.	>29	>480	<0.1
		Sulfuryl chloride	L	nt	nt	nt	nt
Inorganic acid halides	**360** Inorganic acid halides	Antimony pentachloride	L	nt	nt	>480	0.1
		Phosphorous oxychloride	L	nt	nt	nt	nt
		Phosphorous trichloride	L	nt	nt	20	28.3
		Sulfuryl chloride	L	nt	nt	nt	nt
		Thionyl chloride	L	nt	nt	nt	nt
		Titanium tetrachloride	L	nt	nt	nt	nt
Inorganic acid oxides	**365** Inorganic acid oxides	Sulfur dichloride, 80%	L	nt	nt	nt	nt
		Sulfur dioxide	G	immed.	>29	>480	<0.1
		Sulfur trioxide	L	nt	nt	nt	nt
Inorganic acids	**370** Inorganic acids	Chlorosulfonic acid	L	nt	nt	nt	nt
		Chromic acid	L	>480	<0.1	>480	<0.1
		Fluorosilicic acid	L	nt	nt	nt	nt

Permeation Guide for DuPont Tychem Fabrics. Reprinted with permission from E.I. duPont de Nemours and Company, 1998.
Immed., 10 minutes or less; ND, none detected; nt, not tested; >, greater than; <, less than; S, solid; L, liquid; G, gas; M, mixture; sat., saturated solution in water; nm, not measured.
*Actual breakthrough time. No normalized breakthrough time available.
NOTE: Numbers reported are averages of samples tested by the ASTM F739 test method. Sample results do vary and therefore averages for these results are reported.
Tyvek, Barricade, and Tychem are registered trademarks of DuPont. Tychem SL is a DuPont registered trademark for Tyvek spunbonded olefin laminated with Saranex 23-P, a registered trademark of The Dow Chemical Company.

TYCHEM 7500		TYCHEM 9400 & BARRICADE		TYCHEM 10,000	
Breakthrough Time Normalized (min)	**Perm Rate (µg/cm²/min)**	**Breakthrough Time Normalized (min)**	**Perm Rate (µg/cm²/min)**	**Breakthrough Time Normalized (min)**	**Perm Rate (µg/cm²/min)**
nt	nt	>480	<0.01	>480	0.001
nt	nt	>480	<0.013	>480	<0.1
nt	nt	>480	<0.013	>480	<0.1
nt	nt	>480	<0.03	nt	nt
nt	nt	nt	nt	>480	<0.01
nt	nt	immed.*	>50	91	139
nt	nt	nt	nt	nt	nt
>480	<0.9	>480	<0.02	>480	<0.17
nt	nt	nt	nt	>480	<0.001
nt	nt	nt	nt	nt	nt
nt	nt	>480	<0.0002	>480	<0.001
nt	nt	>480*	<0.28	nt	nt
nt	nt	>480*	<0.49	nt	nt
nt	nt	>480*	<0.51	nt	nt
nt	nt	nt	nt	nt	nt
nt	nt	nt	nt	nt	nt
nt	nt	104	1.7	360	0.18
nt	nt	nt	nt	nt	nt
nt	nt	>480*	<0.3	nt	nt
125	0.5	45	0.69	>480	<0.07
nt	nt	nt	nt	nt	nt
nt	nt	nt	nt	>480	<0.001
nt	nt	330	0.1	290	0.26
nt	nt	nt	nt	nt	nt
>480	<0.9	>480	<0.2	>480	<0.17
nt	nt	nt	nt	>480	<0.001
nt	nt	45	96.0	immed.	11.4
nt	nt	>480	<0.1	>480	<0.028
195	0.33	>480	<0.1	>480	<0.1
nt	nt	135	6.7	>480	<0.1
nt	nt	nt	nt	35	0.55
nt	nt	>480	<0.01	>480	<0.001
nt	nt	nt	nt	nt	nt
nt	nt	90	>1.1	nt	nt
nt	nt	>480	0.001	nt	nt
nt	nt	>480	<0.1	>480	0.002
nt	nt	>480	<0.01	280	>0.1
nt	nt	>480	<0.1	>480	<0.1
nt	nt	nt	nt	nt	nt
nt	nt	>480	<0.1	>480	0.053
nt	nt	>480	<0.1	nt	nt
nt	nt	>480	<0.1	>480	<0.1
nt	nt	35	2495	>480	<0.1
nt	nt	>480	<0.1	>480	0.071
nt	nt	70	6.0	>480	<0.1
nt	nt	>480	<0.01	280	>0.1
nt	nt	90	696	70	>50
nt	nt	180	98.4	>480	0.047
nt	nt	nt	nt	nt	nt
nt	nt	>480	<0.1	>480	<0.1

contamination. They require a suitably attired assistant. Throughout the procedures, both responder and assistant should avoid any direct contact with the outside surface of the suit.

Chemicals that have begun to permeate clothing during use may not be removed during decontamination and may continue to diffuse through the material toward the inside surface. This presents a hazard of direct skin contact to the next person who uses the clothing. Where such potential hazards may develop, clothing should be checked inside and out for discoloration or other evidence of contamination. This is especially important for multiuse, fully encapsulating suits, which are generally subject to reuse because of their cost. Level A suits must be pressure-tested before each reuse.

Clothing reuse

At present, little documentation exists about clothing reuse. Reuse decisions must consider both permeation rates and toxicity of the contaminants. In fact, unless extreme care is taken to ensure that clothing is properly decontaminated and that the decontamination does not degrade the material, it is not advisable to reuse CPC that has been contaminated with toxic chemicals. This is the major reason why limited-use protective clothing is becoming popular. The lower cost of limited-use garments makes disposal after each incident a viable alternative. All equipment, such as SCBAs, that will be reused must be carefully decontaminated.

Clothing Maintenance

CPC should be inspected when it is received from the factory, periodically while in storage, and before and after each use. Detailed inspection procedures are usually available from the manufacturer.

The technical depth of maintenance procedures varies. Manufacturers frequently restrict the sale of certain PPE parts to individuals or groups who are specially trained, equipped, and authorized by the manufacturer to purchase them. Procedures should be adopted to ensure that the appropriate level of maintenance is performed only by individuals having this specialized training and equipment.

Clothing and respirators must be stored properly to prevent damage or malfunction resulting from exposure to dust, moisture, sunlight, damaging chemicals, extreme temperatures, and impact. Many equipment failures can be directly attributed to improper storage.

Different types and materials of clothing and gloves should be stored separately to prevent issuing the wrong type or material by mistake. Protective clothing should be stored according to manufacturers recommendations.

Detailed records should be maintained on each item of PPE and clothing. This is especially true of reusable items. Records should contain the item's purchase date, inspection records, decontamination information, and the chemicals to which the item has been exposed.

Summary

Selection of PPE is a complex task and should be performed by personnel with training and experience. If the chemical has been identified, the following items should be considered:

- State of matter (solid, liquid, vapor) of the chemical
- Chemical and physical properties of the chemical
- Level of protection required (vapor or splash protection)
- Type of fabric that will provide the longest breakthrough time
- Type of activities to be performed
- Potential for heat stress

If the chemical(s) have not been identified, the task of proper equipment selection is much more difficult. Additional indicators that should be assessed include:

- Visible IDLH indicators (e.g., visible vapors, smoke, or particles; incapacitated victims or animals; dead vegetation)
- Positive readings on direct-reading instruments
- Indicators of gases or highly toxic substances (e.g., placards, labels, specific containers, signs)
- Poorly ventilated or enclosed areas

Under all conditions, equipment is selected by evaluating the performance characteristics of the equipment against the requirements and limitations of the scene- and task-specific conditions.

It is unlikely that most EMS responders will ever need to wear Level A PPE. Entrance into the contaminated area and rescue of patients from this area usually is carried out by the HAZMAT response team. Patient care activities are limited by the Level A suit. In rare cases, EMS responders may be called on to perform triage in the contaminated area. Patients who are trapped may need care during extrication. EMS responders should have an understanding of PPE. At locations where EMS activities may be needed in the hot zone, training with Level A suits should be conducted. Under no circumstances should responders wear any PPE without proper training, practice, and fit testing as necessary.

CHAPTER REVIEW QUESTIONS

1. What are the limitations of body substance isolation equipment when dealing with a hazardous materials incident?
2. List five adverse effects that can be caused by wearing PPE.
3. List three types of respiratory-protective equipment and discuss the limitations of each.
4. List the PFs of half-face APRs, full-face APRs, and pressure-demand SCBAs.
5. Identify the types of respiratory-protective equipment that can be used in an IDLH environment.

6. Identify the EPA's protective-equipment levels, and discuss the use and limitations of each.
7. List the three ways that CPC can fail.
8. List at least five factors that should be considered in selecting PPE.
9. Name at least six signs that indicate the failure of PPE.
10. Describe the difference between limited-use and multiuse CPC.

BIBLIOGRAPHY

Agency for Toxic Substances and Disease Registry: *Managing hazardous materials incidents, emergency medical services: a planning guide for the management of contaminated patients,* Atlanta, Ga, 1992, US-DHHS.

Andrews LP, editor: *Emergency responder training manual for the hazardous materials technician,* New York, 1992, Van Nostrand Reinhold.

Bowen JE: *Emergency management of hazardous materials incidents,* Quincy, Mass., 1995, National Fire Protection Association.

Bronstein AC, Currance PL: Module 4: emergency medical operations. In Ayers S, Christopher J, editors: *Medical Response to Chemical Emergencies,* Washington, DC, 1994, Chemical Manufacturers Association.

Carroll TR: *Contamination and decontamination of turnout clothing,* Emmitsburg, Md, 1993, Federal Emergency Management Agency, US Fire Administration.

Currance PL: *Hazmat for EMS,* St Louis, 1995, Mosby, videotape and guidebook.

DOT: *1996 North American emergency response guidebook,* Office of Hazardous Materials Transportation, Research and Special Programs Administration, Washington, DC, 1996, US Department of Transportation.

EPA: *EPA standard safety operating guidelines,* Washington, DC, 1984, US Government Printing Office.

Forsburg, Krister, Keith: *Chemical protective clothing permeation and degradation compendium,* Boca Raton, Fla, 1993, Lewis Publishers.

Guidelines for public sector hazardous materials training: 1998 ed, HMEP Curriculum Guidelines, Emmitsburg, Md, 1998, National Emergency Training Center.

Hazardous materials response training program, New Jersey/New York, 1988, Hazardous Materials Worker/Training Program.

National Fire Protection Association: *NFPA 471, Recommended practice for responding to hazardous materials incidents,* Quincy, Mass, 1992, The Association.

National Fire Protection Association: *NFPA 1991, Vapor-protective suits for hazardous materials emergencies,* Quincy, Mass, 1992, The Association.

National Fire Protection Association: *NFPA 1992, Liquid splash protective suits for hazardous materials emergencies,* Quincy, Mass, 1992, The Association.

National Fire Protection Association: *NFPA 1993, Support function protective garments for hazardous materials emergencies,* Quincy, Mass, 1992, The Association.

NIOSH/OSHA/USCG/EPA: *Occupational safety and health guidance manual for hazardous waste site activities,* Washington, DC, 1985, DHHS (NIOSH) Publication No 85-115, US Government Printing Office.

Noll GG, Hildebrand MS, Yvorra JG: *Hazardous materials: managing the incident,* ed 2, Stillwater, Okla, 1995, Fire Protection Publications.

OSHA: 29 CFR 1910.120, Hazardous waste operations and emergency response; Final rule, March 6, 1989; Washington, DC, US Government Printing Office.

Strong CB, Irvin TR: *Emergency response and hazardous chemical management: principles and practices,* Delray Beach, Fla, 1996, St. Lucie Press.

Tokle G, editor: *Hazardous materials response handbook,* ed 2, Quincy, Mass, 1993, National Fire Protection Association.

Varela J, editor: *Hazardous materials handbook for emergency responders,* New York, 1996, Van Nostrand Reinhold.

9

Air Monitoring and Detection Equipment

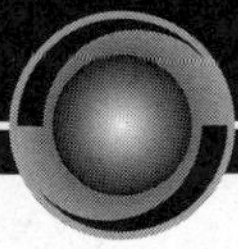

Phil Currance

CHAPTER OBJECTIVES

At the conclusion of this chapter the student will be able to:

- Discuss the need for air monitoring and detection equipment at hazardous materials incidents.
- Discuss the limitations of field instruments.
- Describe how instruments are rated as intrinsically safe.
- Describe the function, use, and limitations of combustible gas indicators.
- Describe the function, use, and limitations of oxygen meters.
- Describe the function, use, and limitations of specific gas sensors.
- Describe the function, use, and limitations of colorimetric indicator tubes.
- Describe the function, use, and limitations of radiation detectors.
- Describe the function, use, and limitations of photo and flame ionization devices.
- Describe the function, use, and limitations of infrared spectrophotometer devices.
- Describe the function, use, and limitations of test strips and field test kits.

CASE STUDY

Hazardous materials (HAZMAT) team, fire, and Emergency Medical Services (EMS) responders are called to an aircraft manufacturing plant because of a release of nitric acid liquid and vapor that occurred during transfer of 1000 gallons from a truck to a fixed-facility tank. The vapor cloud has drifted across the plant site and into the surrounding community. Numerous employees and citizens were exposed while trying to evacuate. EMS/HM Level I and Level II responders are on scene. The EMS/HM Level I responders are treating patients after decontamination. The HAZMAT team has deployed responders with air monitoring equipment to assess the extent and severity of the release (Fig. 9-1). The incident commander is consulting with the EMS/HM Level II responder regarding the extent of patient exposure and need for further evacuation. In addition, the number of patients who were possibly exposed is overwhelming the capability of EMS and hospital resources. High concentrations of nitric acid can cause skin and eye burns, and severe upper and lower airway damage that may be delayed. Lower concentrations can result in airway, skin, and mucous membrane irritation. The permissible exposure limit (PEL) of nitric acid is 2 ppm, and the Immediately Dangerous to Life or Health (IDLH) value is 25 ppm.

- Can data from air monitoring equipment be used to assist with evacuation decisions?

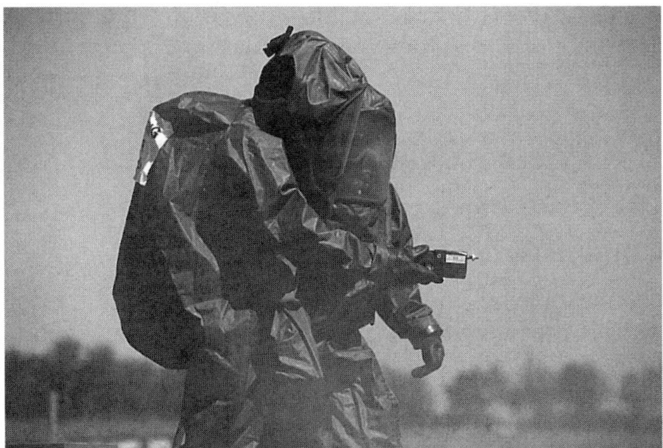

FIG. 9-1 Responders in Level A protective equipment monitoring air.

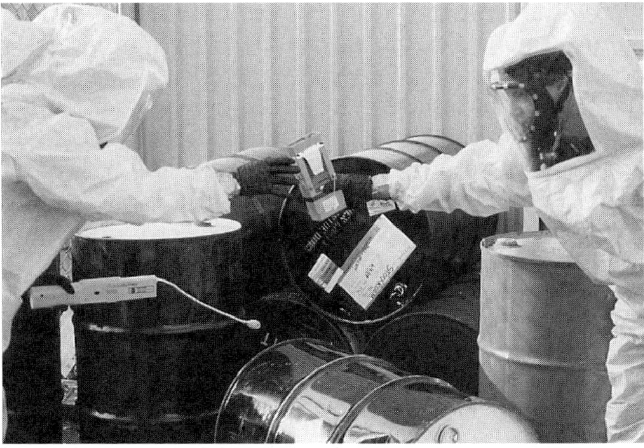

FIG. 9-2 Responders should not rely on visual assessment alone.

- Can this data assist with triage decisions (who was exposed and level of exposure)?
- Which air monitoring devices will detect nitric acid?
- What limitations must be considered when assessing data supplied by air monitoring devices?

At an incident involving hazardous materials, decisions must be made regarding the identity and amount of the released material, the extent of spread of the material, and the types of personal protective equipment (PPE) that responders will need to accomplish their goals. The identity of the chemical and the extent of exposure must be determined so specific medical treatment may be provided. Responders must not rely on a visual assessment alone. Many gases and vapors are invisible to the eye, and those that are visible are usually in very high concentrations. Detection and air monitoring equipment can aid in these decisions by supplying data (Fig. 9-2). This data can be used to:

- Determine the extent of release
- Establish boundaries of the hot zone
- Assist in identifying unknown products
- Define the source of a release
- Assist in the selection of PPE
- Assess changes in conditions and ensure proper safety of responders
- Guide specific medical treatment modalities

This chapter will look at common portable equipment used by HAZMAT teams to detect, identify, and monitor environments containing chemical hazards. EMS responders must be able to identify the limitations associated with these devices to use the data accurately to make decisions and guide treatment. Air monitoring should be an on-going process throughout the response. Conditions may change without warning and present extreme hazards.

Direct-reading instruments often are complex electronic devices. Before using such instruments, training is essential to understand their limitations, select the proper instrument, ensure proper use and calibration, and interpret the data generated.

Limitations

To derive maximum benefit from monitoring instruments, responders must be aware of the instruments' capabilities and limitations. Some responders refer to the use of the monitoring equipment as *air sampling.* Air monitoring and air sampling are vastly different, however. Air sampling is done to ascertain the identity and quantity of the sample. To carry this out, laboratory analysis is required. Because emergency responders need immediate information, sampling has limited application. On the other hand, direct-reading air monitoring instruments are designed to supply immediate information by way of a readout or gauge. The information may not be totally accurate and in some cases, exact identification of the product cannot be established.

Over the years, as monitoring devices have become more sophisticated, we often have incorrectly assumed that they are able to tell us exactly what and how much of a chemical is present. In reality, direct-reading air monitoring devices are extremely limited in their scope. Some monitors will only assess flammability, whereas others may monitor oxygen (O_2) concentration or toxicity levels. Some devices will work only with organic compounds. EMS responders must understand these limitations and use appropriate caution when assessing the data supplied by direct-reading air monitoring and detection equipment. Also, using more than one type of instrument will improve the quality of data used for hazard assessment.

Selection

Air monitoring equipment used for emergency response situations must meet certain criteria (Box 9-1).

A major concern is that the instrument not present an ignition source if used in the presence of flammable gases or vapors. Instruments operated in these areas should be certified as intrinsically safe or explosion-proof. Minimum standards for inherent safety in hazardous atmospheres have been defined by the National Fire Protection Association (NFPA) in the National Electric Code (NEC). Categories of hazardous atmospheres are defined by class, group and division. Instruments are certified as being intrinsically safe for specific classes and groups of flammable atmospheres by Factory Mutual Research Corp. (FM) (Fig. 9-3) or Underwriter's Laboratory, Inc. (UL).

An important consideration is the suspected or known contaminant. Does the material present a flammable, toxic, radioactive, or corrosive hazard? At an emergency response scene, answers to these questions may not be readily available, therefore extra caution must be taken. Corrosive atmospheres may damage the instrument. Some vapors and gases may adversely affect the sensors, resulting in false readings or no response at all. The more information obtained about the suspected materials, the better the selection of monitoring equipment and the more useful the information gathered from the monitoring program. It is essential that the correct monitoring instrument be used for a specific situation. At present, no single instrument is able to cover all situations.

BOX 9-1

CRITERIA FOR AIR MONITORING EQUIPMENT

Easy to use
Accurate
Reliable
Able to generate a fast response
Easy to interpret
Portable
Able to withstand weather conditions
Approved for HAZMAT team use
Easy to decontaminate

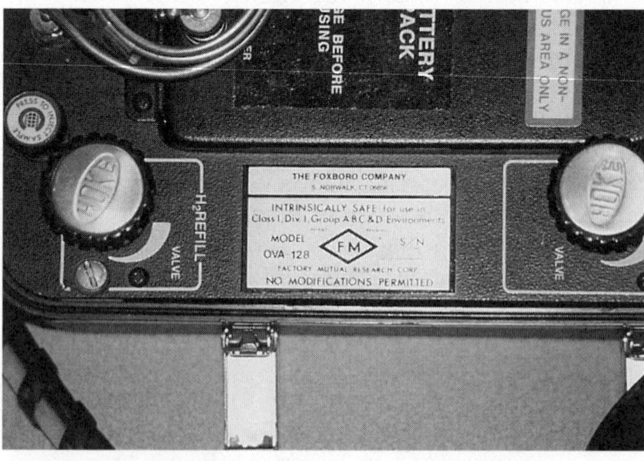

FIG. 9-3 FM label on monitoring device.

Overview of Commonly Used Instruments

Combustible Gas Indicators

Combustible gas indicators (CGI) are some of the most widely used field instruments found in emergency response operations (Fig. 9-4). CGIs also are known as *explosion meters* or *lower explosive limit (LEL) monitors.* Most of these instruments are of the heated catalytic filament type. The LEL monitor uses a circuit called a *wheatstone bridge* (Fig. 9-5). Air is drawn into a sensor chamber containing two filaments. Both filaments are at the same temperature and have the same electrical resistance. One filament is coated with a catalyst, often platinum, and the other filament is uncoated. The catalyst-coated filament can burn flammable vapors at lower concentrations than normally required in open air. The amount of vapor burned on the filament changes the resistance on that side of the circuit. The degree of imbalance in resistance is translated to a percentage of the LEL.

The catalytic filament can be damaged by contami-

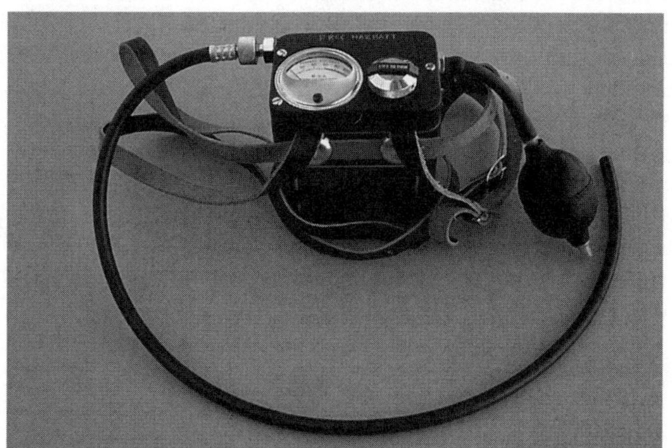

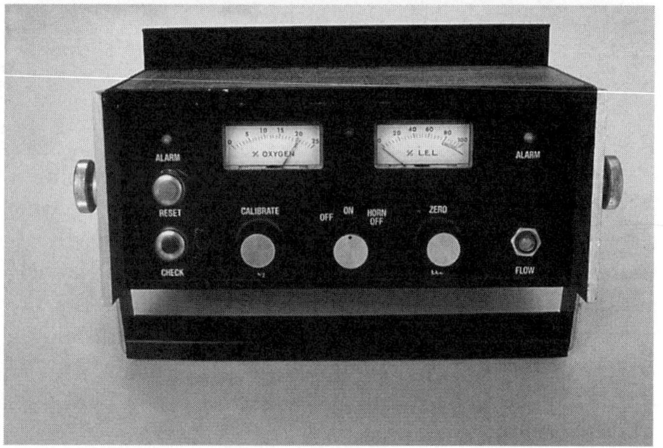

FIG. 9-4 **A** and **B,** Combustible gas indicators.

nants such as sulfur compounds, heavy metals (especially lead), and silicon compounds. Often, these materials form fumes that coat the filament and interfere with the burning process. Oxidizers, halogenated hydrocarbon compounds, and corrosive vapors also can damage the filaments.

It is important to note that the majority of CGIs read in percentage of LEL, not in percentage of gas in air. Because of this, they cannot be used to determine if an atmosphere is too rich to burn. Therefore an LEL meter reading of 100% means that 100% of the LEL has been reached, not the percentage of the gas in the air. This instrument will allow the user to select LEL readout or percentage of gas in air. An LEL readout monitor will only determine whether an air concentration is below or above the LEL. A percentage gas monitor will determine the percentage of gas in air and can be used to determine whether concentrations are above the upper explosive limit (UEL). These devices also use two filaments. One filament is exposed to the gas, and the other one is sealed so its temperature remains constant. The high concentration of vapors cools the exposed filament and creates the imbalance. There is no combustion in this sensor. Most percentage gas monitors are calibrated to methane and are only accurate with that gas. These may be useful to EMS responders at confined-space emergencies. If high percentages of methane exist, there is a corresponding decrease in oxygen levels, leading to hypoxia in the victims. A third type of CGI gives readouts in ppm. Both of these devices are rare and are not commonly used for emergency response because of the difficulty of interpretation in situations where the gas is unknown.

CGI readings are relative to the calibration gas used. Pentane, methane, propane, and hexane are common calibration gases. The device will be accurate only when sensing the gas for which it was calibrated. Methane is commonly used for instruments that will be used for confined-space entry, whereas pentane usually is used to calibrate instruments used for gasoline spills. A common practice is to use propane as a calibration gas because the number of carbon atoms it contains (three) falls between the number contained in methane (one) and pentane (five), giving a calibration that is somewhat more accurate for each of these common gases. When measuring a different gas, the instrument works the same but the LEL will not be accurate. The change in resistance is in direct relationship to the heat produced by the sample being burned. If a vapor burns at a greater temperature than the calibration gas, then lower concentrations are needed to produce a given change. If less heat is produced, then greater concentrations are needed to produce a given change. Most manufacturers provide a graph or table showing the response of their instruments to various gases and vapors. This response curve is vital for interpretation of the monitoring data. Calibration should be carried out daily. With some units, calibration checks are done daily, and full calibration is performed monthly (follow the manufacturers instructions).

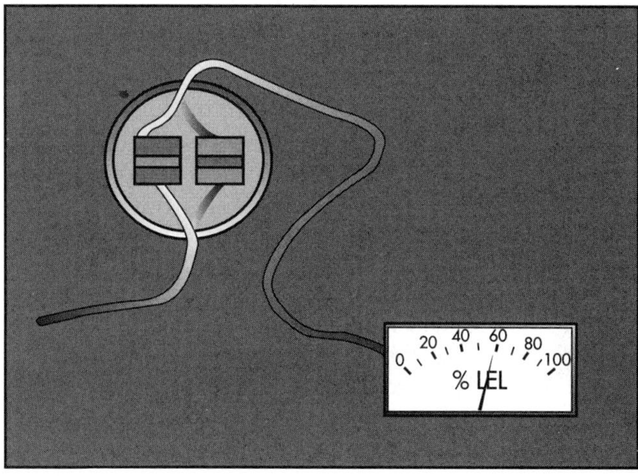

FIG. 9-5 Wheatstone bridge.

When an atmosphere contains sufficient levels of flammable vapors, the catalyzed filament will respond first, followed by the second filament. The result is that the resistance will balance. With some CGIs this results in the meter reporting 100% LEL, then returning to 0% LEL. If operators are not paying close attention to the readout, they may miss this occurrence and find themselves in a flammable atmosphere. Some devices have a latching device, which will lock the display or produce a warning alarm.

Because the CGI operates by burning gases, appropriate levels of O_2 are required for accurate results. Most models require at least 10% O_2 for accurate readings, and some hydrocarbons require at least 14% O_2 to burn; low O_2 concentrations will produce falsely low values. Additionally, O_2-enriched environments (O_2 concentrations greater than 25%) will enhance combustion and result in falsely high readings.

Because of the inherent inaccuracy of CGIs and the presence of possible mixtures of gases or vapors, action levels should be established. At the action level, personnel must evacuate the area or take special precautions. The action level usually referred to for CGIs in outdoor operations is 20% to 25% LEL. The Occupational Safety and Health Administration (OSHA) has established 10% LEL as the action limit in confined spaces.

Oxygen Meters

Many conditions may be encountered in which O_2 concentrations are abnormal. High concentrations of other gases may displace O_2, or combustion and/or chemical reactions may deplete the O_2 supply. Chemical reactions, chemicals that act as oxidizers, and a release from an O_2 supply, such as a welders torch, may increase the level of O_2. Oxygen levels must be determined to select PPE, ensure proper operation of CGIs, assess the flammability hazard, and determine the possible mechanism of injury. Oxygen meters determine the percentage of O_2 in the air and are usually calibrated to detect concentrations between 0% and 25% O_2; some may go to 50% (Fig. 9-6).

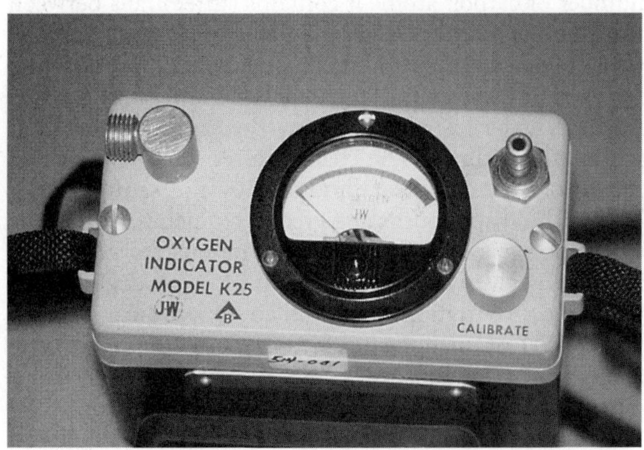

FIG. 9-6 Oxygen meter.

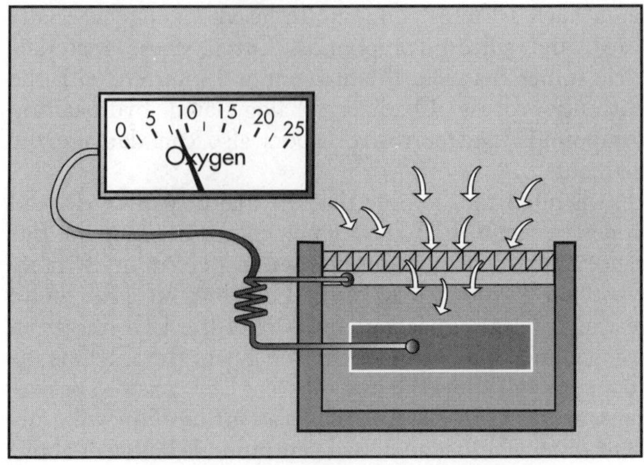

FIG. 9-7 Oxygen sensor.

In many cases, the CGI and O_2 meters are combined in a single meter.

Air is drawn into a detector cell by a pump or by diffusion (Fig. 9-7). The O_2 molecules diffuse though a membrane of the O_2-detection cell containing an electrolyte. A chemical reaction between the O_2 and electrolyte within the cell produces a small current that is proportional to the sensor's O_2 content. The current passes through an electronic circuit, and the resulting signal is displayed on a readout.

Certain vapors can damage the detection cell. Carbon dioxide (CO_2) concentrations greater than 0.5% can permanently affect the detector cell. When oxidizers in the atmosphere are being monitored, they react with the sensor in addition to O_2, resulting in an above-normal O_2 response.

Elevation above sea level affects both efficiency and accuracy of the meter because of atmospheric pressure changes on the membrane. Less air pressure reduces both the rate and amount of diffusion, thus giving both slow and false readings. Extreme temperatures also will affect the accuracy. It is important to calibrate these instruments for local conditions.

The electrolyte in the O_2 meter begins to wear out from the time the unit is first used. The sensor should be replaced according to the manufacturers recommendations.

OSHA has established 19.5% as the minimum O_2 concentration in ambient air that is safe for workers. Below 19.5%, air-supplied respirators (self-contained breathing apparatus [SCBA] or air line with escape bottle) must be used. Because of increased flammability in high O_2 concentrations, 25% is considered the upper safe limit. Oxygen-enriched environments must be vented before workers can enter. In confined spaces, OSHA has established 19.5% as the minimum and 23.5% as the maximum allowable concentrations of O_2.

Environments low in O_2 are caused by several situations. In some cases O_2 is displaced by another gas, often a toxic or flammable gas. Because O_2 constitutes only one fifth of air, approximately 5% of a displacing gas is needed to drop the O_2 concentrations by 1%. This is equal to 50,000 parts per million (ppm). EMS responders must remember that toxic conditions may exist long before the O_2 level reaches 19.5%.

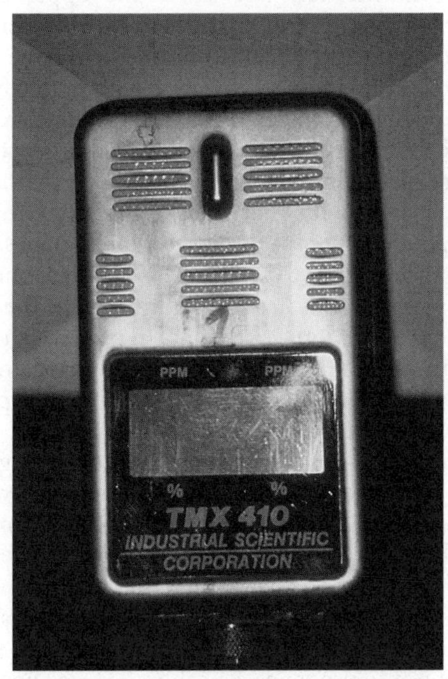

FIG. 9-8 Gas-specific sensor.

Gas-Specific Sensors

Many gas-specific monitors are available (Fig. 9-8). These monitors commonly are found combined within the same instrument containing a CGI and O_2 monitor. Monitors are available that include CGI/O_2 and one, two, three, or four specific gas sensors. Specialized instruments can detect vapors such as chlorine, ammonia, hydrogen sulfide, and carbon monoxide (CO). In most cases these instruments function similarly to the O_2 meter. Chemically reactive sensors produce electrical signals

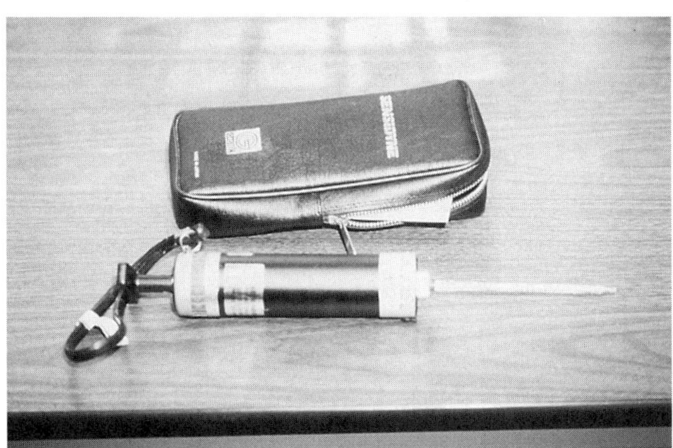

FIG. 9-9 Colorimetric indicator tube.

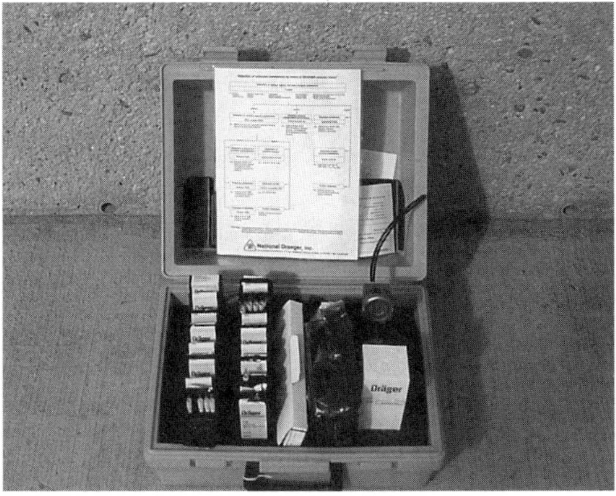

FIG. 9-10 Tubes in kit form, with a decision tree.

that are converted to vapor concentration on the monitor. Use caution when interpreting data supplied by these monitors. Other gases or vapors may interfere with the device, resulting in an inaccurate reading. For example, in a confined workspace, a combination monitor that measures combustible gas and O_2, CO, and hydrogen sulfide (H_2S) levels (the latter two gases are common toxic gases in confined spaces) is commonly used. If other toxic gases are present, this device probably will not provide adequate warning or information.

Gas-specific sensors measure products in ppm. They are not useful in interpreting flammability. Because these devices are designed to measure a specific gas, they are not useful in the identification of unknown chemicals. The identity of the released chemical should be ascertained so that the proper device may be selected. As with O_2 sensors, these devices should be calibrated under local conditions.

The action level for gas-specific sensors may be set at the specific chemical's permissible exposure limit/threshold limit value (PEL/TLV), immediately dangerous to life or health (IDLH) limit, or level of concern (LOC).

Colorimetric Indicator Tubes

Colorimetric indicator, or detector, tubes are a type of gas-specific monitor (Fig. 9-9). The tubes are specific for a certain compound or family of chemicals. Approximately 400 types of tubes are manufactured. The tubes contain chemically treated granules that react with the contaminant to produce a stain or color change. The tubes are marked with a scale to indicate the approximate concentration of vapor that is drawn through the tube.

This air monitoring system consists of a hand-operated piston or bellows pump and detector tubes. Battery-powered pumps also are available. Following selection of the appropriate tube, the glass tips at both ends are broken off and the tube is inserted into the pump. The tube must be inserted in the correct direction, which is indicated by an arrow on the tube. The arrow should point toward the pump.

Many manufacturers market a special selection of tubes in kit form that may be helpful in assessing unknown chemicals. A selection of tubes is used, and results are compared with a decision tree (Fig. 9-10). The test may be able to identify the family of chemicals involved and allow for more effective patient assessment/treatment and a better selection of responder PPE.

HAZMAT team responders who are using colorimetric tubes must be properly trained. Each type of tube requires a certain number of pump strokes and a minimum amount of time between each stroke. Many pumps are equipped with an end-of-stroke indicator, signaling when a full stroke has been completed. Manufacturers instructions must be followed carefully to ensure that the proper volume of air is drawn through the tube. If responders do not use these tubes properly, the data will not be accurate.

Tubes from different manufacturers are not interchangeable. Calibration of colorimetric tubes is not necessary, but the pump must be checked periodically for leaking valves. This often is accomplished by inserting an unbroken detector tube into the pump orifice and attempting to aspirate air through the pump. If air is drawn in, the pump leaks. Additionally, the pump should be volumetrically calibrated regularly.

Colorimetric tubes have a shelf life that is marked on the box in which they are packaged. Storage under hot conditions may reduce this shelf time. Expired tubes should not be used. If stored in a refrigerator, tubes should be allowed to reach ambient temperature before use. Temperature and humidity may affect the tubes' accuracy.

The length of the color change within the tube corresponds to the gas concentration. This color change should be examined immediately. The length of the color stain may change after just a few minutes, causing responders to misread the results and severely compromise the quality of the data. Tubes are marked in either percentage or ppm. Often it is easier to read the tube by comparing the exposed tube with an unexposed tube of the same type. Unfortunately, the color change commonly is not a straight line but a jagged or faded edge. This makes determining exactly where the color change

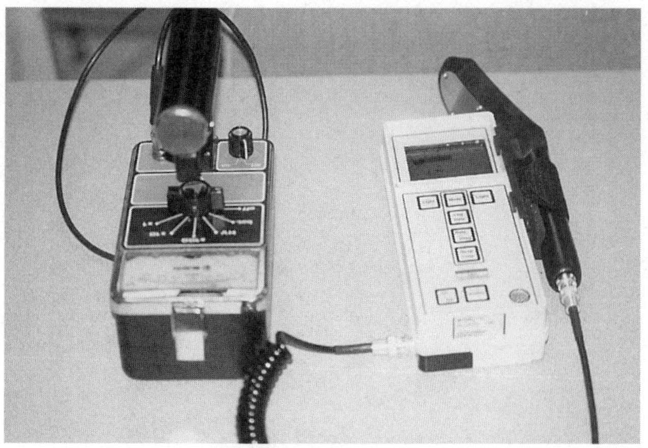

FIG. 9-11 Various types of radiation meters.

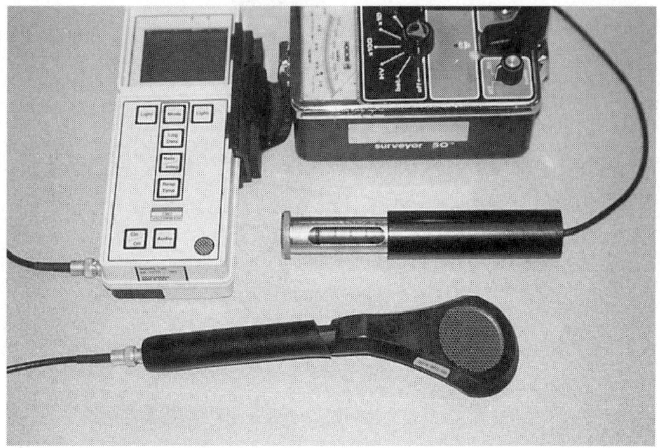

FIG. 9-12 Various probes.

ends difficult. Estimates should always indicate the worst-case scenario.

If detector tubes are used when more than one gas is present, cross-sensitivity may occur. This means that a gas other than the one of interest may cause a color change within the tube. Possible cross-sensitivity problems are identified on the instruction sheet that accompanies the tubes.

The limitations just discussed substantially affect the accuracy of colorimetric tubes. The error factor generally can range from 25% to 50%.

As with specific gas monitors, the action level may be set at the specific chemical's PEL/TLV, IDLH, or LOC.

Radiation Meters

Whenever radioactive materials might be encountered, a radiation survey meter should be used to detect the type of radiation (generally alpha, beta, and gamma) and its level (Fig. 9-11). Using this information, patient and equipment decontamination efficiency, safe work practices, and PPE needs can be determined. In addition to survey instruments, personal dosimeters commonly are used in radioactive environments to determine an individual's dose of radiation.

Radiation survey instruments measure ionizing radiation. Detectors containing an ionizable detection medium commonly are used. The ions produced in the medium are counted electronically, and a relationship is established between the number of ions and the amount of radiation present. Different probe types may be used to determine the type of radiation present (Fig. 9-12).

Pancake or end-window probes with a mica window are used for alpha radiation. For beta and gamma radiation the most common type of probe is the Geiger-Mueller. A side window allows beta radiation to pass through, and a movable metal shield is used to cover the window and allow for gamma-radiation monitoring.

Radiation survey instruments are factory calibrated and usually returned to the factory or manufacturer for recalibration. Calibration checks can be performed using a cesium-137 source, which can be obtained from the manufacturer.

Radiation usually is measured in milliroentgens (mRs) per hour. This unit expresses an exposure rate, or the amount of radiation that an individual would be exposed to at the point of measurements. Many meters also have a scale that reads in counts per minute; both counts per minute and mRs are functionally related. When interpreting the data, keep in mind that the Geiger counter may be sensitive to radio waves, microwaves, magnetic fields, and electrostatic fields. The radiation level depends on distance from the source. What is considered a safe level may be unsafe as the responder moves closer to the source. Thus, when radioactive materials are suspected, a systematic and thorough search of the area must be made.

Generally, when the radiation level increases to three to five times the background level, responders should withdraw and assess the need for special procedures. OSHA regulations state that when radiation exceeds 0.2 mR per hour protective measures must be taken.

The instruments described so far are common to most HAZMAT teams. A few well-equipped teams or industrial locations may have other instruments available. These may include general survey meters such as photo ionization detectors (PIDs) and flame ionization detectors (FIDs) and infrared (IR) spectrophotometers. Military units may use a device known as a *chemical agent monitor (CAM)* to detect the presence of nerve and blister agents. Test strips and sophisticated test kits for assessing liquid and solid chemicals also are available. The rest of this chapter will address these specialized instruments.

Photo Ionization Detectors

PIDs are used to determine the concentration of ionizable vapors in the air (Fig. 9-13). PIDs will detect most organic and a few inorganic vapors. They are used for general monitoring, characterizing plumes, and detecting situations in which PPE is needed.

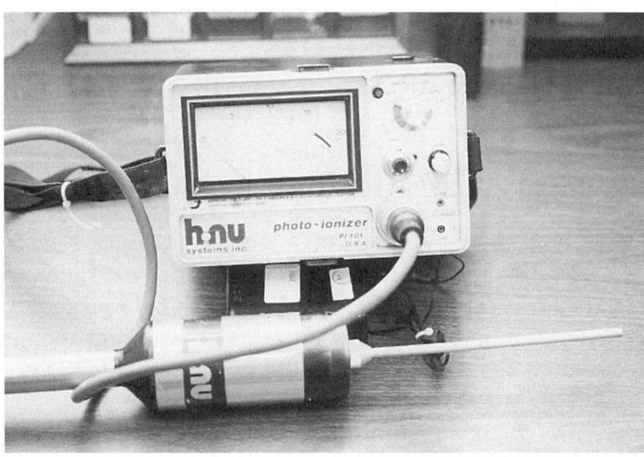

FIG. 9-13 Photo ionization detectors will detect most organic and a few inorganic vapors.

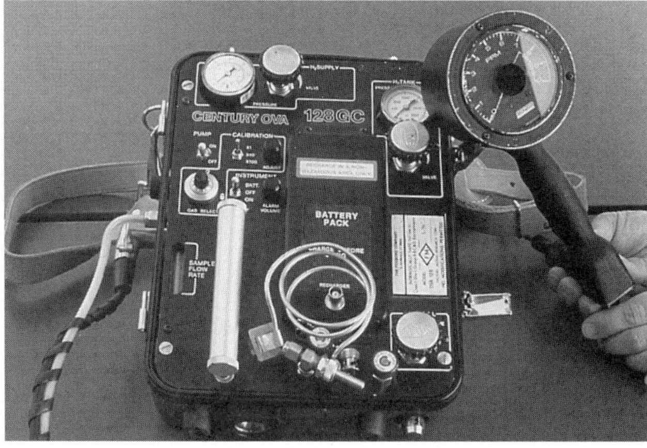

FIG. 9-15 Flame ionization detector.

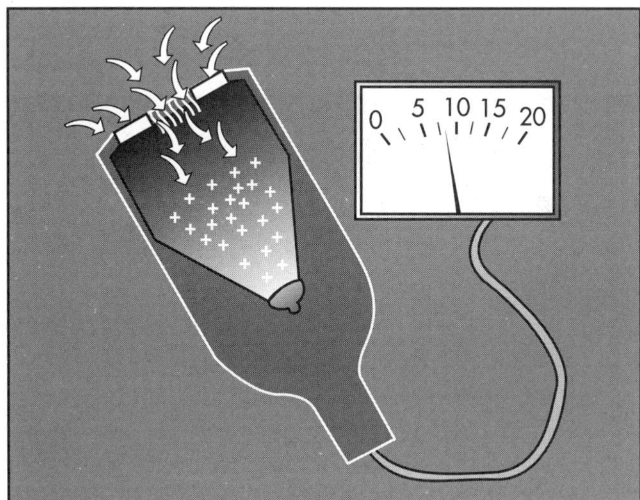

FIG. 9-14 Photo ionization detector chamber, ultraviolet light, and grid.

Air is pumped into an ionization chamber, which is flooded with ultraviolet (UV) light (Fig. 9-14). The light provides the energy to split uncharged molecules into charged ions. The ions are attracted to a metal grid within the ionization chamber. The grid conducts a small amount of current, and the ions attracted to the grid produce a change in current. This change is displayed as a ppm equivalent.

A PID usually is calibrated to isobutylene. Its ability to accurately detect other gases depends on how closely these other gases resemble isobutylene in terms of ionization. Most PID units have a span setting, which can electronically change the reading to correspond to other gases. All ionizable molecules collected will produce a reading, so the reading will represent the total ionizables present.

Anything that interferes with light transmission can affect PID readings. When water vapor is present in the ionization chamber, it acts like a fog and scatters and reflects the UV light back toward the source. Also, gases that cannot be ionized act in a similar manner.

The PID measures all ionizable vapors within the range of the energy supplied by the UV light source. Therefore, the instrument can ionize only those vapors that have an ionization potential (IP) (measured in electron volts [eV]) equal to or less than the eV emitted by the UV lamp. For example, a PID having a UV lamp of 10.3 eV will not detect any vapors that have an ionization potential greater than 10.3 eV. The interchangeable UV lamps in PIDs generally range from 9.6 to 11.7 eV. Most organic vapors have a low ionization potential, so the PID is an excellent instrument for detection of most, but not all, organic vapors. Ionization potentials can be found in the *NIOSH Pocket Guide to Chemical Hazards.* Some simple compounds, such as methane, cannot be detected by a PID. A reading of 0 ppm on the monitor should never be interpreted as meaning that no chemicals are present. Toxic chemicals may be present that the monitor cannot ionize.

The PID detects all vapors within its ionization range; it cannot isolate specific vapors or tell the operator which vapor is present. Therefore, the PID is of greatest use when the specific chemical has been identified. Some PIDs are equipped with a gas chromatograph feature. The gas chromatograph, in the hands of an experienced operator, may be able to identify specific chemicals.

Once the chemical has been identified and the PID properly calibrated, the action level may be set at the specific chemical's PEL/TLV, IDLH, or LOC.

Flame Ionization Detectors

FIDs, sometimes called *organic vapor analyzers (OVA),* are similar to PIDs in that they detect ionizable vapors (Fig. 9-15). The operational theory of an FID is similar to a PID, with one important difference. The energy source for an FID is a hydrogen flame that generates 15.3 eV, which is enough energy to ionize any compound containing carbon.

Gases are pumped into a detection chamber containing a hydrogen flame. The ions that are produced are attracted to a grid within the detector. An electrical current is generated proportional to the ionic concentration. The change then is displayed as a ppm equivalent.

The FID detects only organic compounds. Additionally, there must be sufficient O_2 in the air to support combustion. The instrument also must be intrinsically safe. As with PIDs, 0 ppm on the monitor should never be interpreted as meaning that no chemicals are present.

The FID typically is calibrated to methane. Like the PID, this instrument has a span setting that can electronically recalibrate the instrument for a specific gas.

The FID measures total ionizable vapors that the hydrogen flame can ionize. Most instruments are unable to distinguish what type of vapor is detected. Similar to PIDs, some FIDs are equipped with a gas chromatograph feature, which will identify specific compounds (Fig. 9-16).

Like PIDs, FID action levels are set at the specific chemical's PEL/TLV, IDLH, or LOC.

Infrared Spectrophotometer

Chemicals will absorb infrared (IR) light at certain distinct wavelengths. IR units use an infrared sensor to monitor specific chemicals (Fig. 9-17). It can be selective based on the wavelength of IR light used. The unit has twin, parallel chambers through which IR light is projected. Some of the IR light is absorbed by the chemical, and the rest is transmitted through. The unit measures the amount of light transmitted, which is compared with manufacturers data, and is expressed as ppm.

Because many chemicals absorb IR light at similar wavelengths, interference may occur when multiple chemicals are present. These instruments are fragile and require flat, level surfaces free of vibration or movement for proper operation.

Action levels for IR units are set at the specific chemical's PEL/TLV, IDLH, or LOC.

Chemical Agent Monitors

The chemical agent monitor (CAM) is a device that is used by military units to detect the presence of chemical warfare agents (Fig. 9-18). The CAM can be used to detect chemical nerve and blister agents. It is a point monitor used to determine if patients or equipment is contaminated with these agents. It is not capable of determining the amount of agent present in the air. The CAM operates similarly to the PID and FID except its ionization source is nickel-63. The readout on the CAM monitor is in units (bars), which represent an increasing level of hazard. Because of its function, the CAM can show false-positive readings with numerous organic compounds.

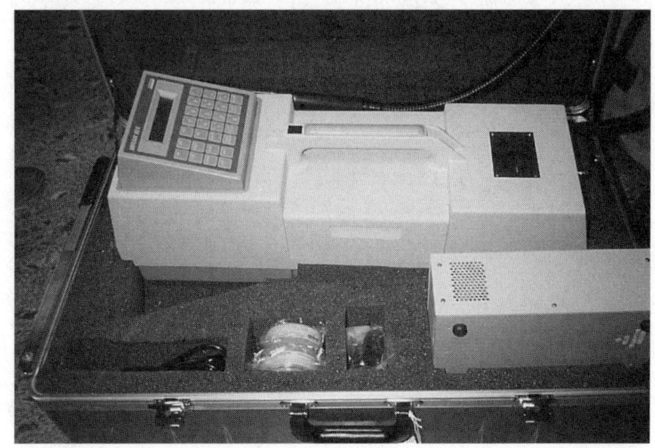

FIG. 9-17 Infrared monitor.

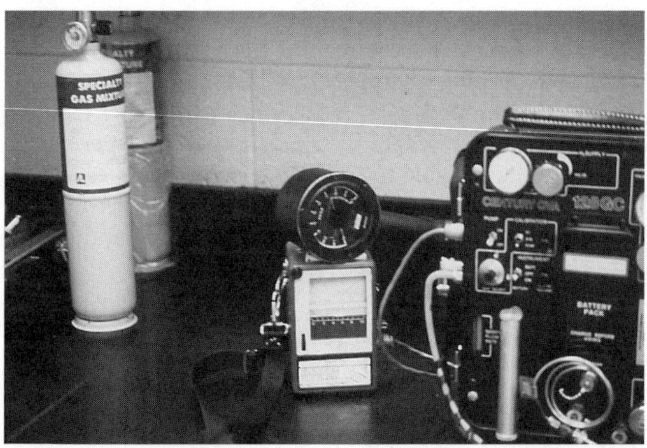

FIG. 9-16 Some flame ionization devices, equipped with a gas chromatograph feature, can identify specific compounds.

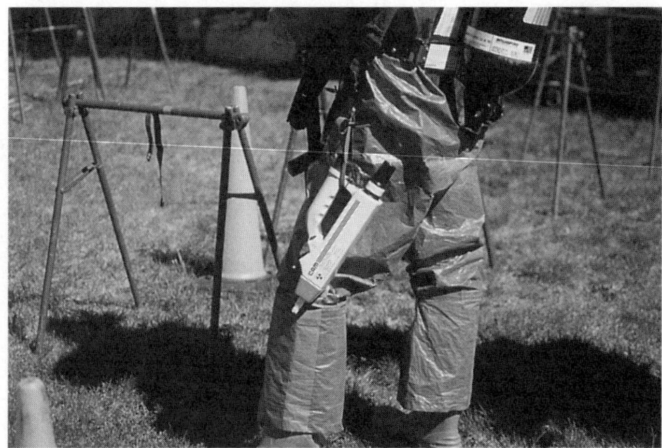

FIG. 9-18 Responder with CAM.

Because of the extreme toxicity of these agents, any reading should be considered as a sign of possible contamination if the use of chemical warfare agents is suspected.

A new instrument, the advanced portable detector (APD) 2000, recently has become available. The APD functions exactly like the older CAM but is capable of screening out most false-positive readings and also will monitor for gamma radiation at the same time.

Test Strips and Field Test Kits

All of the instruments discussed so far have been air monitoring devices. Often, emergency responders must determine the identity of solids or liquids. Numerous devices, ranging from simple paper test strips (Fig. 9-19) to sophisticated categorization kits (Fig. 9-20) are available to help in identification of solids or liquids. Paper test strips are available for measuring pH and other values. The accuracy of paper test strips depends on the ability of the user to determine the color change compared with standard color charts. Handheld meters are available for testing pH, temperature, and oxidation-reduction potential. Field test kits are available for determining the concentration of specific liquids. Hazard categorization kits, designed for identification of unknown products, are useful for identifying liquids and some solids. To use any of these devices the responder must come into direct contact with the chemical. Because the product has not been identified, PPE may not be adequate. Extreme caution must be used.

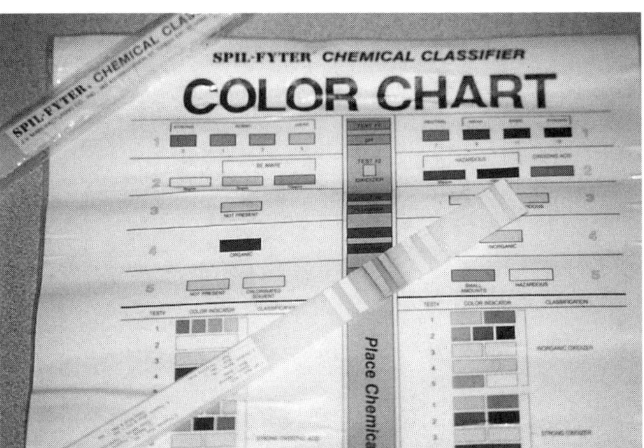

FIG. 9-19 Chemical test strips.

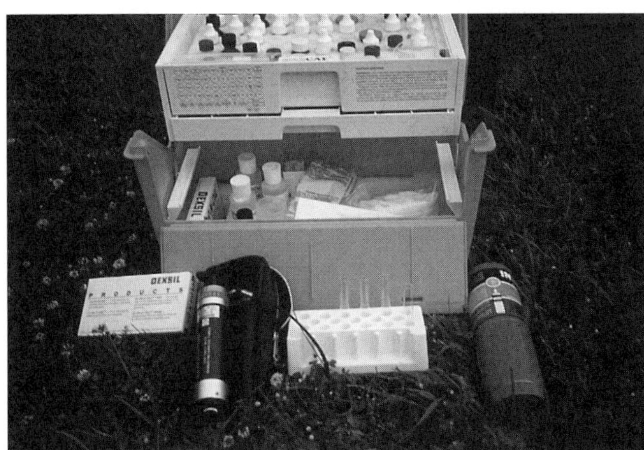

FIG. 9-20 Chemical test kit.

Summary

Detection and air monitoring equipment allow responders to make decisions regarding the identity and amount of the released material, the extent of spread of the material, and the types of PPE needed. EMS responders can use the data supplied by direct-reading air monitoring equipment to assist in triage and patient management. To accomplish this the appropriate device must be chosen, the instrument must be used properly, and the results must be properly and accurately assessed. Typically, responders will use a minimum of Level B PPE and combustible gas monitors, oxygen meters, and radiation survey instruments in an initial survey. If organic vapors are suspected, PIDs or FIDs also may be used. If chemical warfare agents are suspected, a CAM or APD can be used to determine the efficiency of decontamination. Remember that PIDs, FIDs, CAMs, and APDs have major limitations and may not detect the presence of certain gases or vapors. Once the suspected chemical is identified, PIDs, FIDs, CAMs, APDs, colorimetric tubes, or specific gas monitors may be used to quantify the amount and monitor for change. If solid or liquid contaminants are present, detector strips or field test kits may be helpful.

Remember that each instrument has limitations. Never interpret a monitor's failure to detect anything as evidence that nothing is present. Different types of detectors may need to be used to detect certain gases. Multiple detectors should always be used to verify results. Gases may form into pockets or stratify in low-lying areas. Accessory pumps and long tubes can be used to draw air from remote distances. Weather conditions, radios, and cellular telephones may affect monitoring devices. Instruments must be properly calibrated, and their accuracy depends on how the detected gas reacts compared with the calibration gas.

Detection instruments can provide invaluable information to emergency response personnel only if they are used properly and in conjunction with adequate risk assessment procedures.

CHAPTER REVIEW QUESTIONS

1. List at least six factors that may be determined by the use of field detection devices.
2. Explain what "intrinsically safe" means.
3. List the action levels used with combustible gas indicators.

4. Why are combustible gas indicator readings often inaccurate?
5. What gases are detected by O_2 meters?
6. List the action levels used with O_2 meters.
7. Identify the major limitations of specific gas sensors and colorimetric indicator tubes.
8. Which types of radiation can be detected with a Geiger-Mueller radiation detector?
9. Explain why PIDs may not show any reading, even in a high concentration of gas.
10. What kind of chemicals can be detected with an FID?

BIBLIOGRAPHY

Andrews LP, editor: *Emergency responder training manual for the hazardous materials technician,* New York, 1992, Van Nostrand Reinhold.

Bowen JE: *Emergency management of hazardous materials incidents,* Quincy, Mass, 1995, National Fire Protection Association.

EPA: *EPA standard safety operating guidelines,* Washington, DC, 1984, US Government Printing Office.

Guidelines for public sector hazardous materials training. 1998 ed, HMEP Curriculum Guidelines, Emmitsburg, Md, 1998, National Emergency Training Center.

Hazardous materials response training program, New Jersey/New York, 1988, Hazardous Materials Worker/Training Program.

Maslansky CJ, Maslansky SP: *Air monitoring instrumentation,* New York, 1993, Van Nostrand Reinhold.

National Fire Protection Association: *NFPA 471, Recommended practice for responding to hazardous materials incidents,* Quincy, Mass, 1992, The Association.

NIOSH/OSHA/USCG/EPA: *Occupational safety and health guidance manual for hazardous waste site activities,* Washington, DC, 1985, DHHS (NIOSH) Publication No 85-115, US Government Printing Office.

Noll GG, Hildebrand MS, Yvorra JG: *Hazardous materials: managing the incident,* ed 2, Stillwater, Okla, 1995, Fire Protection Publications.

OSHA: 29 CFR 1910.120, Hazardous waste operations and emergency response; Final rule, March 6, 1989; Washington, DC, US Government Printing Office.

Strong CB, Irvin TR: *Emergency response and hazardous chemical management: principles and practices,* Delray Beach, Fla, 1996, St. Lucie Press.

Tokle G, editor: *Hazardous materials response handbook,* ed 2, Quincy, Mass, 1993, National Fire Protection Association.

Varela J, editor: *Hazardous materials handbook for emergency responders,* New York, 1996, Van Nostrand Reinhold.

10

EMS/Hazardous Materials Response Practices and Scene Management

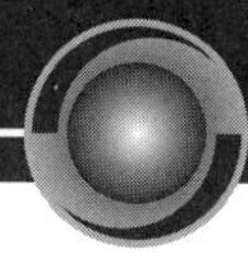

Phil Currance

CHAPTER OBJECTIVES

At the conclusion of this chapter the student will be able to:

- Identify safe locations when responding to a hazardous materials emergency.
- Identify priorities when responding to a hazardous materials emergency.
- Discuss the need for and the use of an incident management system.
- Identify duties and responsibilities of the incident commander.
- Identify duties and responsibilities of the incident safety officer.
- Explain the need for a safety briefing at a hazardous materials incident.
- Identify common topics of a safety briefing.
- Explain the need for Emergency Medical Services (EMS) involvement at a hazardous materials emergency.
- Discuss the need for an incident-specific safety plan.
- Discuss the need for site security at a hazardous materials incident.
- Identify the exclusion (hot), contamination reduction (warm), and support (cold) zones at a hazardous materials incident, and describe the EMS actions performed in each zone.
- Explain the buddy system.
- Discuss the need for internal and external communications at a hazardous materials emergency.
- Identify the need for an emergency signal at a hazardous materials incident.
- Identify special EMS/hazardous materials equipment that may be useful.

CASE STUDY

EMS responders are called to a lawn and garden store for a report of numerous people ill after a case containing glass jars of the pesticide malathion falls from a shelf, breaking the glass. Workers tried to clean up the spill, but they soon became ill. On arrival, EMS responders are met by the store manager, who states, "Since this is an over-the-counter pesticide, it shouldn't be that hazardous." Fire department personnel are en route but have not yet arrived.

- ◆ What is the EMS responders' first priority?
- ◆ Is it safe to go into the store to check things out?

- Is it safe to treat the patients immediately?
- Where should the EMS responders stage their equipment?

Hazardous materials incidents are among the most dangerous that EMS responders must face. The combination of chemical and physical threats compounded by the uncontrolled nature of emergency responses mandate that precautions be taken to ensure the safety of response personnel. When hazardous materials incidents involve victims, EMS agencies may be the first called and first to arrive. The presence of hazardous materials may not have been determined yet. Responders should always be alert for clues to the presence of hazardous materials on any and every response. It may sound like overkill, but remember that hazardous materials are everywhere. Hazardous materials may have caused the problem initially or may have been released because of the incident. Planning, safe response practices, site-control measures, and administration procedures can reduce potential hazards and allow responders to focus on mitigation of the incident.

Safe Response and Work Practices

Safe Response Practices

Many responders are injured during the initial approach to a hazardous materials incident. Clues that hazardous materials are involved, such as what the site is being used for, container shape, markings/colors, placards/labels, shipping papers, senses, and multiple patients with the same complaint, must be recognized and should be actively assessed (Box 10-1). Responders must determine if a release of hazardous materials has occurred.

Response must be to a safe area away from obvious and foreseeable dangers. Areas that are upwind, uphill, and upstream from the incident are best. Initial priorities always are to ensure that responders are in a safe area and isolation of the incident. At the first hint that a hazardous material is involved, responders should stop a safe distance from the contaminated area. The *North American Emergency Response Guidebook* (NAERG) gives dis-

BOX 10-1

FACTORS IN ASSESSING SITE OF HAZARDOUS MATERIALS INCIDENT

Are there any visual clues to the presence of hazardous materials?
What type of material has been released, and what impact is it having on the area?
Has more than one material been released?
What are the chemical and toxicological threats posed by the material(s)?

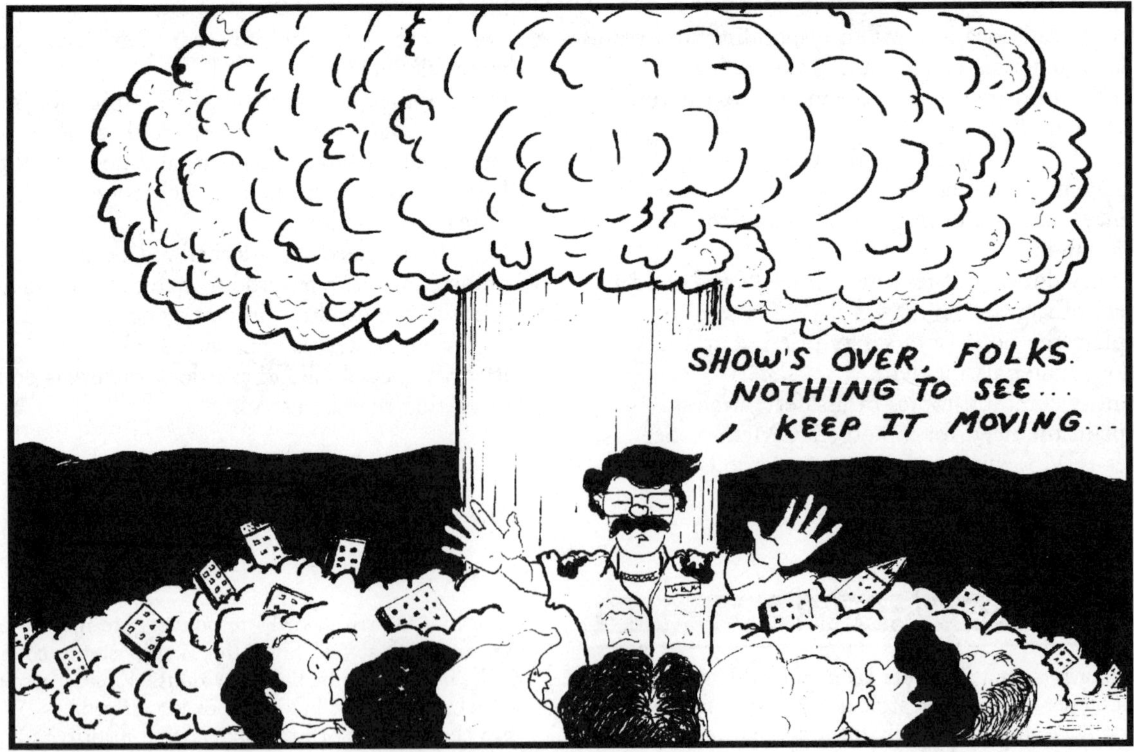

Reprinted with permission from Steve Berry's *I'm Not an Ambulance Driver* cartoon book series.

tance suggestions (Fig. 10-1). If no other personnel are on site, EMS responders will need to establish a command post and set up an incident management system (IMS). Ensure that other emergency personnel are responding to a safe area. If an IMS already is established, EMS responders should report to the incident commander or staging area as directed.

The first priority is to protect responders. Rescues from contaminated areas should not be attempted until the chemical has been identified and properly trained responders with appropriate personal protective equipment (PPE) are available. This is difficult to do when it is obvious that people are in distress and need help. However, if untrained and unprotected responders enter the area to carry out a rescue, they are likely to become victims themselves and become part of the problem, not part of the solution. The hazard area should be isolated and secured from entry by unauthorized personnel. A safe zone that is upwind, uphill, and upstream from the incident should be established. Because gases and vapors will spread the fastest and go the farthest, upwind is the most important factor in selection of a safe zone. Because most vapors are heavier than air, they will accumulate in low areas. Therefore, all low-lying areas should be avoided. If the incident has occurred inside a structure, avoid areas around the building's ventilation exhaust. Isolation and evacuation distances will vary depending on chemical/product, weather, and situation. Suggested evacuation and protective distances can be found in the NAERG, and CHEMTREC (see Chapter 6) may be able to provide more detailed information.

Never assume that the scene is safe because the substance does not have any apparent odor or obvious color. Many chemicals are colorless, odorless, and tasteless. Some chemicals have warning properties that are not detectable until a dangerous level is reached. Some chemicals, such as hydrogen sulfide (H_2S), may cause fatigue of the olfactory nerve, resulting in an inability to sense the chemical by smell.

Assistance (e.g., police, fire, hazardous materials

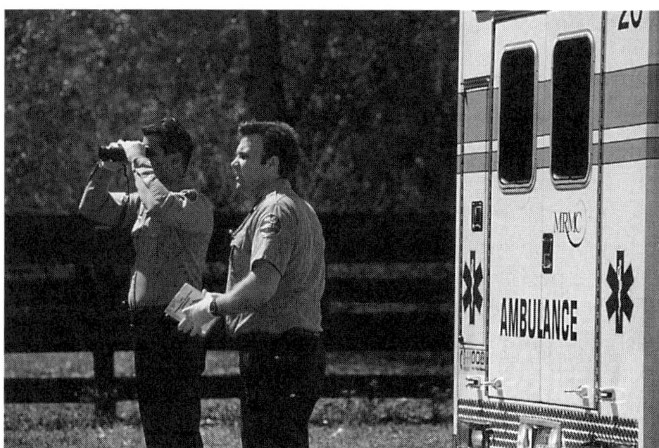

FIG. 10-1 EMS responders should stop at a safe distance from the contaminated area.

(HAZMAT) team, local or state health department) should be requested as soon as possible. HAZMAT teams may have long response times, so prompt notification is vital. Effective response practices and proper patient treatment modalities depend on identification of the product. Responders should attempt to identify the product(s) involved by using identification clues or discussions with on-scene witnesses. Binoculars can be used to assess the scene from a safe distance. Witnesses should be interviewed, but remember that they may or may not have a complete understanding of the incident or the chemical that is involved. Evaluate the witness's level of expertise before taking his or her information as 100% correct. If in doubt, check other references to back up the validity of the information.

Personnel should never attempt to recover a manifest or bill of lading unless wearing proper PPE. To enter a possibly contaminated area, responders will need to wear positive-pressure self-contained breathing apparatus (SCBA) and appropriate PPE that are specified in reference sources. Selection must be made by a knowledgeable individual. To use this type of equipment, personnel must have adequate training and fit-testing. If PPE is not available or responders are not trained in its proper use, response activities should be limited to scene isolation and identification from a safe distance. Once the substance has been identified, responders should consult written or computer references, or contact CHEMTREC, MEDTREC, the regional poison center, or medical control for more detailed information.

Remember that bystanders, witnesses, and well-meaning individuals who stopped to assist may be exposed or contaminated. These people need to be screened for possible exposure and injuries. If a possibility of contamination exists, decontamination will be necessary. The level of decontamination will depend on the degree of contamination. Names and addresses should be noted in case future information indicates an exposure.

Incident safety plan

Each incident should be handled using an incident-specific safety plan (Box 10-2). The safety of all responders and many EMS activities are directed by the safety plan.

The incident-specific safety plan must be user friendly and should be a guide or checklist for mitigation of the incident. It also serves to document the response activities and serves as a briefing tool for responders. The safety plan is a dynamic document that should change as scene conditions change. Checklists can be established to assist in the development of the safety plan (Box 10-3).

Safety briefing

A safety briefing should be held before all entry activities (Fig. 10-2). Entry/backup team members and all essential response personnel, including all EMS personnel, should be included in the briefing. The briefing ensures that hazards are identified and that the team is focused on the same objectives (Box 10-4).

BOX 10-2

Incident-specific Safety Plan

At a minimum, this plan should do the following:

- Identify the incident location, surrounding topography, and possible exposures
- Identify the chemical and physical hazards that exist at the incident
- Document current and forecasted weather conditions
- Document initial site conditions
- Keep track of scene organization (incident management system)
- Identify scene control areas
- Identify PPE requirements
- Identify decontamination requirements, including patient and equipment decontamination
- Identify work or response activities for each entry team
- Identify air monitoring requirements
- Identify communications procedures, including emergency evacuation signals
- Describe emergency procedures and evacuation routes

BOX 10-3

Typical Checklist Forms Used to Develop an Incident-specific Safety Plan

Chemical evaluation forms
Entry team checklists
Incident briefing forms
News release worksheets
Staging area logs
Decontamination logs
Hot-zone entry logs
Incident management sector checklists

Safe Work Practices

The incident commander must identify, to the extent possible, all hazardous substances or conditions present and appropriately address the following:

- ◆ Scene analysis
- ◆ Use of engineering controls
- ◆ Maximum exposure limits
- ◆ Hazardous substance handling procedures
- ◆ Use of new technologies

Based on the hazardous substances and/or conditions present, the incident commander should implement appropriate emergency operations and ensure that the PPE worn is appropriate.

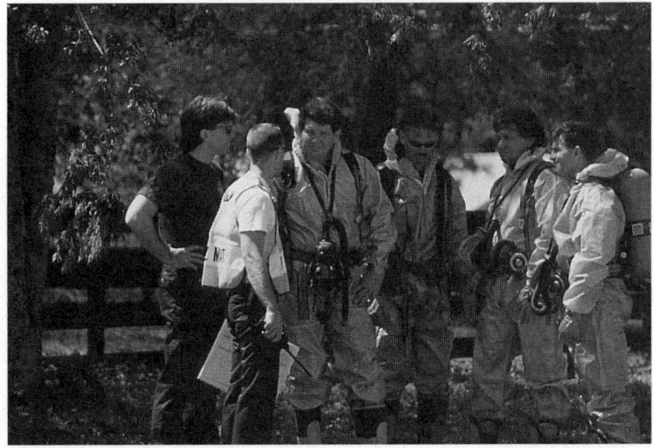

FIG. 10-2 The briefing ensures that both hazards and team objectives are identified.

BOX 10-4

Briefing Topics

Expected hazards
Signs and symptoms of exposure
Work plan
Communication systems
Emergency signals and evacuation routes
Safe work practices
Decontamination plan

Personal protective equipment

Employees engaged in emergency response and exposed to a potential inhalation hazard must wear positive-pressure SCBA until the incident commander determines, through the use of data supplied by air monitoring equipment, that a decreased level of respiratory protection will not result in a hazardous exposure.

Limited site access

The incident commander should limit the number of emergency response personnel at the emergency site (those areas of potential or actual exposure to incident or site hazards) to those who are actively performing emergency operations. However, operations in hazardous areas must be performed using the buddy system and in groups of two or more. Backup personnel should be standing by with equipment and ready to provide assistance or rescue as needed (Fig. 10-3). EMS should also be standing by with medical equipment and transportation capability to a designated medical facility. Plans should be established for emergency rescue and decontamination of victims and responders who are injured in the hot zone. Patients

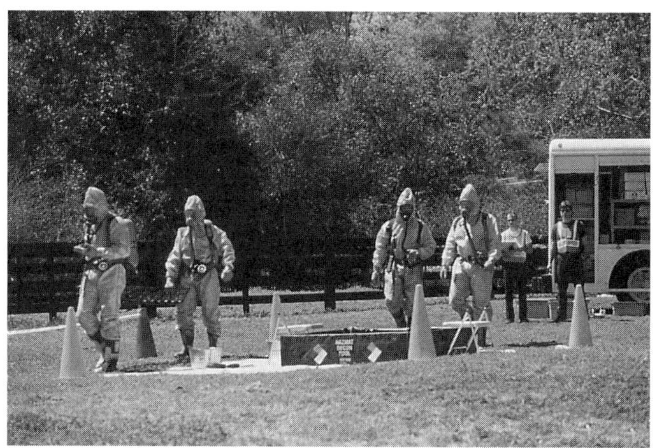

FIG. 10-3 The backup team should be standing by, ready to assist.

should not be turned over to EMS until they have been decontaminated.

Safety officer

The incident commander should designate a safety officer, who is knowledgeable in the operations being implemented at the emergency response site. This individual is specifically charged with identifying and evaluating hazards, and providing direction with respect to the safety of operations for the emergency at hand. At minor incidents the incident commander may also serve as the safety officer. When the safety officer judges activities to be immediately dangerous to life or health (IDLH) or to involve an imminently dangerous condition, that officer must have the authority to alter, suspend, or terminate those activities. The safety officer should immediately inform the incident commander of any actions needed to correct hazards at the emergency scene.

Buddy system

Activities in contaminated or hazardous areas should be conducted using the buddy system (Box 10-5). This means that responders must work in teams of at least two people and that a backup team must be ready.

The buddy system alone may not be sufficient to ensure that help will be provided in an emergency. At all times, responders in the hot zone should be in line-of-sight of or have verbal communication with backup personnel in the warm or cold zone. In some cases, closed-circuit television may be used to establish line-of-sight with entry teams inside structures.

Communications systems

Two sets of communications systems should be established during a response: internal communication among response personnel on site and external communication between on-site and off-site personnel. Effective internal communication is critical for safe operations. Both a primary and a backup system should be established. Radio communication is the most effective. However, using standard, handheld radios with SCBA and chemical-protective equipment can significantly hinder the clarity of verbal communication. Special radios can have microphones mounted in the SCBA face piece, bone microphones on top of the responders' head, or throat microphones. Even if radio communication is available, a backup system should be in place. Writing boards can be a useful communication device between entry-team members in high-noise atmospheres or between the entry team and personnel in the warm and cold zones. The entry team can write chemical information or requests for equipment on the board, which then can be read with binoculars from the cold zone.

Chemical-protective suits can be marked with the responder's name, color coding, or numbers to allow them to be identified from a distance. Hand signals also are a useful communication tool for responders at a hazardous materials incident. Typical hand signals include the following:

- Both hands over the head: emergency help needed
- Hands gripping throat: low/out of air
- Thumbs up: OK/yes/I understand
- Thumbs down: no/negative
- Grip partner's wrist or both hands around waist: leave area immediately

Emergency communication also should be established. An emergency signal should be designated that will warn people to leave the hot zone immediately and be on the lookout for potential problems. Air-powered fog horns or personnel-alert sirens work well. In high-noise areas, a visual signal, such as a strobe light, may need to be added. All communications devices used in a potentially explosive atmosphere must be intrinsically safe and should be checked daily to ensure proper operation.

The primary means of external communication will be radio and mobile/cellular telephone (Box 10-6). It should be remembered that radio and mobile/cellular communications are not secure and can be monitored by the news media and public.

BOX 10-5

BUDDY SYSTEM

A buddy is necessary to:
- Provide his or her partner with assistance
- Observe his or her partner for signs of chemical or heat exposure
- Periodically check the integrity of his or her partner's PPE
- Notify the incident commander or safety officer if emergency help is needed

BOX 10-6

Reasons to Establish External Communication Between On-site and Off-site Personnel

Coordinate emergency response
Request additional assistance
Obtain detailed chemical information
Contact medical control
Inform hospitals of scene conditions and patient information

Scene Management

Scene Control

Scene-control activities are very important to the safety of response personnel. Scene control is accomplished by site security, control zones, and safe response practices.

Site security

Site security is necessary to limit scene access to properly trained and equipped response personnel. Hazardous materials incidents are newsworthy events and attract a lot of attention. Bystanders and news media personnel may easily end up in the wrong area and become unwilling participants.

Control zones

Control zones should be established during an incident to reduce the chances of accidental spread of hazardous substances by responders from the contaminated area to the clean area. Different types of operations will occur within these zones, and the flow of personnel in and out of the zones can be controlled (Fig. 10-4).

Control zones are necessary to ensure that response personnel and the public are protected against hazards, contamination is confined to the appropriate areas, and personnel can be accounted for and evacuated if necessary. Typically, three zones are established: the hot zone, warm zone, and cold zone.

THE HOT ZONE. The *hot,* or *exclusion, zone* is the area in which contamination exists. Activities in this zone include scene characterization and mitigation activities. Entrance into this zone will require proper training and appropriate PPE, given the identified or suspected threat (Fig. 10-5). Entry teams must consist of two or more responders, and backup teams must be available. All people exiting this area must be decontaminated.

Because this area is contaminated, the most obvious patient management technique is patient removal. EMS units do not usually operate in the hot zone, but responder involvement will depend on area needs, standard operating procedures, training, and specific incident considerations. These issues must be dealt with as a part of preplanning. Awareness-level EMS responders are restricted to the cold zone, and operations-level–trained responders may work in the warm zone. EMS responders who work in the hot zone must be trained to a technician or specialist equivalent.

In multi/mass casuality incidents, triage activities may be required. If patients are trapped in the hot zone, they may require EMS treatment during extrication activities (Box 10-7). Patient care activities in this area should routinely include rapid patient removal, with attention to possible spine injuries. If the patient is trapped or pinned, stabilizing care may be required (medical procedures must be carried out by qualified personnel). Airway control and isolation of the spontaneously breathing patient's airway with an escape mask or SCBA will limit any further inhalation exposure. If the patient needs ventilatory support, it should be provided with demand valve or bag-valve-mask with reservoir and oxygen. Rapid spine immobilization should be carried out as necessary, and the patient should be removed rapidly from the area. Because of the difficulties of assessing and treating patients while wearing PPE, patient care in this zone is extremely limited. *Remember that any activity, including rescue, will require proper preplanning, training, and appropriate PPE.*

THE WARM ZONE. The *warm zone,* also called the *contamination reduction zone (CRZ),* is the transition area between the contaminated and clean areas (Fig. 10-6). It is designed to reduce the probability that the clean areas will become contaminated or affected by scene hazards. This is an area of potential contamination and must be adequately controlled.

The distance between the hot zone and clean areas and decontamination procedures limit the physical transfer of hazardous substances into clean areas. Decontamination procedures take place in a designated area within the warm zone called the *contamination reduction corridor,* or *decon corridor.* The number of personnel allowed in this area is kept to a minimum, and they must be properly trained (operations level) and wearing appropriate PPE. The level of protection in this zone usually is one level below that of the entry team but may be the same level, depending on the hazards that are present. All personnel must be decontaminated before exiting this area. No eating, drinking, or smoking is allowed in this zone. In special circumstances, such as an extended warm zone established because of possible explosions, a forward safe haven may be established. This is a safe location established in the warm zone in which support functions may be carried out.

Similar to actions in the hot zone, warm-zone EMS activities will require special preparation. Somebody with medical training should be available to manage the patient's medical needs during decontamination. EMS involvement again will depend on area needs, standard operating procedures, training (preplanning concerns), and specific incident considerations. As a preplanning concern, identify personnel (either a HAZMAT team or fire department responder with medical training or EMS responder with PPE training) to be available to perform

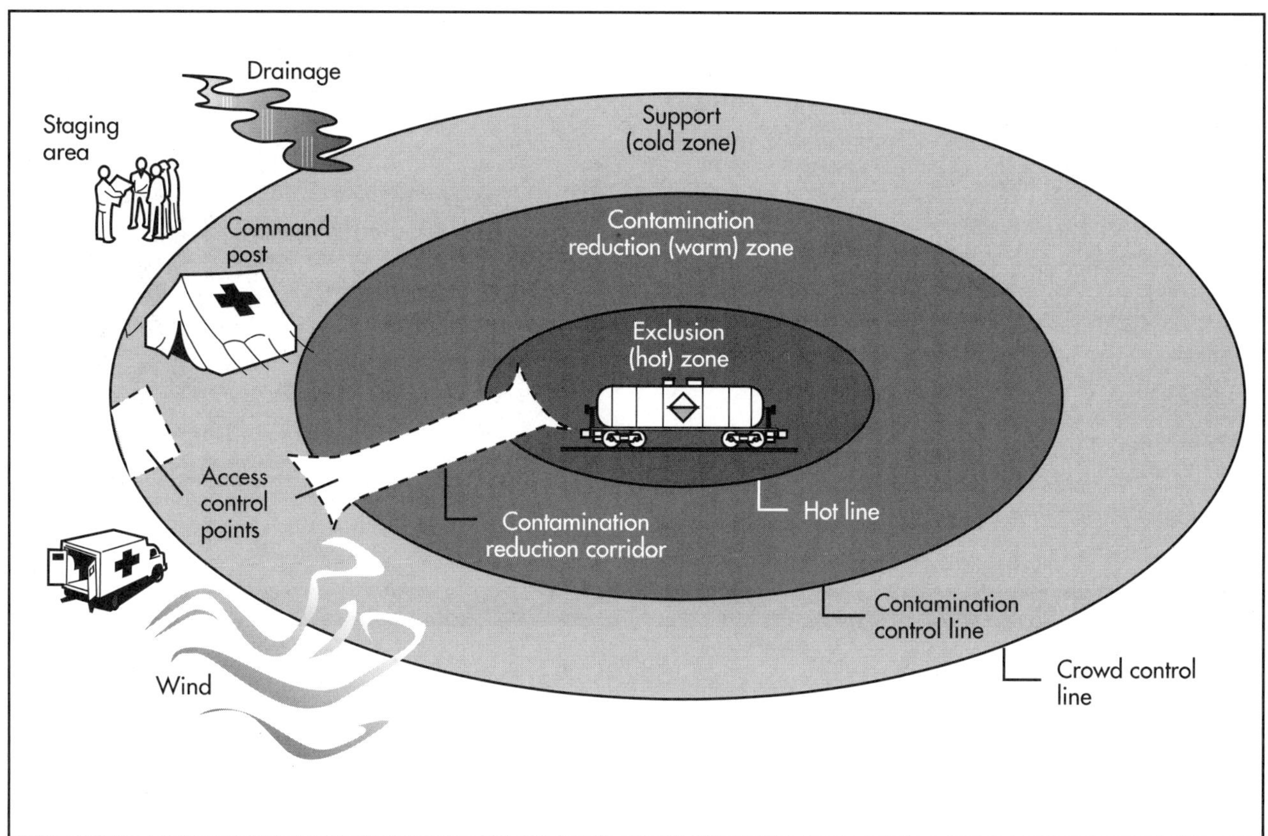

FIG. 10-4 Response zones.

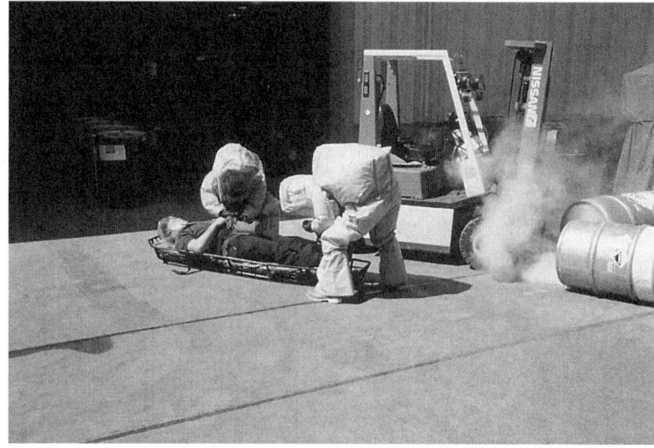

FIG. 10-5 Entrance into the hot zone requires training and appropriate PPE.

BOX 10-7

PATIENT CARE ACTIVITIES IN THE HOT ZONE*

- Rapid patient removal, with attention to possible spinal injuries
- If patient is trapped or pinned, medical/trauma stabilization care may be required (medical procedures must be carried out by qualified personnel). Because of the contaminated environment, invasive procedures must be kept to an absolute minimum
- Airway control
- Isolation of spontaneously breathing patient's airway with an escape mask or SCBA
- Ventilatory support with demand valve or bag-valve-mask with reservoir and oxygen as needed
- Rapid removal when extrication procedures are complete

*Activities in this zone require proper preplanning, training, and PPE.

warm-zone patient management. Patient care should be available during decontamination. Ambulatory patient self-decontamination should be supervised and assisted as necessary by properly trained personnel. In multicasualty incidents, triage for decontamination priority may be needed as patients are removed from the hot zone. Qualified personnel also should be available to provide immediate care of injured team members during decontamination. Usual patient care activities provided in the warm zone include basic life support during decontamination. Airway, breathing, circulation, cervical-spine (c-spine) immobilization, decontamination, and evaluation for systemic toxicity (ABC^2DE) should all be considered priority items (Box 10-8). Spinal immobilization and oxygen

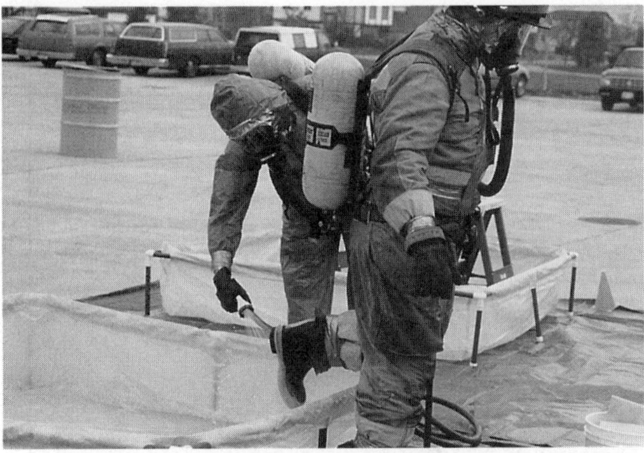

FIG. 10-6 The warm zone is the transition area between the contaminated and clean areas.

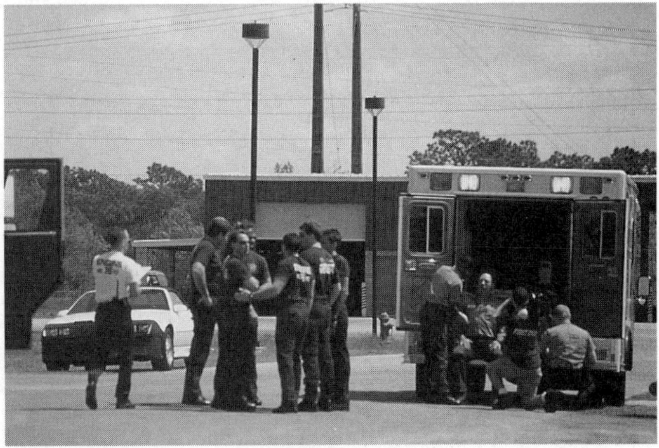

FIG. 10-7 Support and rehabilitation functions are located in the cold zone.

BOX 10-8

*Patient Care Activities in the Warm Zone**

Medical care during decontamination
ABC^{2}DE
- *A*irway
- *B*reathing
- *C*irculation (hemorrhage control)
- *C*-spine stabilization
- *D*econtamination
- *E*valuation for systemic toxicity

Oxygen administration
Limited invasive procedures
CPR as necessary

*Activities in this zone require proper preplanning, training, and PPE.

BOX 10-9

*Patient Care Activities in the Cold Zone**

Ensure that adequate decontamination has been performed.
Transfer patient from decontamination personnel to medical care givers to limit contamination spread.
Place patient on a clean backboard.
Perform basic and advanced life support functions as required.

*Activities in this area will require proper preplanning, training, and minimal PPE.

administration should be ensured and continued. As in the hot zone, ventilatory support should be carried out with demand valve or bag-valve-mask with reservoir and oxygen as needed. Invasive procedures, such as starting intravenous (IV) lines, should be limited until complete decontamination can be ensured. Cardiopulmonary resuscitation (CPR) should be performed as necessary during decontamination. *As in the hot zone, any activity in this area will require proper preplanning, training, and appropriate PPE.*

The cold zone. The *cold,* or *support, zone* is an area under responder control but is located safely away from the emergency (Fig. 10-7). All support and rehabilitation functions are located in the cold zone.

The command post and staging area are located in this zone. The command post should be situated in a secure location, away from the danger area. A view of the incident scene is nice but not essential. Adequate communication must be available for the command post. A staging area also should be established in a safe location. Responding units can be amassed in the staging area, which should allow easy access to all sides of the incident so units can be dispatched easily as needed. The person in charge of the staging area must have reliable communication with the incident commander or operations officer.

At a hazardous materials incident, EMS personnel will be most active in the cold zone. Patients who have been decontaminated and are as clean as reasonably possible will be cared for in the cold zone (Box 10-9). They should be passed to clean care givers, on a clean backboard, to limit contamination spread. All patient care equipment that was used in the warm zone should be considered contaminated and must remain in the warm zone. As in the other zones, responder involvement will depend on area needs, standard operating procedures, training (preplanning concerns), and incident-specific considerations.

Trained and informed EMS responders also can act as a liaison to the incident commander or planning sector officer on the potential toxicological, physical, and/or environmental health concerns of the incident. Triage and

BOX 10-10

Considerations When Establishing Control Zones

Visual survey of the immediate environment
Determination of locations of hazardous substances and possible movement patterns
Evaluation of data from air monitoring equipment
Distances needed to prevent an explosion or fire from affecting personnel outside the hot zone
Distances that personnel must travel to and from the hot zone
Physical area necessary for site operations
Meteorological conditions and predictions

patient care areas must be established. Once patients have passed through decontamination they will need to be triaged for transport priority. Patient management and transportation of clean patients is initiated from the cold zone. The EMS system should be especially knowledgeable in planning patient destination in multicasuality incidents.

The control zones can be established in any configuration necessary to control the incident (Box 10-10). For example, for an incident inside a building, the hot zone may be the building itself. A warm zone may surround the building, with the decontamination area set up immediately outside the door. The cold zone would be an area further out but still surrounding the building. The line separating the hot and warm zones is called the *hot line.* It should be clearly marked by cones, signs, barrier tape, or existing landmarks. The line separating the warm and cold zones is designated the *contamination control line* and also should be clearly marked. Access-control points should be established to regulate the flow of personnel into the warm and hot zones and help verify that proper procedures for entering and exiting are followed. The entrance and exit to the hot zone should be located at the decontamination corridor. In addition to the primary exit, an emergency exit should be established in case personnel cannot reach the primary exit during an emergency evacuation.

Scene Preparation

Once a hazard is identified, most responders try to determine how to protect against it. A better tactic is to direct efforts to reducing as many hazards as possible. Incidents may involve both physical and chemical hazards, and it is almost impossible to protect against every hazard. As many hazards as possible should be eliminated by scene preparation (see Box 10-11). In industrial settings this is known as *using engineering controls.*

Because many response activities involve multiple hazards, the identification of all possible hazards is vital. As many hazards as possible should be mitigated. PPE can then be used to protect against the hazards that cannot be mitigated.

BOX 10-11

Examples of Scene Preparation

Eliminate physical hazards from the response area as much as possible
Stabilize vehicles, if necessary
Deenergize machinery close to the operational area and lock out controls/power supplies
Ventilate and control vapors in an enclosed structure before the team enters
Eliminate ignition sources
Identify, eliminate, or avoid as much as possible, all sharp or protruding edges, such as glass, nails, and torn metal, which can puncture PPE and inflict puncture wounds
Identify, eliminate, or avoid as much as possible debris and loose or unstable footing, which can cause slips and falls
Identify and secure unsecured items, such as gas cylinders, that may fall
Suppress volatile/flammable vapors with foam to reduce the chance of fire and exposure
Use nonsparking tools and intrinsically safe equipment
Use air monitoring equipment to guide response activities
Where portable electrical tools and appliances are used, three wire-grounded extension cords with an in-line ground fault interrupter should be used
Provide adequate illumination for work activities

Useful EMS/Hazardous Materials Equipment

EMS units usually do not carry specific hazardous materials management equipment. They do carry certain items, such as PPE designed for body substance isolation (Fig. 10-8), that will provide adequate protection for carrying out patient treatment on decontaminated patients in the cold zone (Box 10-12). It is important to note that the respirators used for protection from tuberculosis will not provide protection from chemical gases or vapors.

Special PPE is required (Box 10-13) for EMS personnel to operate in the warm zone providing treatment during patient decontamination, or in the hot zone conducting triage or patient management for trapped patients. This equipment consists of special respiratory protective equipment such as an air-supplied respirator (SCBA or air line) or an APR with the appropriate cartridge (Fig. 10-9). Chemical-resistant protective clothing also will be necessary to provide skin protection. Use of this type of

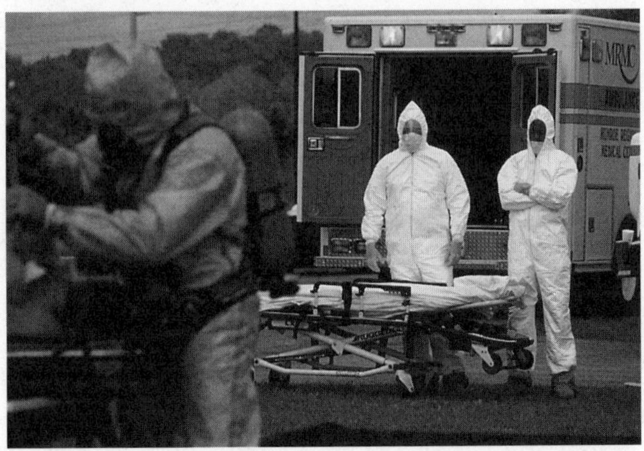

FIG. 10-8 Body substance isolation equipment will provide protection for treating decontaminated patients.

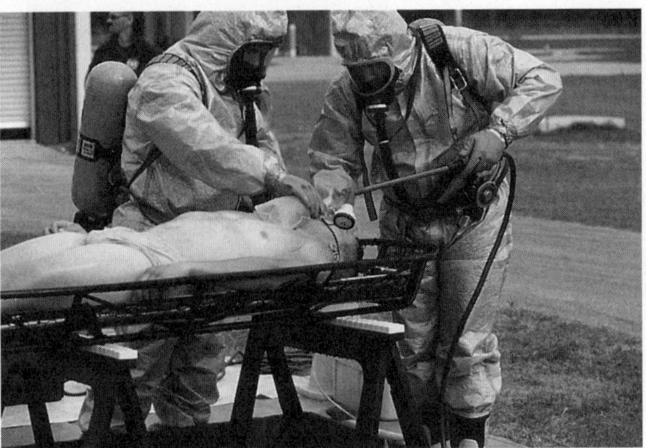

FIG. 10-9 For EMS responders to operate in the warm or hot zone, special protective equipment is required.

BOX 10-12

Body Substance Isolation Equipment for Cold Zone Operations

Eye protection
Mask
Gloves (latex under gloves and chemical-resistant outer gloves)
Fluid-resistant gowns or suits
Fluid-resistant shoe covers
Rain gear

BOX 10-13

Specialized PPE for Warm or Hot Zone Operations

Self-contained breathing apparatus
Air-purifying respirators
Chemical-resistant gloves (with latex under gloves)
Chemical-resistant suits
Boots or shoe covers

equipment requires extensive training. Responders should not attempt to utilize PPE without proper preplanning, training, medical examinations, and fit testing as required. Selection of equipment by a knowledgeable individual using appropriate reference sources is essential. Having equipment is not enough. The equipment must be compatible with the chemical. Chemical-protective equipment usually does not provide protection against fire or heat. Repeated training and practice with the equipment is essential for safe and effective use.

Certain other equipment may need to be added to the ambulance inventory for hazardous materials response activities, including reference sources, patient management equipment, and support equipment. The basic reference source that should be in every ambulance is the NAERG. The major limitation of the NAERG is that it does not supply detailed information, such as chemical and physical properties, or in-depth patient treatment information. Many other written and computer references are available that supply this information (Box 10-14). Remember that also available are telephone references, such as CHEMTREC (see Chapter 6), and your regional poison center.

BOX 10-14

Examples of Useful, Quick Information Sources

NAERG
Material Safety Data Sheets (MSDSs)
National Institute of Occupational Safety and Health (NIOSH) *Pocket Guide to Chemical Hazards*
United States Coast Guard *CHRIS* manual
Mosby's *Emergency Care for Hazardous Materials Exposure*
Chemical Manufacturers Association (CMA), CHEMTREC ([800] 424-9300)
Regional poison center

Besides references, EMS responders will find certain support equipment useful (Box 10-15). Binoculars or a spotting scope will allow responders to assess the incident from a greater distance and should be part of every ambulance's inventory. Plastic bags and basins of various sizes should be available to isolate the patient's clothes and vomitus, and protect equipment from contamination. Because many hazardous materials incidents involve multiple casualties, oxygen supplies should be upgraded for

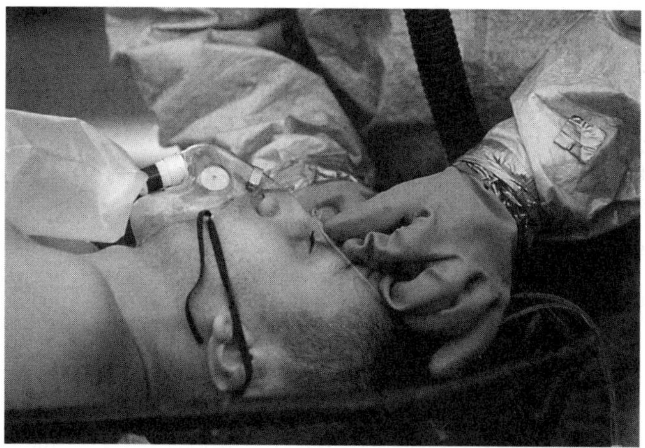

FIG. 10-10 A nasal cannula can be used for eye irrigation.

prolonged or multiple-patient care situations. Numerous devices are available that allow multiple patients to be treated with oxygen from one regulator. Morgan Therapeutic Eye Irrigation Lenses provide effective ocular irrigation. IV solutions of normal saline and setups also can be used with nasal cannulas to irrigate eyes (Fig. 10-10). The cannula is placed over the bridge of the patient's nose, and the irrigation fluid flows from the cannula across each eye.

Disposable medical equipment, such as blood pressure cuffs, stethoscopes, suction units, and laryngoscopes, will save expensive equipment that may not be able to be decontaminated.

Patient isolation systems are available that will encapsulate the patient during transport. Some are specifically designed for this task, whereas some EMS agencies and HAZMAT teams use zip-front body bags or simply wrap the patient in blankets. Although these do add a margin of safety for EMS providers during transport, they will add to patient exposure if decontamination procedures are inadequate. Some authorities argue that if field decontamination is complete, patient isolation procedures are not necessary. In reality, each situation will differ. Numerous situations, such as cold weather, multiple patients, and unusual chemical agents, may make it difficult or impossible to obtain *complete* decontamination in the field. In these cases, decontamination that is as effective as possible and patient isolation equipment may be necessary.

Large quantities of blankets, towels, and patient gowns should be stockpiled and readily available in case many ambulatory patients must be decontaminated. In addition, stockpiles of backboards or stretchers should be identified in case many nonambulatory patients need to be moved. At least one military-type stretcher being manufactured is designed for chemical use and decontamination.

For EMS/hazardous materials Level 2 responders certain medications may be useful for patient management (Box 10-16). Patient treatment modalities, especially the use of specialized medications, will require approval from local medical control.

Although EMS units do not have to carry decontamination equipment, responders should know the location of such equipment in their area. Most HAZMAT teams will carry equipment to carry out this function, but EMS responders need to verify this in preplanning. Special considerations may need to be made for decontamination of large numbers of ambulatory patients.

BOX 10-15

Minimum Suggested Equipment for EMS Response Units

Binoculars
Body substance isolation equipment
North American Emergency Response Guidebook
Expanded oxygen and IV supplies

BOX 10-16

Suggested Specific Physiological Antagonists (Antidotes) for Field Use

Activated charcoal
Atropine (multidose vials)
Calcium gluconate
Calcium gluconate gel
Cyanide antidote kit
Fomepizole
Methylene blue
Naloxone

Summary

Hazardous materials incidents are among the most dangerous emergencies that EMS responders face. Because of the multiple hazard potential at these incidents, scene management procedures become essential. Scene control procedures, such as establishment of hot, warm, and cold zones, are essential to responder safety. All hazards must be identified and as many as possible mitigated with scene preparation and safe work practices. Proper planning, active scene safety procedures, and administrative support will allow EMS personnel to safely and effectively respond to these emergencies.

CHAPTER REVIEW QUESTIONS

1. What clues should alert EMS responders to the presence of hazardous materials?

2. What immediate actions should be taken on arriving at a scene involving hazardous materials?
3. Why is proper identification of the hazardous substance so important?
4. What items should be included in an incident-specific safety plan?
5. What subjects should be addressed in a preentry briefing?
6. What EMS activities usually take place in the hot, warm, and cold zones?
7. What factors should be considered when establishing the control zones?
8. What actions can be taken to lessen safety risks at a hazardous materials emergency?
9. What types of communications systems should be established at a hazardous materials emergency?
10. What types of items can be added to the ambulance inventory to improve hazardous materials response capabilities?

BIBLIOGRAPHY

Agency for Toxic Substances and Disease Registry: *Managing hazardous materials incidents, emergency medical services: a planning guide for the management of contaminated patients,* Atlanta, Ga, 1992, USDHHS.

Andrews LP, editor: *Emergency responder training manual for the hazardous materials technician,* New York, 1992, Van Nostrand Reinhold.

Bowen JE: *Emergency management of hazardous materials incidents,* Quincy, Mass, 1995, National Fire Protection Association.

Bronstein AC, Currance PL: *Emergency care for hazardous materials exposure, ed 2, 1994,* St Louis, Mosby.

Bronstein AC, Currance PL: Module 4: emergency medical operations. In Ayers S, Christopher J, editors: *Medical response to chemical emergencies,* Washington, DC, 1994, Chemical Manufacturers Association.

Currance PL: *Hazmat for EMS,* St Louis, 1995, Mosby, (videotape and guidebook).

DOT: *1996 North American emergency response guidebook,* Office of Hazardous Materials Transportation, Research and Special Programs Administration, Washington, DC, 1996, US Department of Transportation.

EMS sector standard operating procedures. In Tokle G, editor: *Hazardous materials response handbook,* ed 2, Quincy, Mass, 1993, National Fire Protection Association.

EPA: *EPA standard safety operating guidelines,* Washington, DC, 1984, US Government Printing Office.

Guidelines for public sector hazardous materials training. 1998 ed, HMEP Curriculum Guidelines, Emmitsburg, Md, 1998, National Emergency Training Center.

Hazardous materials response training program, New Jersey/New York, 1988, Hazardous Materials Worker/Training Program.

NIOSH/OSHA/USCG/EPA: *Occupational safety and health guidance manual for hazardous waste site activities,* Washington, DC, 1985, DHHS (NIOSH) Publication No 85-115, US Government Printing Office.

NFPA: *NFPA 471, Recommended practice for responding to hazardous materials incidents,* Quincy, Mass, 1992, National Fire Protection Association.

NFPA: *NFPA 473, Standard for professional competence of EMS responders to hazardous materials incidents,* Quincy, Mass, 1992, National Fire Protection Association.

Noll GG, Hildebrand MS, Yvorra JG: *Hazardous materials: managing the incident,* ed 2, Stillwater, Okla, 1995, Fire Protection Publications.

OSHA: 29 CFR 1910.120, Hazardous waste operations and emergency response; Final rule, March 6, 1989; Washington, DC, US Government Printing Office.

Strong CB, Irvin TR: *Emergency response and hazardous chemical management: principles and practices,* Delray Beach, Fla, 1996, St. Lucie Press.

Summit County hazardous materials standard operating procedures. In Tokle G, editor: *Hazardous materials response handbook,* ed 2, Quincy, Mass, 1993, National Fire Protection Association.

Varela J, editor: *Hazardous materials handbook for emergency responders,* New York, 1996, Van Nostrand Reinhold.

11

Hazardous Materials Response Team Medical Support

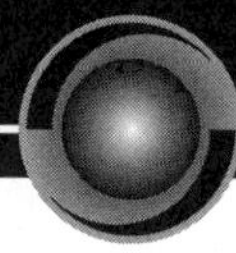

Phil Currance

OBJECTIVES

At the conclusion of this chapter the student will be able to:

- Identify the need for Emergency Medical Services (EMS) involvement at a hazardous materials incident.
- Discuss how the use of chemical-protective clothing (CPC) can increase the risk of heat-related injuries.
- List the parts of a preentry evaluation.
- Discuss the medical criteria for restricting the use of CPC or entrance into the hot zone.
- Identify the ways to detect heat stress or dehydration in the hazardous materials (HAZMAT) team member.
- Discuss the need for a rehabilitation area at a hazardous materials incident.
- Identify steps that EMS responders at a hazardous materials incident can take to prepare for emergencies.
- Describe items that should be included in a post-exit evaluation.
- Discuss the importance of team member rehydration at a hazardous materials incident.
- Identify ways to reduce the risk of heat-induced injuries.
- Discuss the importance of Wet Bulb Globe Temperature and adjusted temperature.
- Identify the temperature at which heat-stress monitoring and prevention should begin.

CASE STUDY

EMS has been requested to respond with the fire department and HAZMAT team to an overturned truck, which is leaking chemicals. The temperature outside is 68° F (20° C), and the sky is overcast. The HAZMAT team commander has requested that EMS responders "check out the HAZMAT team before they get into protective equipment."

- ◆ Is heat-stress monitoring and prevention necessary?
- ◆ What items should be included in a preentry evaluation?
- ◆ When should a responder be restricted from wearing chemical-protective equipment?
- ◆ What can be done to prevent heat stress?

A trained EMS contingent should respond to every hazardous materials incident. Under federal Occupational Safety and Health Administration (OSHA) and Environmental Protection Agency (EPA) standards, medical support with transportation capabilities to a designated medical facility must be standing by at hazardous materials emergencies. EMS should be present to treat any victims of the incident and ensure safety of the response team during emergency hazardous materials response and remediation operations (Fig. 11-1).

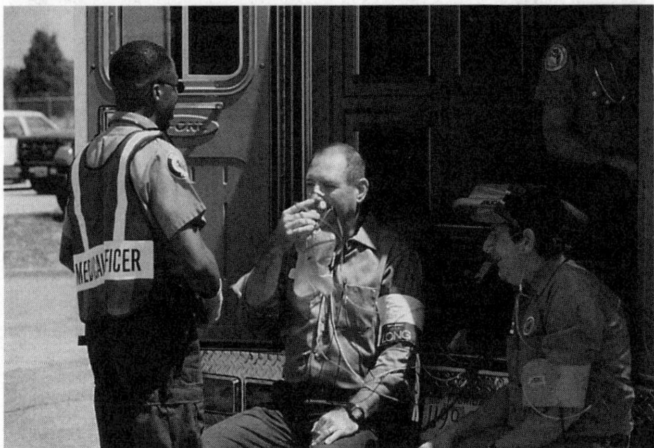

FIG. 11-1 EMS responders should be present to treat and transport any victims of the incident.

Team members should be monitored to prevent heat- or cold-related problems. If a HAZMAT team member is exposed, EMS activities can limit the chemical effects by providing timely management. Knowledgeable and informed medical responders can supply information to the incident commander and HAZMAT team on expected toxicological health effects, including signs and symptoms, onset times, and required treatment. They also can debrief HAZMAT team members on delayed signs and symptoms of exposure.

Chemical exposure and heat stress are prime threats to HAZMAT responders. Temperature-induced problems are especially common when incidents have a prolonged duration or when temperature extremes are present. Working in CPC or firefighting gear reduces the efficiency of the body's heat loss mechanisms and adds weight and bulk, thereby increasing the chance of heat-induced injuries. In this chapter we will discuss how to prevent and monitor for the effects of heat stress. In Chapter 12 we will discuss in depth the mechanism of these illnesses and their treatment.

IT'S FROM THE PARAMEDICS...SAYS THEY'LL BE DOWN THE STREET IF WE NEED THEM.
BERRY 95 ©

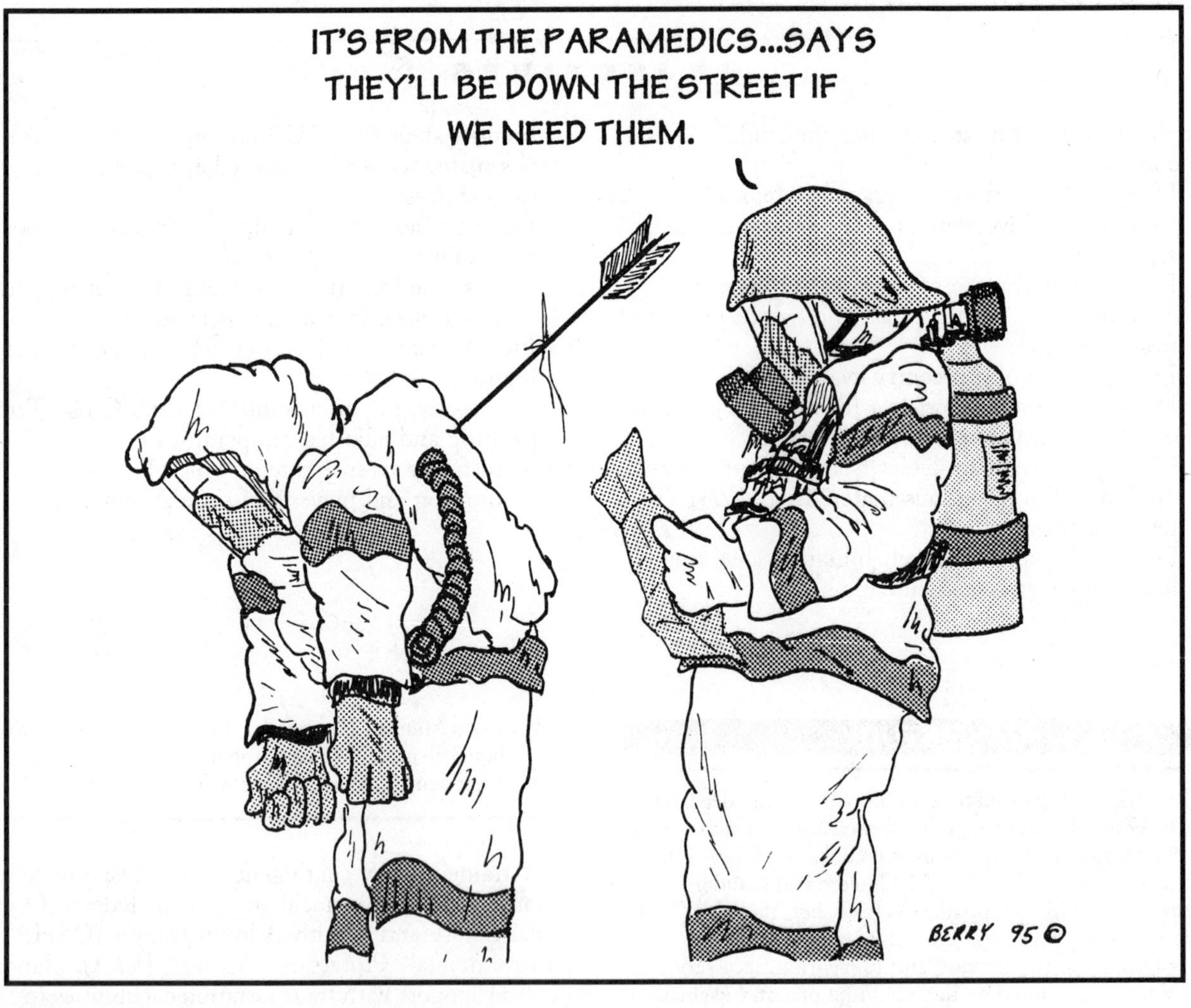

Reprinted with permission from Steve Berry's *I'm Not an Ambulance Driver* cartoon book series.

Preentry Evaluation

Baseline information is needed on every team member who wears CPC or firefighting gear, or who may possibly be exposed to chemicals. In cases of heat stress or chemical exposure, this information may prove vital. Many approaches have been taken to provide this baseline information. Some HAZMAT teams require that members periodically fill out a baseline information form. Although this does provide an in-depth history, the information is soon out of date. Typically, these forms are not updated in a timely fashion, leaving many holes in the team member's baseline profile. A better approach is to conduct a rapid evaluation before HAZMAT teams are deployed into the hot zone (Fig. 11-2). This evaluation will provide the baseline information needed in case of heat stress or chemical exposure and also will help to prevent injury by catching potential problems before team members don personal protective equipment (PPE). Criteria for restricting team members' use of chemical/firefighters clothing or entrance into the hot zone must be established. Commonly used criteria will be addressed in the following sections; however, the exact criteria should be established by working with your local medical control physician and HAZMAT team leaders.

Baseline Information

The preentry evaluation should begin with a set of baseline vital signs. Pulse, blood pressure, respiratory rate, and body temperature should all be assessed (Box 11-1). If the event is expected to last longer than 3 hours, body weight also should be measured and recorded. The pulse is one of the most important of the baseline vital signs. Because the pulse will increase as the team member becomes dehydrated, it will be one of the earliest indicators of heat stress and dehydration. Hot-zone entry or protective clothing use should be restricted if the team member's pulse is irregular (without prior history or previous medical clearance) or if the pulse is greater than 110 beats per minute (bpm). EMS personnel should take the excitement of the situation into consideration when assessing tachycardia. However, the effects of adrenaline on a normally functioning system should be limited, and excitement-induced tachycardia rarely exceeds 20 to 30 minutes. A decrease in blood pressure also can be an indicator of heat stress, but will not show up early and usually is evident when dehydration is advanced. Assessing blood pressure also will prevent problems caused by hypertension. Hot-zone entry or protective clothing use should be restricted if the team member's blood pressure is greater than 150 systolic or 100 diastolic. The team member's respiratory rate should be established. A rapid respiratory rate may indicate an abnormal lung condition and will result in a decrease in the duration of the work time in self-contained breathing apparatus (SCBA). Hot-zone entry or protective clothing use should be restricted if the team member's respiratory rate is greater than 24 breaths/min.

Body temperature is probably the best indicator of heat stress. Historically, assessing temperature under field conditions has been a problem. Obtaining a reading with an oral thermometer takes time, and any oral hydration with cool water nullifies the result. Tympanic membrane thermometers, if used properly, provide accurate readings and can easily be used under field conditions. They provide extremely rapid readings, and oral hydration can be carried out at the same time. Manufacturers instructions must be followed to obtain accurate readings. The professional versions of these thermometers will provide readings in core temperature, oral temperature equivalent, or rectal temperature equivalent. To give an accurate assessment of core temperature, they assess the temperature of the blood in the tympanic membrane. The tympanic membrane shares a common blood supply with the hypothalamus, the temperature control center of the body. Hot-zone entry or protective clothing use should be restricted if the temperature is greater than 37.8° C/100° F (oral) or 38° C/100.4° F (core).

Body weight can be used during prolonged events to provide information on the team member's hydration level. Team members should be weighed in at the beginning of the day, at regular intervals during the day, and again at the end of the day. A scale that is accurate to ± 0.25 pounds should be available. The team members must be dressed in the same clothes for each assessment. Although this procedure may not be practical in all emergency response situations, it commonly is conducted in

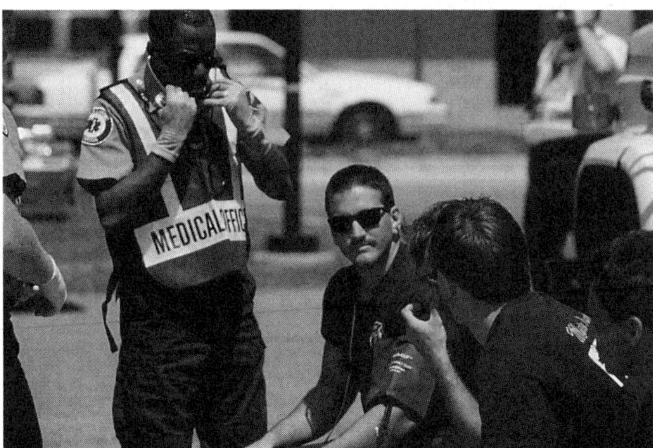

FIG. 11-2 To keep baseline information updated, an evaluation should be conducted before HAZMAT teams deploy into the hot zone.

BOX 11-1

BASELINE VITAL SIGNS

Pulse
Blood pressure
Respiratory rate
Temperature
Body weight

hazardous materials remediation work. If team members lose more than 1.5% of their total body weight (TBW), they should increase their fluid intake and not be allowed to wear chemical/firefighters protective clothing for the rest of the day or the next day.

Physical Examination

A basic physical examination also should be performed. This examination should include breath sounds, evaluation of skin condition, mental status evaluation, and an electrocardiogram (ECG), if indicated (Box 11-2). Because inhalation is the quickest route of exposure and the respiratory system is one of the most vulnerable systems in the body, a baseline evaluation of the lungs is extremely important. In addition to respiratory rate, lung sounds should be assessed. Hot-zone entry or protective clothing use should be restricted if any abnormal lung sounds (wheezing, rales, or rhonchi) are present. If protective clothing should fail, the skin is the last level of defense. Any skin damage will increase the speed and rate of absorption. Team members should be quickly assessed for skin damage. Large areas of dermatitis, sunburn, or skin damage (e.g., lacerations, burns, abrasions) are reasons to restrict hot-zone entry. Any indications of an irregular pulse found during the baseline vital signs check should be investigated with an ECG. Any cardiac rhythm other than a sinus arrhythmia should be cleared with medical control before allowing the team member to don PPE. A mental status evaluation should be carried out. Team members who are not alert and oriented to person, place, and time should never be allowed to don PPE or enter the hot zone.

Medical History

In addition to a set of baseline vital signs and a basic physical examination, a specific medical history should be obtained (Box 11-3). This will provide EMS personnel with an updated history for each team member rather than relying on outdated information from a form. A past medical history to identify preexisting medical conditions should be obtained. Many resources provide information on medical problems that may be aggravated by specific chemical exposure. Team members with these medical conditions should not be placed into a situation in which they could be chemically exposed. Because heat stress can be aggravated by dehydration, any recent history of illness, fever, vomiting, or diarrhea should be identified. Any recent onset of medical problems should be a reason to restrict the use of protective clothing or entry into the hot zone. Many chemicals can synergize or potentiate with other chemicals in the body. Therefore, any evidence of recent chemical exposure is an important finding. Alcohol use affects judgment and reaction time, and acts as a diuretic, leading to dehydration. Team members should not use PPE or be allowed to enter the hot zone if there has been heavy alcohol consumption in the past 24 hours or any alcohol consumption in the past 6 hours. An important part of the history is a list of prescription and over-the-counter medications that the team member is taking. Because of the chance of chemical exposure synergizing or potentiating with medications, all prescription and over-the-counter medication use should be cleared by medical control. Allergies to medications also should be identified.

The preentry evaluation must be performed efficiently. HAZMAT teams must be able to suit up and move into action rapidly. Ways to streamline this process include a scribe to record the information from the evaluation or a small cassette recorder. The recorder probably is the best way to accomplish the task. The EMS responder can hand the recorder to the HAZMAT team member, and he or she can record their name, age, weight, and answers to the medical history questions. After the baseline vital signs and examination, the EMS responder can record the results and move on to the next team member. Once the team is functioning, the information then can be transferred to a standard evaluation form. Although standard criteria will remove much of the decision making in this process, there will be unusual cases. Any questionable physical findings or medication questions should be cleared with medical control (Box 11-4). This will require some preplanning to provide medical control with the information and resources needed to answer these questions effectively.

Preentry Briefing

A briefing should be conducted with all team members before entry into the hot zone (Fig. 11-3). Possible briefing topics include expected hazards, work plan, communication systems, emergency signals and evacuation

BOX 11-2

Physical Evaluation

Breath sounds
Dermatitis, sunburn, or skin damage, such as lacerations, burns, or abrasions
ECG, if indicated
Mental status evaluation

BOX 11-3

Medical History

Past medical history
Recent history of illness, fever, vomiting, or diarrhea
Recent chemical exposures
Recent alcohol consumption
Prescription and over-the-counter medications
Allergies to medications

routes, safe work practices, and decontamination plan. EMS responders can contribute to this briefing by ascertaining the identity of any chemicals and evaluating them using appropriate resources. Team members should then be supplied with information on the chemical's toxicological effects and expected signs and symptoms of exposure. HAZMAT team members also should be reminded of the signs and symptoms of heat or cold exposure as necessary.

Rehabilitation Area

Before the HAZMAT team enters the hot zone, EMS personnel should ensure that procedures are in place

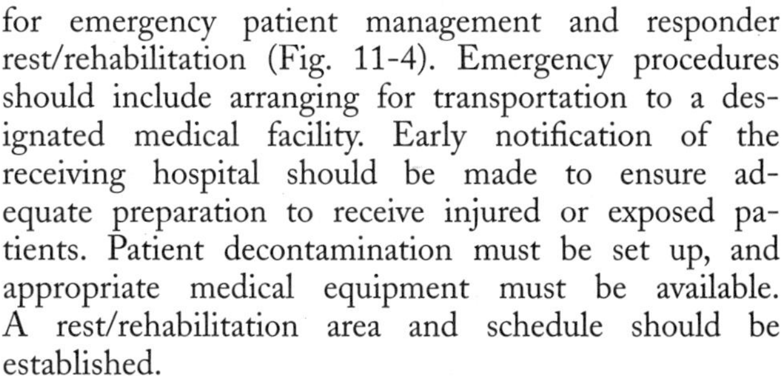

for emergency patient management and responder rest/rehabilitation (Fig. 11-4). Emergency procedures should include arranging for transportation to a designated medical facility. Early notification of the receiving hospital should be made to ensure adequate preparation to receive injured or exposed patients. Patient decontamination must be set up, and appropriate medical equipment must be available. A rest/rehabilitation area and schedule should be established.

BOX 11-4

Medical Considerations in Evaluating Fitness to Use Protective Clothing or Enter the Hot Zone

Pulse irregular (without prior history or previous medical clearance)
Pulse greater than 110 bpm
Temperature greater than 37.8° C/100° F (oral) or 38° C/100.4° F (core)
Blood pressure greater than 150 systolic or 100 diastolic
Respiratory rate greater than 24 breaths/min
Abnormal lung sounds (wheezing, rales, or rhonchi)
Recent onset of medical problems
Recent history of vomiting, diarrhea, or dehydration
Heavy alcohol consumption in past 24 hours or any alcohol consumption in past 6 hours
Skin lesions; dermatitis; or large, sunburned areas
New prescription medications (not cleared by medical control) or over-the-counter medication use

Location

The rehabilitation area should be a safe location within the cold zone and should be large enough to accommodate numerous personnel. The area should be easily reached from the decontamination area and easily accessible to EMS units for patient loading. It should provide protection from environmental conditions (i.e., a cool, shaded area in warm weather and a warm, dry area in cold weather). A structure or large vehicle (e.g., bus, truck) located in the cold zone could be used.

Supplies

Certain supplies and equipment should be available in the rehabilitation area, including fluids for oral replenishment (e.g., cool water, electrolyte solutions) and food (for incidents that last more than 3 hours). Fruit, stew, soup, or broth will be digested faster than solid food such as sandwiches. Fats and salty foods should be avoided. Medical equipment will be necessary, including oxygen, blood pressure cuffs and stethoscopes, thermometers, cardiac monitors, intravenous (IV) fluids/administration sets, and advanced cardiac life support (ACLS) medications and antidotes. Support equipment includes tarps and awnings for shade, fans for warm weather and heaters for cold weather, lights for night operations, and extra clothing.

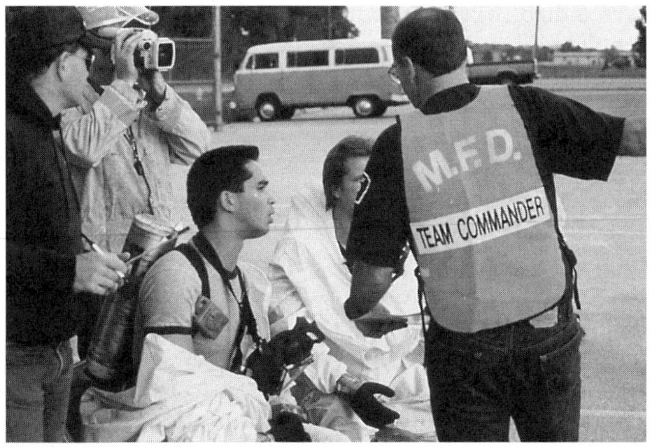

FIG. 11-3 A preentry briefing should be conducted with all team members.

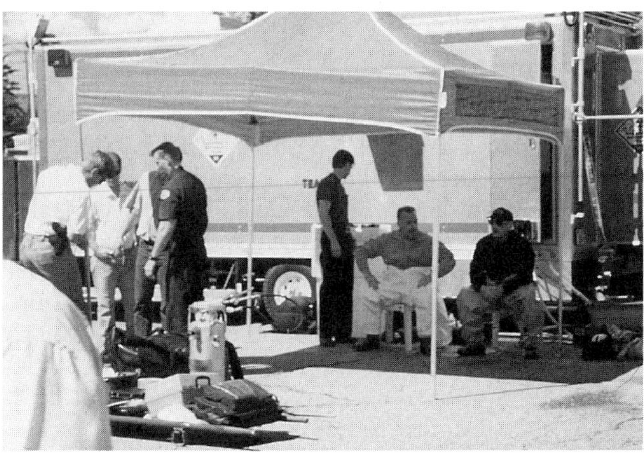

FIG. 11-4 Rest/rehabilitation area.

Schedule

A fixed rehabilitation schedule needs to implemented. Numerous variables must be taken into account when establishing this schedule. The number of technician-trained team members eligible for hot-zone deployment, type of emergency, associated risk factors, level of PPE, and weather conditions must all be considered. A rule of thumb often used by HAZMAT teams is to take a rest period after each SCBA bottle is used. This will be approximately every 20 to 30 minutes. A rehabilitation schedule also should be established for decontamination team members and support personnel. During the rehabilitation time, team members should move to a safe area and replenish fluids.

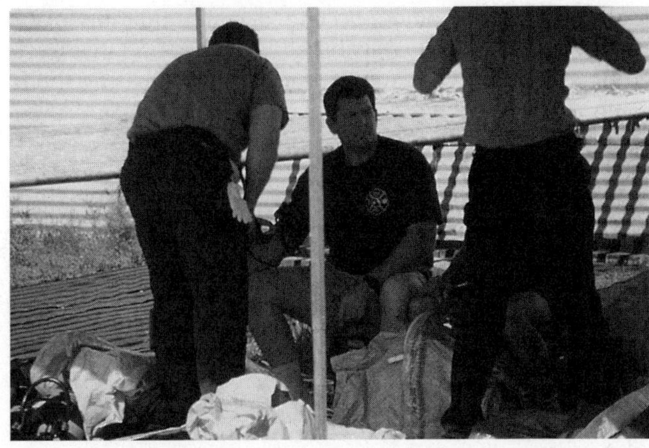

FIG. 11-5 EMS responders should perform a postexit examination on HAZMAT team members.

Decontamination and Postexit Evaluation

Everyone exiting the hot or warm zones must be decontaminated. After decontamination they should undergo a postexit evaluation (Fig. 11-5). This evaluation repeats the vital signs and basic examination conducted in the preentry evaluation. The focus of this evaluation should be to identify signs of heat stress and/or chemical exposure. If signs of chemical exposure are present, the team member should be treated as appropriate according to protocol and transported for further care or medical follow-up.

Heat Stress

Each team member should be evaluated for signs of heat stress before being allowed to return to service. Heart rate is an excellent indicator of body heat stress. If the team member's age-adjusted heart rate ($220 - \text{age} \times 0.7$) is exceeded or the heart rate does not return to within 10% of the baseline rate by the end of a rest period, heat stress is indicated. The team member should not be allowed to return to service until the heart rate is reduced to no more than 10% above the baseline rate. The next work period in protective clothing should be shortened by one third.

Hydration

Fluid loss must be replaced with oral rehydration. The team member's temperature also should be evaluated. If the temperature rises 0.8° C/1.5° F above baseline, the next work period in protective clothing should be decreased by one third. Fluids should be replaced orally, and temperature reevaluated. Team members should not be allowed to work in protective clothing if their oral temperature exceeds 37.8° C/100° F (core temperature 38° C/100.4° F). Team members also can be weighed to determine risk of heat stress. If body water loss (BWL) exceeds 1.5% of baseline TBW, heat stress is indicated, and the team member should not continue to wear protective clothing. Again, fluids should be replaced orally.

Fluid replacement plays a vital part in preventing heat stress. EMS personnel can help prevent the effects of heat stress by ensuring that HAZMAT team members stay hydrated. Aggressive fluid replenishment is necessary. During hot-weather response activities, HAZMAT team members should consume a minimum of 1 liter of fluid per hour. Hydration starts by having each team member drink a minimum of 16 oz of water or an electrolyte solution before donning PPE. A minimum of 12 oz of fluid should be ingested at every rest break. This hydration schedule should be followed rigidly. Thirst is not an adequate indicator of hydration level. Fluid replacement also is needed in cold weather. Heat stress and fluid loss still occur when PPE is worn. Fluids should be cooled to approximately 4.4° C (40° F) to make them more palatable. Ice-cold liquids should be avoided because they require time to warm before they can be absorbed across the gastrointestinal membranes. Some authorities suggest that electrolyte solutions should be diluted to 3 parts water to 1 part solution. Caffeinated beverages will constrict blood vessels and should be avoided. Likewise, carbonated beverages should not be used because of slower absorption rates. Alcoholic beverages should never be used for rehydration. Because most people receive enough salt in their normal diet, salt tablets generally are contraindicated.

Cooling Devices

Cooling devices also can be used to prevent heat stress. They include ice vests, fixed-line cooling units, and body-cooling suits. In some cases, these devices can add bulk or weight and contribute to heat stress, so caution must be used. Ice vests can provide cooling, but depending on design, may not make a major difference in core temperature. Vests that provide a cooling surface over the entire anterior and posterior torso are the most effective. They also add bulk and weight. Fixed-line cooling units provide adequate cooling because they remove hot air from the suit and replace it with cool air. However, because of

TABLE 11-1

SUGGESTED ACCLIMATION SCHEDULE

ACCLIMATION TIME	WORK AND ENVIRONMENTAL DESCRIPTION
Day 1-3	Light work during the morning or late afternoon, not to exceed 2 hrs
Day 4-6	Light work during the morning or late afternoon, not to exceed 3 hrs
Day 6-8	Light work during the morning or late afternoon, not to exceed 4 hrs
Day 8-10	Moderate work during the morning and afternoon, approximately 4 hrs
Day 10-12	Moderate work during the middle of the day, approximately 5 hrs
Day 12-14	Moderate work during the middle of the day, approximately 6 hrs
After day 14	Full days of moderate work

the line, which must be dragged around, they are cumbersome for emergency response operations. Body-cooling suits resemble thermal underwear, with cooling lines running throughout the suit. The cooling lines hook up to a lightweight, cold-water reservoir and pump unit worn at the team member's hip, under the protective clothing. Body-cooling suits probably are the most efficient cooling devices with the least bulk. However, these suits are expensive, and their use at this time is somewhat limited.

A very effective way to prevent heat stress is through acclimation to hot environments. Acclimation takes time and is an important factor in remediation work in hot environments. In most cases it is not feasible for emergency operations. Table 11-1 demonstrates the acclimation time required for full-day work in hot environments.

Other acclimation schedules include either a 4- or 7-day period. Regardless of the schedule used, unless emergency response team members work daily in a hot environment they will not remain acclimated.

Detection of Dangerous Temperatures

Many sources have tried to predict the temperature at which heat stress will become a major factor and therefore the temperature at which to begin monitoring and prevention procedures. Standard thermometers, known as *dry bulb thermometers,* report only ambient temperature. This may not give an accurate picture of the risk of heat-induced illness. The temperature at which to begin heat stress monitoring and prevention should take into consideration the ambient temperature, humidity, radiated heat, and cloud cover (solar load). The wet bulb globe temperature (WBGT) and the adjusted temperature take these into account. WBGT uses a

BOX 11-5

Calculation of Adjusted Temperature

Adjusted temperature = dry bulb temperature + 13 × (% cloud cover factor).

Cloud cover factor:

No clouds	= 1.0
25% clouds	= 0.75
50% clouds	= 0.5
75% clouds	= 0.25
100% clouds	= 0.0

combination of a dry bulb thermometer for ambient temperature, a wet bulb thermometer for humidity, and a black globe thermometer for radiated temperature. In some cases HAZMAT teams may have an on-board weather station for this information. Responders also can obtain the WBGT by calling the meteorology department at their local television or radio stations. Meteorologists calculate the WBGT by using the following formula:

$$\text{WBGT} = 0.7\,(\text{wet bulb temperature}) + 0.2\,(\text{black globe temperature}) + 0.1\,(\text{dry bulb temperature})$$

If the WBGT is not available from local sources, an estimate can be calculated from the following equation:

$$\text{WBGT} = (0.567T_{db}) + (0.393P_a)$$

T_{db} = dry bulb temperature

P_a = water vapor pressure

The adjusted temperature is calculated by taking a standard thermometer temperature (dry bulb temperature) and adding the sum of 13 multiplied by a constant representing the percentage of cloud cover (Box 11-5).

Most sources agree that heat stress prevention and monitoring techniques should be instituted when either WBGT or adjusted temperature reaches 23.9° C/75° F (Level C PPE work environments). Some authorities have suggested 21° C/70° F for Level A or B PPE. Both WBGT and adjusted temperature should be considered and the higher value utilized.

Emergency responders also need to be protected from cold hazards. Cold procedures (warm area, dry clothing, warm liquids, and food) should be instituted when the wind chill index is below −12° C/10° F. The wind chill index should be available from local weather stations.

Summary

EMS responders can play an integral part in the health and safety of personnel at a hazardous materials emergency. Their assessment skills and knowledge of anatomy and physiology, coupled with an understanding of heat stress and PPE, makes them the ideal choice to manage these concerns at a hazardous materials emergency. The effects of heat stress and cold exposure can result in severe injuries to response personnel. A preentry and post-exit monitoring plan will reduce the chance of injury. EMS responders should work with their local medical control and HAZMAT team to establish entry and exclusion criteria. Measures can be undertaken to prevent or lessen the effects of temperature stress. Measures, such as adequate fluid replacement, cooling devices, and proper rehabilitation, should all be in place at a hazardous materials emergency.

CHAPTER REVIEW QUESTIONS

1. Why should EMS respond to every hazardous materials incident?
2. Why are temperature-induced problems especially common at hazardous materials incidents?
3. Why is the collection of baseline information vital before HAZMAT responders enter the hot zone?
4. List four medical criteria for restricting responders' use of PPE or entry into the hot zone.
5. List three items that should be included in a preentry examination.
6. List three criteria for choosing the location of a rehabilitation area.
7. List at least three ways to help prevent heat stress.
8. List at least three items that indicate heat stress in a HAZMAT team member.
9. Explain why heat acclimation may not be useful for emergency responders.
10. Explain the difference between dry bulb temperature and wet bulb globe temperature, and identify the temperature at which heat stress monitoring/prevention should begin.

BIBLIOGRAPHY

Agency for Toxic Substances and Disease Registry: *Managing hazardous materials incidents, emergency medical services: a planning guide for the management of contaminated patients,* Atlanta, Ga, 1992, US-DHHS.

Bowen JE: *Emergency management of hazardous materials incidents,* Quincy, Mass, 1995, National Fire Protection Association.

Bronstein AC, Currance PL: *Emergency care for hazardous materials exposure,* ed 2, 1994, St Louis, Mosby.

Bronstein AC, Currance PL: Module 4: emergency medical operations. In Ayers S, Christopher J, editors: *Medical response to chemical emergencies,* Washington, DC, 1994, Chemical Manufacturers Association.

Currance PL: *Hazmat for EMS,* St Louis, 1995, Mosby (videotape and guidebook).

EMS sector standard operating procedures. In Tokle G, editor: *Hazardous materials response handbook,* ed 2, Quincy, Mass, 1993, National Fire Protection Association.

EPA: *EPA standard safety operating guidelines,* Washington, DC, 1984, US Government Printing Office.

FEMA: *Emergency incident rehabilitation,* Washington, DC, 1992, Publication No FA-114, USFA Publications.

Guidelines for public sector hazardous materials training. 1998 ed, HMEP Curriculum Guidelines, Emmitsburg, Md, 1998, National Emergency Training Center.

Keffer WJ: So you want to start a haz mat team! In Tokle G, editor: *Hazardous materials response handbook,* ed 2, Quincy, Mass, 1993, National Fire Protection Association.

National Fire Protection Association: *NFPA 471, Recommended practice for responding to hazardous materials incidents,* Quincy, Mass, 1992, The Association.

National Fire Protection Association: *NFPA 473, Standard for professional competence of EMS responders to hazardous materials incidents,* Quincy, Mass, 1992, The Association.

NIOSH: *Hot environments,* Cincinnati, 1980, DHHS (NIOSH) Publication No 80-130, US Government Printing Office.

NIOSH/OSHA/USCG/EPA: *Occupational safety and health guidance manual for hazardous waste site activities,* Washington, DC, 1985, DHHS (NIOSH) Publication No 85-115, US Government Printing Office.

Noll GG, Hildebrand MS, Yvorra JG: *Hazardous materials: managing the incident,* ed 2, Stillwater, Okla, 1995, Fire Protection Publications.

OSHA: 29 CFR 1910.120, Hazardous waste operations and emergency response; Final rule, March 6, 1989; Washington, DC: US Government Printing Office.

Sullivan JB, Kreiger GR, editors: *Hazardous material toxicology: clinical principles of environmental health,* Baltimore, 1992, Williams & Wilkins.

Summit County hazardous materials standard operating procedures. In Tokle G, editor: *Hazardous materials response handbook,* ed 2, Quincy, Mass, 1993, National Fire Protection Association.

Teele BW, editor: *NFPA 1500 handbook,* Quincy, Mass, 1993, National Fire Protection Association.

Tokle G, editor: *Hazardous materials response handbook,* ed 2, Quincy, Mass, 1993, National Fire Protection Association.

12

Heat and Cold Stress at Hazardous Materials Incidents

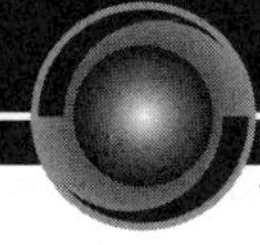

Phil Currance

CHAPTER OBJECTIVES

At the conclusion of this chapter the student will be able to:

- Identify how heat and cold stress can occur at a hazardous materials incident.
- Discuss the factors that contribute to heat stress at a hazardous materials incident.
- Discuss how the use of protective clothing can increase the risk of heat stress.
- Identify the ways that the body reduces heat.
- Explain how the use of protective clothing interferes with the ways that the body reduces heat.
- Identify the predisposing factors that can increase the severity of heat stress.
- Identify the types of heat-related illness.
- Explain the difference between classical and exertional heat stroke.
- Describe the proper treatment for each type of heat-related illness.
- Describe the signs and symptoms of both superficial and deep frostbite.
- Describe the proper treatment for both superficial and deep frostbite.
- Describe the signs and symptoms of hypothermia.
- Describe the proper treatment for hypothermia.

CASE STUDY

The sprayer tank on a crop-duster airplane has been damaged and is leaking herbicide onto a hot asphalt runway. Hazardous materials (HAZMAT) responders are wearing Level A protective clothing as they try to off-load the herbicide tank. During the second entry, one of the team members collapses. His buddy signals for help, and the backup team enters the hot zone to perform a rescue. The responder is decontaminated, and the protective clothing is removed (Fig. 12-1). He is handed over to Emergency Medical Services (EMS) responders for care. The patient is semiconscious and responds to noxious stimuli by withdrawal. His skin feels warm/hot to the touch, but he appears to be sweating profusely. His pulse rate is 120; his blood pressure is 92/50.

- Are these signs of herbicide exposure or heat stress?
- If heat stress is the causative event, is the patient in heat exhaustion or heat stroke?
- What is the proper treatment for this patient?

In Chapter 11 we discussed the importance of EMS support to HAZMAT teams. One of the greatest risks to hazardous materials responders working in personal protective equipment (PPE) is heat stress. The body's ability to regulate heat may be impaired by chemical exposure

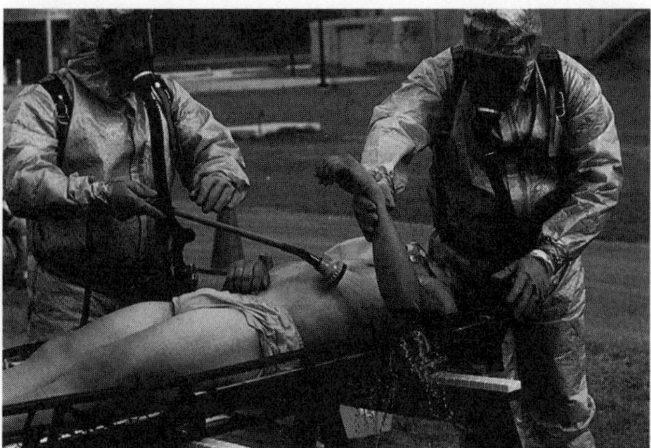

FIG. 12-1 The responder is decontaminated, and his protective clothing is removed.

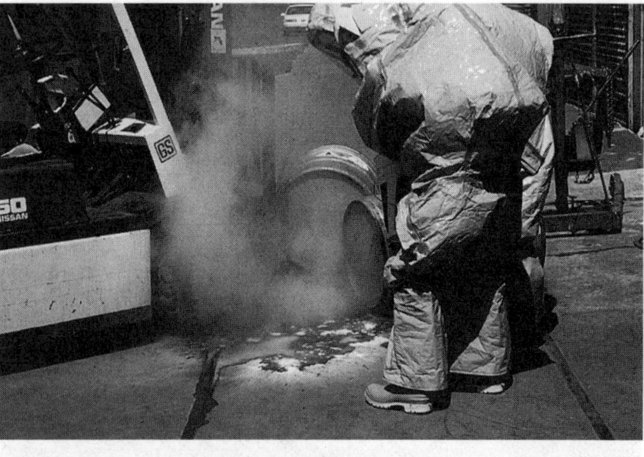

FIG. 12-2 Protective equipment can put an additional strain on the body's thermal response mechanism.

and the wearing of PPE. This overloads the individual's thermal response mechanism and at the same time increases heat production by adding bulk and weight, which increases the work necessary to perform required activities (Fig. 12-2). Certain chemical exposures may aggravate the body's response to heat stress. Cold exposure also may cause problems for patients and emergency response personnel. Frostbite is possible when dealing with cryogenic liquids or rapidly expanding liquified gases that are escaping from their containers. Hypothermia may occur when HAZMAT team members remove chemical-protective clothing (CPC) in cool weather. Hypothermia is always a risk when performing patient decontamination procedures in cooler weather conditions.

Heat Stress Contributing Factors

The amount of heat stress that responders face depends on many factors. The environmental temperature obviously is a prime factor in heat stress threat, but other factors also must be considered. The amount of heat that is radiated from the surface will directly affect the heat load placed on the body. The type and color of surface is important. Darker surfaces, such as black asphalt, will absorb much heat. The higher temperature of these surfaces will result in much radiant heat, increasing the risk of heat stress. The level of moisture in the air will affect the cooling mechanisms of the body. At higher humidity levels, less sweat will evaporate, and the level of body cooling will decrease. PPE is a major factor in the amount of heat stress that can be expected. Protective clothing will reduce the efficiency of body cooling mechanisms and will add more heat to the body.

Personal Protective Equipment

CPC, firefighters protective clothing, and respiratory-protective equipment such as the self-contained breathing apparatus (SCBA) all add weight and bulk. The weight causes muscles to work harder and produce more heat energy. In addition, this weight increases energy expenditure and causes responder fatigue. The bulk of firefighters gear or CPC causes a hobbling effect. Muscles have to work harder to move against the bulk of the clothing, causing a significant increase in heat production.

The use of firefighters gear or CPC reduces the efficiency of the body's normal heat-exchange mechanisms. The body can lose heat in four ways. In *radiation heat loss*, infrared (IR) energy is radiated directly into the environment. *Conduction* occurs when the body touches a cooler surface. Heat is transferred to the cooler object. *Convection* occurs when air moves over the body surface and carries away heat. *Evaporation* occurs when the water in perspiration changes from a liquid to a gas state. At lower environmental temperatures (less than 92° F [33.3° C]) the body commonly uses radiation and convection as cooling mechanisms. When wearing PPE, radiation heat loss is extremely limited. The bulk and insulation of firefighters clothing and the dead airspace within CPC trap any heat lost by radiation. In convection, the body loses heat by heating up an air curtain around the body. As air circulates or as a person moves, the air curtain around the body is stripped away. The process is then repeated. Convection is the reason why we can cool ourselves with a fan even though the air is not cooled or why we feel cooler in windy conditions. This process becomes less efficient when the air temperature reaches or exceeds skin temperature (approximately 92° F [33.3° C]). At this point, the body ceases to lose heat by convection. No matter what the environmental temperature is, once firefighters or HAZMAT responders don and work in protective clothing, the temperature inside the clothing will quickly exceed skin temperature. Encapsulated CPC, such as Environmental Protection Agency (EPA) Level A and Level B protective clothing (see Chapter 8), present the greatest threat (Fig. 12-2). The dead airspace inside the suit will quickly be heated to at least body temperature. Because of environmental temperature, radiant heat, and the absorbed heat of the suit, the temperature inside the suit often is higher than body temperature, causing an additional heat load. In hot weather it is common to find in-suit temperatures as much as 10° higher than the environmental temperature.

As the environmental temperature rises above skin temperature and radiation and convection start to fail as effective body-cooling measures, perspiration starts and evaporation takes over. Perspiration will only be effective if it evaporates. Body heat production and heat loss are measured in kilocalories (kcal). Basal metabolism produces 65 to 85 kcal/hour with normal body temperature. With elevated body temperature, from exertion or fever, the heat production increases approximately 13% for every degree Fahrenheit rise in temperature. Exertion also adds heat. Moderate work can produce 300 kcal/hour, and strenuous work can generate up to 1000 kcal/hour. As sweat evaporates, heat is lost. For every 1.7 cc of sweat evaporated, approximately 1 kcal of heat is lost. In summer conditions, with normal clothing, adults have an approximate sweat rate of 1.5 to 2 L/hour. Theoretically, that would mean a maximum heat loss of 900 to 1200 kcal/hour is possible. Because some sweat will soak into clothing or drip from the body and not evaporate, an average heat loss of 600 kcal/hour is realistic. When wearing encapsulated, impermeable PPE, a sweat rate as high as 3.5 L/hour is possible, allowing a maximum heat loss of approximately 2000 kcal/hour. The problem is that, in high-humidity atmospheres, sweat does not evaporate readily. HAZMAT responders wearing encapsulated PPE use air from the breathing apparatus and then release moist, exhaled air at body temperature into the suit. A hot atmosphere, with 100% humidity inside the suit, results and severely limits the amount of sweat evaporation. Realistic heat loss from evaporation when wearing impermeable PPE is probably well below 600 kcal/hour. Conduction heat loss, like radiation, is diminished because of the insulating value of the clothing. Heat may actually be gained when the skin touches CPC that has been heated by the sun. It is easy to see why using this type of equipment will cause heat stress. The responder is producing approximately 1100 kcal/hour and off-loading half that much.

Predisposing Factors

Many predisposing factors can increase the severity of heat stress. Because we all have approximately the same amount of body surface area to off-load heat, the amount of bulk makes a major difference. Obese people will generate much more heat than thin people and are more susceptible to heat injuries. As discussed in Chapter 11, acclimation will make a major difference in the responder's ability to adapt to heat stress. When people are acclimated to the heat, their entire body handles the stress more effectively. Their sweat composition also changes. More water and less sodium is released by the sweat glands. Because the body retains more sodium, fluid replenishment is much more effective. Age also is a variable in response to heat stress. Older people have a decreased work capacity, slightly higher body temperature, and lower sweat rates. As such they are at greater risk for heat-related illness. Any condition that results in dehydration also will make the patient more susceptible to heat stress. Alcohol use, infection, and diarrhea are examples of conditions that will result in dehydration.

Medications

Certain medications also will increase the severity of heat-related injuries. Atropine, belladonna, antihistamines, diuretics, thyroid hormone, and aspirin are prime examples. Exposure to certain chemicals may cause an increase in body temperature and severity of heat injuries. Exposure to compounds, such as pentachlorophenol, dinitrophenols, 2,4-D, and 2,4,5-T, may cause disturbances in body temperature regulation and exacerbate heat stress conditions.

Heat Stress Syndromes

Heat Stroke

As body temperature increases, so does the sweat rate. If the body is not cooled and lost body fluid is not replaced, heat stress syndromes can result. Heat stroke is the most serious effect of heat stress and can occur with little or no warning. Heat stroke occurs when the body's system of temperature regulation fails, the sweating mechanism stops, and the body's temperature rises to critical levels. Heat stroke eventually will result in multisystem organ failure and is life threatening. Immediate action must be taken to cool the body before serious injury and death occur. Heat stroke can present as either classical or exertional. Classical heat stroke, common in heat waves, usually involves an elderly or debilitated patient who is exposed to an extended period (many hours or even days) of high temperatures. Their ability to respond to the heat stress often is compromised by cardiovascular problems, medications, or alcohol use. Heat stroke has a slow onset, and victims may have been sweating profusely for a prolonged time. They commonly are dehydrated and present with hot, red, dry skin. Emergency responders in PPE are more likely to develop exertional heat stroke, which occurs in younger, usually physically fit patients. Because of exposure to severe external heat and exertional heat production, the body's heat loss mechanisms are overwhelmed. Intensifying the situation is the reduction of heat loss mechanisms resulting from the use of PPE. These victims do not have an advanced degree of dehydration and in many cases are wet with perspiration. Whereas classical heat stroke presents over time, exertional heat stroke has a rapid onset. With dry or wet skin, patients with heat stroke will have a markedly elevated body temperature. The core body temperature is often above 104° F (40° C).

Heat stroke involves multiple systems in the body (Box 12-1). *Mental status abnormalities are the most important indicator of heat stroke.* The patient will present with an altered mental status, such as confusion or irrational behavior, or may be comatose. Paralysis and seizures may result. Effects on the cardiovascular system can include congestive heart failure, pulmonary edema, and cardiovascular collapse. Liver damage also may occur. The patient often will be hyperventilating. Tachycardia usually is present, and T-wave changes on an electrocardiogram (ECG) may be seen. Treatment should include moving the patient to a cool environment. Ensure that decontamination is rapidly carried out, if necessary, and remove all clothing. An adequate airway, respiratory rate, and circulation must be established. Intubation may be necessary to control the airway. For patients in heat stroke, rapid cooling is essential. The most effective way to cool the body is enhancement of evaporation. A water mist can be applied to the skin from a handheld spray bottle or other device. Air is then circulated over the moist body surface with a fan, dramatically increasing the evaporation rate and cooling the body quickly. This procedure will work better in low-humidity rather than in high-humidity weather conditions. Other methods include cold-water–soaked sheets placed on the body, cold water poured over the skin surface, and ice packs in areas, such as the neck, underarm, and groin, where major blood vessels are close to the skin surface.

Immersion in cold water probably should be avoided because of the difficulty in caring for the patient and the chance that peripheral vasoconstriction will inhibit the body's ability to lose heat. To avoid overcooling and the chance of shivering, slow or modify cooling measures when the patient's temperature reaches 100° to 102° F (37.8° to 38.9° C). High-flow oxygen should be administered by nonrebreather mask. If advanced-level EMS personnel are on scene, they should start an intravenous (IV) solution of normal saline (NS) or lactated Ringers (LR) and should titrate it to maintain an adequate blood pressure. If EMS personnel are qualified, the patient's cardiac rhythm should be monitored, and arrhythmias should be treated as necessary according to advanced cardiac life support (ACLS) or local protocol. Seizures should be anticipated and treated as necessary. Antiseizure medication can be used by advanced-level EMS responders. The patient should be evaluated to rule out toxic exposure or other medical conditions. The patient must be transported rapidly to an appropriate medical facility.

Heat Exhaustion

Heat exhaustion is caused by an excessive loss of fluid and/or electrolytes through excessive perspiration (Box 12-2). As fluid is lost through the sweating mechanism, plasma moves across the blood vessel membrane, and vascular volume is decreased, resulting in a relative state of hypovolemia. Patients are awake and have little or no alteration in mental status. They most often will be

BOX 12-1

Heat Stroke

SIGNS AND SYMPTOMS

Heat regulatory process fails; life threatening
Decreased level of consciousness, seizures, and coma
Tachycardia
Hyperventilation
Skin may be wet or dry
Core body temperature elevated greater than 104° F (40° C).
T-wave ECG changes may be seen

TREATMENT

ABC_2DE. Intubate as necessary
Oxygen administration (10 to 15 L/min) by nonrebreather mask
IV fluids (NS or LR) titrated to maintain adequate blood pressure (BP)
Cardiac monitoring with treatment of arrhythmias as necessary
Rapid cooling
Treatment of hypotension and seizures
Assessment for toxic exposure or other causes
Rapid transport to appropriate medical facility

BOX 12-2

Heat Exhaustion

SIGNS AND SYMPTOMS

Ill-defined precursor of heat stroke
Caused by excessive loss of fluid and/or electrolytes through perspiration
Postural vital sign changes
Nausea and vomiting
Little or no change in mental status
Elevated core temperature up to 104° F (40° C)
Suspect heat stroke

TREATMENT

ABC_2DE
Administer oxygen (10 to 15 L/min) by nonrebreather mask
Remove from exposure
Rapid cooling as necessary
Cardiac monitoring with treatment of arrhythmias as necessary
IV fluids (NS or LR) titrated to maintain adequate BP
Assessment for toxic exposure or other causes
Transportation to appropriate medical facility

sweating profusely, and the skin will be cool and pale. The pulse rate commonly is increased, and the blood pressure is decreased. Patients often will show postural vital sign changes. They usually complain of nausea and may have vomited. In heat exhaustion, the core body temperature may be elevated to 104° F (40° C). Remember that in exertional heat stroke, the skin may still be wet and pale. Heat stroke should be suspected if the level of consciousness is decreased. Treatment for heat exhaustion should include decontamination as necessary and moving the patient to a cool environment. An adequate airway and respiratory rate must be established. Administer oxygen and, if qualified, establish an IV line of NS or LR and titrate its flow to maintain an adequate blood pressure. If the patient's temperature is elevated, rapid cooling procedures are warranted. If advanced-level EMS personnel are on scene, the patient's cardiac rhythm should be monitored and arrhythmias treated as necessary. The patient must be assessed for signs of toxic exposure or other causes. The patient in heat exhaustion should be transported to an appropriate medical facility.

Heat Syncope

Heat syncope, or fainting, is caused by the pooling of blood in dilated vessels of the skin and lower body (Box 12-3). The vessel dilation probably is caused by stimulation of the vagus nerve. The risk of heat syncope increases with conditions that cause dehydration. In most cases, heat syncope is self-limited in nature. When the victim falls to a supine position, the blood is redistributed, and the victim regains consciousness. The victim may be injured in the fall and, for HAZMAT responders, PPE may be damaged, resulting in chemical exposure. Heat syncope also may accompany heat exhaustion. Treatment for heat syncope starts with moving the victim to a cooler area. Ensure that the victim has been decontaminated, if necessary. Loosen the victim's clothing and elevate his or her feet 6 to 8 inches. Evaluate the victim for other possible causes for the syncope, signs of heat exhaustion, chemical exposure, and injuries sustained in the fall. Fluids should be replaced orally. If the patient's symptoms are severe or recur, advanced-level EMS personnel should provide oxygen and IV fluids (NS or LR). The patient then should be transported to a medical facility.

Heat Cramps

Heat cramps commonly occur in physically fit individuals who are not used to working in hot environments (Box 12-4). Most often these cramps occur during a rest period or after work. Heat cramps usually affect the major muscle groups that are being used. Common sites for heat cramps include the calves and upper back muscles. Although the exact cause of heat cramps is unclear, it is believed to result from a loss of electrolytes caused by heavy sweating. This, in turn, leads to contraction of the larger muscle groups and cramps. Symptoms of heat cramps include painful muscle cramping and spasms. Victims usually are sweating profusely. They commonly are nauseated and may have vomited. Victims usually will have a normal pulse and blood pressure. Treatment for heat cramps includes rest in a cool climate and oral fluid replenishment. Salt tablets are contraindicated for this or any other heat stress condition. Most people receive enough salt in their normal diet. Gentle hand pressure to the affected area may ease the cramps. If symptoms are not relieved by oral rehydration and rest, oxygen should be administered and IV fluids (NS or LR) given by qualified personnel. The patient should be transported to a medical facility. Every patient with heat cramps should be evaluated for signs or symptoms of heat exhaustion.

BOX 12-3

Heat Syncope

SIGNS AND SYMPTOMS

Self-limited in nature
Probably vasovagal in origin
Increased risk with conditions causing dehydration

TREATMENT

ABC_2DE
Place patient in supine position
Raise legs 6-8 inches
Rule out other causes
Oral fluid replacement if no airway compromise
IV fluid replacement as necessary
Assess for toxic exposure or other causes
Transport to medical facility as necessary

BOX 12-4

Heat Cramps

SIGNS AND SYMPTOMS

Strikes physically fit individual who is not accustomed to working in hot climates
Occurs during or after work
Affects most major muscle groups

TREATMENT

Rest
Cool climate
Oral fluid replacement
Gentle hand pressure to affected area
Evaluate for signs of heat stroke
Transport to hospital as necessary

BOX 12-5

Heat Fatigue

SIGNS AND SYMPTOMS

Common effect of prolonged heat exposure
Loss of coordination and alertness
Heat rash, edema, and fatigue

TREATMENT

Rest
Cool climate
Fluid replacement
Transport to hospital as necessary

BOX 12-6

Frostbite

SIGNS AND SYMPTOMS

Superficial frostbite

Red followed by gray, white, or mottled coloring
Stinging, burning, or paresthesia
Affected area is stiff to the touch, but underlying tissues remain soft

Deep frostbite

White, yellow-white, or mottled, bluish-white coloring
Affected area is hard, cold, and insensitive to the touch

TREATMENT

ABC_2DE
Administer oxygen at 10 to 15 L/min by nonrebreather mask.
Handle the affected area gently, and protect it from friction and pressure.
For superficial frostbite, rewarm with body heat.
For deep frostbite or frozen skin, when extensive transport times to the hospital are involved, warm the affected area in a water bath at a temperature of 100° to 105° F (37.8° to 40.6° C).
Prolonged rewarming may be necessary, and the procedure may be painful. Rewarming is best accomplished at the medical facility, unless transport times are excessive.
Check neurological and vascular status both before and after warming.
Place sterile cotton between affected digits.
Apply soft, sterile dressings lightly over affected parts.
Maintain body temperature with blankets. Do not apply external heat.
Assess and treat any other injuries.

Heat Fatigue

Heat fatigue is the least-threatening and most common effect of prolonged heat exposure (Box 12-5). Victims may show a loss of coordination and alertness. Heat fatigue can be accompanied by heat rash in moist areas of the body when sweat glands become clogged and inflamed. Edema of the patient's extremities may be seen, and generalized fatigue is common. Treatment for this condition includes rest in a cool climate and oral fluid replacement. Heat rash can be treated by cleansing the affected area with cool water and applying mild drying lotions or powders.

Cold Exposure

Cold exposure also may affect victims and responders at hazardous materials incidents. Various degrees of frostbite and hypothermia are possible. Frostbite can be caused by contact with leaking liquified gas or cryogenic cylinders. As discussed in Chapter 4, liquified gas, when released, expands to a much larger vapor cloud. For example, propane expands from 1 cubic foot of liquid to 270 cubic feet of vapor. Chlorine expands at a ratio of 450 to 1; anhydrous ammonia expands at a ratio of 850 to 1. This expansion is accompanied by a massive cooling of the vapor. The larger the expansion ratio, the greater the degree of cooling. Persons in close contact with the escaping gas may experience frostbite. Cryogenic liquids are gases that have to be supercooled before they can be liquified. The resulting liquid has a temperature below −130° F (−90° C). Without proper PPE, any contact with cryogenics, either in liquid form or in gases immediately escaping from the container, will result in frozen tissue.

Frostbite

Superficial frostbite of the skin presents with reddening followed by gray, white, or mottled coloring (Box 12-6). Patients report stinging, burning, or numbness/tingling (paresthesia). The affected area is stiff to the touch, but underlying tissues remain soft. Deep frostbite of frozen tissue presents with a white, yellow-white, or mottled, bluish-white–colored skin that is hard, cold, and insensitive to the touch. Treatment for these conditions starts with ensuring that the patient has been decontaminated. All of the patient's clothing, shoes, and jewelry should be removed. If any clothing is frozen to tissue, it should be left in place until after warming. Handle the affected area gently and protect it from friction and pressure. Ensure that the patient has an open airway, and support respirations as necessary. Oxygen should be administered at 10 to 15 L/min by nonrebreather mask. For superficial frostbite, the affected part can be rewarmed with body heat. Dry or radiant heat may cause burns and should not be used. For deep frostbite, prolonged rewarming may be necessary, and the procedure may be very painful. Unless transport times are excessive, rewarming may best be accomplished at the medical facility. For deep frostbite or frozen skin, when extensive transport times to the hospital are involved, the affected area may be warmed in a water bath at a temperature of 100° to 105° F (37.8° to 40.6° C). The temperature of the bath should be monitored to ensure that it remains constant. The affected area should be kept immersed until it is completely flushed in color, is warm to the touch, blanches with tactile pressure, and stays flushed when removed from the bath. Neurological and vascular status distal to the area should be checked both before and after warming. After the part is warmed, sterile cotton should be placed between affected digits, and soft, sterile dressings should be lightly applied over affected parts. Do not allow the affected area to refreeze. As the affected area thaws, fluid will leak out of damaged cells, and blood vessels and the area will swell. If this excess fluid refreezes, damage will be much more extensive. Antibiotic or anesthetic ointments should not be applied to affected areas, and blisters should not be ruptured. Under medical control, paramedics may consider administering morphine sulfate or another analgesic if no respiratory distress or other contraindicating trauma is present. The patient's body temperature should be maintained with blankets. The patient should be assessed for chemical exposure and any other medical conditions or injuries. All cases of frostbite from chemical exposure should be transported to an appropriate medical facility.

Hypothermia

Hypothermia, by definition, is a body core temperature below 95° F (35° C) caused by prolonged exposure to cold environments or abnormal thermoregulation. When patients are wet, even exposure to cool temperatures may result in hypothermia. Patients may develop hypothermia while undergoing prolonged decontamination procedures in cold or even cool environments. Removing PPE in cool environments may lead to rapid cooling when perspiration quickly evaporates from moist skin. Mild hypothermia (90° to 95° F [32.2° to 35° C]) depresses the central nervous system and increases the metabolic rate. Patients in mild hypothermia shiver in an attempt to rewarm themselves. They also may present with difficulty speaking, memory loss, stumbling gait, and apathy. They may complain of paresthesia and pain in the extremities.

The shivering mechanism stops in moderate hypothermia (80° to 90° F [27° to 32.2° C]). At this point, the patient's level of consciousness is decreased. Arrhythmias commonly occur. Atrioventricular block, nodal tachycardia, atrial and ventricular fibrillation, an increased QT interval, and premature ventricular contractions (PVCs) are common arrhythmias seen with hypothermia. The heat production mechanisms start to fail, and a cold sweat is seen. A core temperature less than 80° F (27° C) is considered to be severe hypothermia. These patients will be comatose, with severely depressed vital signs and respirations.

Treatment for hypothermia will include ensuring that the patient is decontaminated as necessary. An adequate airway must be established; however, rough handling and intubation attempts may send the hypothermic patient into intractable ventricular fibrillation. Ventilation should be assisted as necessary, and supplemental oxygen administered. The patient's wet clothing should be removed, and he or she should be protected against wind chill. Passive patient rewarming can be carried out using warm blankets (Box 12-7). Some authorities suggest using warm blankets only on the trunk of the body. They point out that as the extremities start to warm, the cold blood in the extremities will be transferred to the core of the body, causing what is termed *core temperature afterdrop.* In this condition, core body temperature will continue to drop during rewarming, and ventricular fibrillation is common. If advanced-level EMS personnel are on scene, the patient's cardiac rhythm should be monitored, and arrhythmias should be treated according to Advanced Cardiac Life Support (ACLS) or local protocol. Cardiopulmonary resuscitation (CPR) should be performed as necessary. Defibrillation should be limited to three attempts until adequate body temperature is restored. Transportation to the hospital should be rapid. Active core rewarming, including warm IV fluids, warm humidified oxygen, warm peritoneal lavage, esophageal rewarming tubes, and extracorporeal rewarming (heating blood outside the body and returning it), can be carried out at a properly prepared receiving hospital.

Patient decontamination efforts during cold-weather extremes should be carried out with warm water or in heated areas whenever possible to minimize the risk of hypothermia. Warm blankets should be available to cover patients immediately after decontamination.

BOX 12-7

Field Rewarming

ABC_2DE
Remove wet clothing and protect against wind chill.
Place patient in horizontal position.
Cover with warm blankets.
Avoid rough movement and excessive activity.
Monitor cardiac rhythm, if the proper equipment and qualified personnel are available.
Monitor core temperature.

Summary

The use of PPE and exposure to certain chemicals can increase the incidence of heat-related injuries. In fact, heat-related problems are one of the most common responder injuries at a hazardous materials emergency. Frostbite can occur when victims or responders in inadequate PPE come in contact with leaking liquified gas or cryogenics. Hypothermia can result when tired, sweating responders remove protective clothing in cool environments and is always a risk when decontaminating patients in cool/cold weather. EMS personnel who respond to hazardous materials incidents should be able to recognize the signs and symptoms of thermal injuries and be able to provide appropriate treatment. Special structures, such as portable shelters or inflatable buildings, may need to be used to provide shade in hot environments or shelter (with portable heaters) for decontamination or rehabilitation efforts in cold weather.

CHAPTER REVIEW QUESTIONS

1. What factors besides environmental temperature should be considered in assessing heat stress risk?
2. How does the use of protective clothing affect the body's heat loss mechanisms?
3. What types of medications can increase the risk of heat-related illness?
4. What is the difference between classical and exertional heat stroke?
5. How can you tell the difference between exertional heat stroke and heat exhaustion?
6. What is the most effective way to cool the patient in heat stroke?
7. What is the difference between superficial and deep frostbite?
8. Explain why rewarming for deep frostbite is better done as an in-hospital procedure.
9. How does hypothermia occur at a hazardous materials incident?
10. What are the signs and symptoms of moderate hypothermia?

BIBLIOGRAPHY

American Conference of Governmental and Industrial Hygienists: *1997-1998 threshold limit values for chemical substances and physical agents and biological exposure indices,* Cincinnati, 1997, ACGIH.

Bledsoe BE, Porter RS, Shade BR: *Paramedic emergency care,* Englewood Cliffs, NJ, 1991, Brady.

Bronstein AC, Currance PL: *Emergency care for hazardous materials exposure,* ed 2, 1994, St Louis, Mosby.

Caroline NL: *Emergency medical treatment,* Boston, 1982, Little Brown & Co.

FEMA: *Emergency incident rehabilitation,* Washington, DC, 1992, Publication No FA-114, USFA Publications.

Goldfrank LR, et al: *Goldfrank's toxicological emergencies,* ed 4, Norwalk, Conn, 1990, Appleton & Lange.

Guidelines for public sector hazardous materials training. 1998 ed, HMEP Curriculum Guidelines, Emmitsburg, Md, 1998, National Emergency Training Center.

NIOSH: *Hot environments,* Cincinnati, 1980, DHHS (NIOSH) Publication No 80-130, US Government Printing Office.

NIOSH/OSHA/USCG/EPA: *Occupational safety and health guidance manual for hazardous waste site activities,* Washington, DC, 1985, DHHS (NIOSH) Publication No 85-115, US Government Printing Office.

Rosen P, et al, editors: *Emergency medicine: concepts and clinical practice,* ed 3, St Louis, 1992, Mosby.

Stewart CE: *Environmental emergencies,* Baltimore, 1990, Williams & Wilkins.

Walraven G, et al: *Manual of advanced prehospital care,* ed 2, Bowie, Md, 1984, Robert J. Brady.

13

Decontamination Procedures

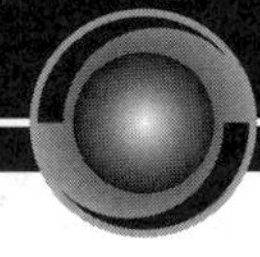

Phil Currance

CHAPTER OBJECTIVES

At the conclusion of this chapter the student will be able to:

- Identify the need for and the contents of a decontamination plan.
- Identify how patients, responders, and equipment may become contaminated.
- Discuss how the decontamination area is established.
- Explain in detail how patient decontamination is carried out.
- Identify chemicals that present a major risk of secondary contamination.
- Describe the differences between ambulatory and nonambulatory patient decontamination procedures.
- Explain how patient decontamination procedures need to be modified in cases of contamination involving radiation or water- or air-reactive materials.
- Describe responder protective equipment/clothing decontamination procedures.
- Discuss how different methods of decontamination (dilution, absorption, physical removal, solidification, isolation/disposal, and chemical neutralization/degradation) are used and their limitations.
- Describe how the dry decontamination process is carried out.
- Identify the need for and describe the process of equipment decontamination.
- Identify the type of protective equipment that should be used by responders carrying out decontamination procedures.
- Identify procedures to determine the effectiveness of decontamination procedures.

CASE STUDY

An unknown chemical has been released in a subway tunnel. There are numerous ambulatory and nonambulatory patients. Using personal protective equipment (PPE), the fire department and hazardous materials (HAZMAT) team have started rescue and decontamination activities. A postdecontamination triage area has been established, and ambulances are ready to transport victims to appropriate medical facilities.

- Which should come first, patient decontamination or primary assessment and airway/breathing/circulation (ABC) management?
- How much patient decontamination is necessary?
- What kind of decontamination procedures will the fire and HAZMAT responders need?
- Will the ambulances need to be decontaminated after they are used for transport?

Decontamination is the process of removing, or rendering harmless, contaminants that have accumulated on personnel, patients, and equipment. It is critical to the health and safety of responders at hazardous materials emergencies and should be a priority. Every agency that

CAR WASH
ENTRANCE
"TELL DISPATCH WE'LL BE OUT DECONTAMINATING THE PATIENT"
BERRY 98©

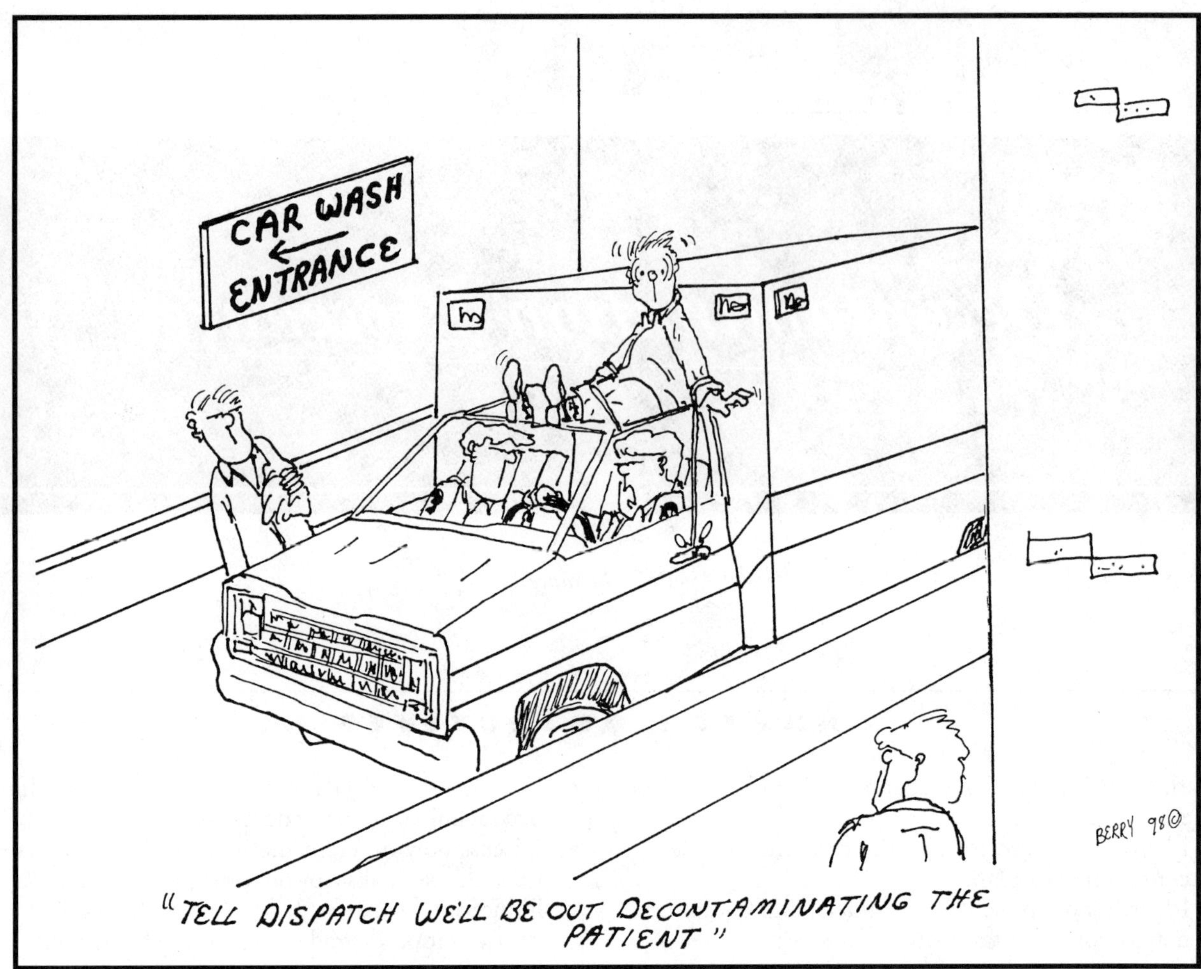

Reprinted with permission from Steve Berry's *I'm Not an Ambulance Driver* cartoon book series.

responds to hazardous materials emergencies should develop a decontamination plan (Box 13-1). Preincident contacts should be made to ensure that each agency's decontamination plan will fit with those of other agencies when they work together at an incident. The plan should guide all decontamination activities at the emergency scene. The best way to decontaminate is never to become contaminated in the first place; therefore, the plan should identify procedures for avoiding contact with hazardous materials. If patients, responders, or equipment become contaminated, the plan should detail the contamination control and decontamination processes.

Contamination occurs when responders, victims, or equipment come in contact with hazardous materials. Direct contact with a hazardous material leaking from a container is an obvious way to become contaminated. However, indirect contact can be much more subtle. People at a hazardous materials emergency scene may become contaminated in a number of ways, including the following:

- Contacting vapors, gases, mists, or particulates in the air
- Being splashed by liquid materials
- Walking through puddles or on contaminated soil
- Using contaminated instruments or equipment
- Contacting contaminated PPE
- Treating contaminated patients

Emergency Medical Services (EMS) responders should be concerned with patient decontamination. If patients are transported before being adequately decontaminated, a risk of secondary contamination of EMS and hospital personnel, ambulances, and the receiving emergency department exists. EMS responders also must know the proper way to decontaminate PPE, equipment, vehicles, and themselves.

Decontamination operations should be established before allowing entrance into the contaminated area, or hot zone, for any reason, including rescue. As victims or personnel exit the hot zone, they must be decontaminated. Contaminated equipment also must be decontaminated as it leaves the hot zone. A contamination reduction corridor, in which decontamination procedures are carried out, should be established in the warm zone. The decontamination corridor should contain separate areas to decontaminate patients, responders, and heavy equipment as necessary. Selection of a decontamination (decon) site should be based on availability, water supply, ability to

BOX 13-1

DECONTAMINATION PLAN

Determine the decontamination equipment needed.
Determine appropriate decontamination methods.
Establish work procedures to minimize responder contact with hazardous substances.
Establish patient decontamination procedures.
Establish responder decontamination procedures.
Establish procedures to prevent contamination of clean areas.
Establish methods and procedures to minimize worker contact with contaminants during removal of personal protective clothing and equipment (PPE).
Establish equipment decontamination procedures.
Establish methods for disposal of clothing and equipment that are not completely decontaminated.

contain runoff, and the proximity of drains, sewers, streams, and ponds. The site should be upwind and uphill from the incident. The site must be a safe distance from the incident but close enough to allow easy access from the hot zone and limit the spread of contaminants. If the decon site must be placed a long distance from the actual work area, transportation will be needed to move personnel and victims. Matters will be complicated if weather or other conditions mandate an off-site decon location. Shelters such as schools, firehouses, garages, and indoor car washes may be used after initial rinse at the scene for thorough decontamination. Remember that transport personnel, vehicles, and the facility used will be contaminated. Another problem associated with indoor facility use is containment of the runoff. If contaminated runoff cannot be contained, contact should be made with local authorities and water treatment plants.

Prehospital decontamination of contaminated patients should be carried out to limit tissue damage and absorption and prevent systemic poisoning (Fig. 13-1). Contamination must be confined in a specified area to prevent secondary contamination of EMS and hospital personnel. Above all, decontamination should be considered an essential part of patient management. If the patient was injured by the effects of the chemical, he or she will not respond to treatment until the exposure is terminated. The patient decontamination procedure should be a planned and practiced event so that it does not take undue time and trouble to implement.

The process of patient decontamination starts with identifying the product, life threat, route of exposure, and need for decontamination. If the exposure is from an unknown material, a worst-case scenario should be considered. The decision to carry out decontamination procedures on an injured patient is not always easy. Whether first to provide patient management or decontamination has always been controversial. Treating the patient before decontamination places EMS personnel at risk. On the

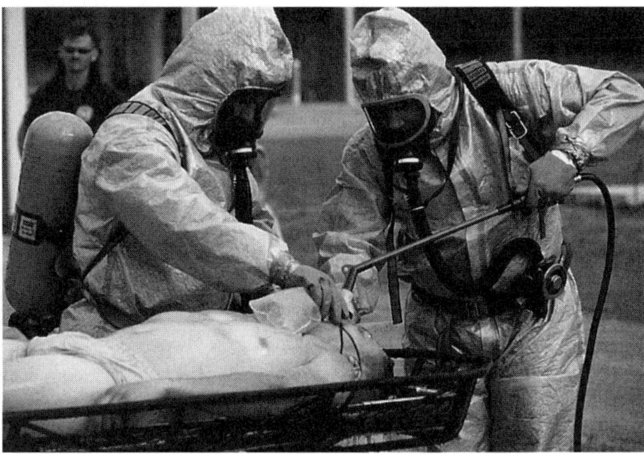

FIG. 13-1 Responders carrying out patient decontamination.

other hand, delaying primary attention to ABC concerns for complete decontamination can severely compromise the patient. Having trained, protected responders manage basic treatment at the same time as decontamination solves part of this problem. Still, the fact exists that extended decontamination procedures delay optimal advanced-care procedures and transport for definitive care. A policy of rapid, primary field decontamination with protected responders providing basic management followed by a detailed secondary decontamination, either at the scene or on arrival at a properly equipped hospital, should be adequate for most situations. In unusual situations, such as mass-casualty incidents, decisions involving patient decontamination can become difficult. Several factors can be used to assist in making these decisions. If known, the nature, state of matter, potential toxicity, and concentration of the chemical should be assessed. Liquids and solids tend to have a longer duration of action because patient exposure is continual. Once the patient is removed from a gas/vapor exposure, the exposure usually stops. In some cases, gases or vapors may be trapped in clothing or turn into solution on moist areas of the patient's skin, necessitating decontamination. Extremely concentrated or high-toxicity agents mandate a higher degree of decontamination.

The route of exposure also must be assessed. Products that attack the body only through inhalation present a minimal risk of further exposure once patients are removed from the area. The duration and extent of exposure also are important considerations. Patients exposed in a peripheral area for a very short time will need minimal, if any, decontamination.

A major consideration in determining the need for decontamination is the risk of secondary contamination of responders, equipment, and hospital staff. Entire systems can be put out of operation by secondary contamination. Gases, such as simple asphyxiants and carbon monoxide (CO), are examples of agents with a low risk of secondary contamination. Some gas exposures may react with skin moisture and create acidic or alkaline conditions (e.g., chlorine, anhydrous ammonia). These exposures may need to be decontaminated for the proper care of the patient. Inhalation-only exposure to volatile liquids or vapors require minimal decontamination. However, responders must be aware of any concurrent liquid or solid exposure. Examples of agents with a high risk of secondary contamination include corrosive products, asbestos, highly toxic products, pesticides/herbicides, high-viscosity liquids, oily or adherent products, dusts, and powders. Patients contaminated with a product that carries a high risk of secondary contamination should always undergo decontamination before transport.

In reality, the decision to decontaminate is not easily made. Consider that several million chemicals are listed in the Chemical Abstract Service (CAS) index, and we have given suggestions for only a handful. In cases of large exposure, if there is a continuing effect, or exposure to an unknown product, decontamination is indicated. Toxicity is not the only concern. Flammable products may cause fire hazards, and patients exposed to these products should be decontaminated. If any visible product or odor remains on the patient, decontaminate. In all cases, *when in doubt, decontaminate!*

Patient Decontamination

To effectively decontaminate patients, a minimum two-step decontamination process should be established (Fig. 13-2). The first decontamination step is clothing removal and water rinse. The second step consists of a soap and water wash and rinse. (A more extensive decontamination process may be necessary. Refer to resource data, medical authorities, and on-scene expertise.)

Decontamination should be carried out in the warm zone, before transport, with simultaneous patient care provided by qualified, trained, and protected responders. Emergency medical decontamination usually is considered a primary decontamination procedure to stop the chemical action on the patient and allow for safe patient care and transport. In other words, the purpose of emergency decontamination is to get the patient as clean as reasonably possible, depending on scene conditions and patient presentation. If time, patient presentation, and scene conditions permit, a secondary, detailed decontamination should be carried out. This secondary process, depending on scene conditions, sometimes may be performed at a prepared and properly equipped hospital emergency department. Hospitals are poor choices for the primary decontamination process. The chemical will continue to affect the patient during transport, and vehicles and personnel may be contaminated.

In inclement weather, a decontamination shelter, the inside of a cargo truck/trailer, or a specially prepared stationary ambulance (in which the walls and floor have been covered by plastic sheeting and nonessential equipment has been removed) can be used for decontamination. As stated previously, other shelters, such as local facilities, may be used for detailed decontamination after an initial rinse at the scene.

Nonambulatory Patients

A procedure for nonambulatory and ambulatory patients should be established as necessary. For the nonambulatory patient, responders must carry out decontamination after removing the patient from the contaminated area. Responders providing initial care or carrying out decontamination operations should wear PPE specified by references such as the *North American Emergency Response Guidebook* or the chemical manufacturer. The patient's clothing, jewelry, and shoes should be removed quickly and isolated for further decontamination or disposal. To reduce the likelihood of a chemical reaction with water, visible solid or particle contaminants should be brushed off as completely as possible before rinsing. Visible liquid contaminants also should be blotted from the body, using absorbent material, before rinsing. Because skin damage increases the chemical absorption rate, use care not to damage the protective dermal barrier. The patient then should be rinsed with copious amounts of water (Fig. 13-3). If possible, warm water (85° F [29.4° C]) should be

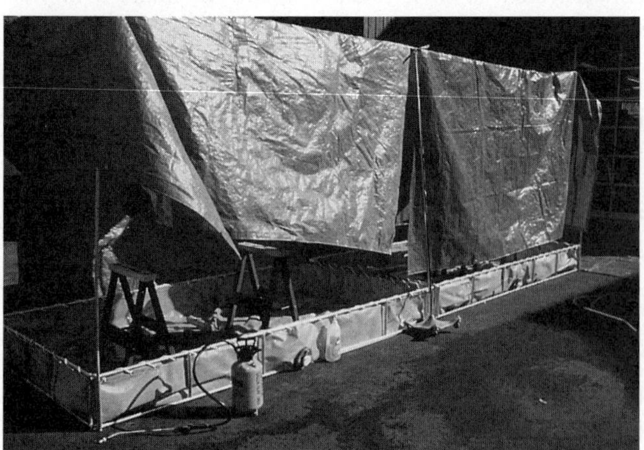

FIG. 13-2 A minimum of two steps should be used in the decontamination process.

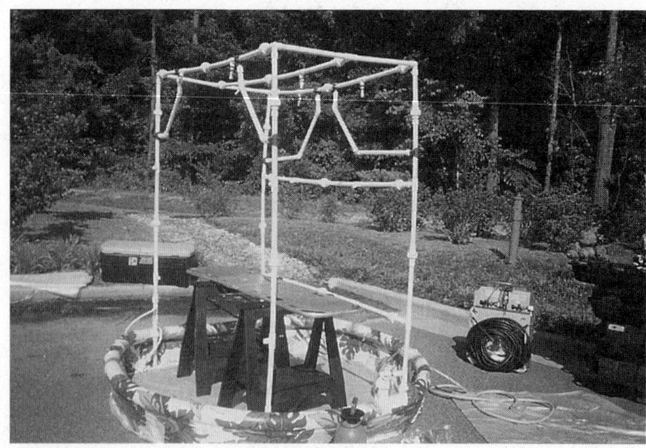

FIG. 13-3 Free-standing, nonambulatory patient shower.

used for extensive washing. Portable heaters that can be connected to the system to supply heated water are available. Hot water should never be used. Hot water will dilate peripheral blood vessels, leading to increased absorption, and may cause further thermal injury to damaged tissue. A high risk of hypothermia exists if cold water is used. Low water pressure and gentle spray nozzles on hose lines should be used to control the spray and avoid aggravating any soft-tissue injuries. Handheld shower massage sprayers work very well. Try to avoid overspraying and splashing. Some teams have designed free-standing shower units to streamline the process. If eye irrigation is necessary, use gentle running water from the nose to the lateral face. If possible, contact lenses should be removed. The patient should be washed with tincture of green soap or a mild liquid soap. In some cases, special decontamination soaps may be necessary. Written/computer resources, the local poison center, and on-scene authorities should be consulted. Liquid soaps dispensed from small squeeze or spray bottles work very well. Bar soaps should be avoided because of the chance of cross-contamination. Special attention should be paid to hair, nail beds, and skin folds. Soft brushes and sponges may be used; however, be careful not to abrade the skin, and use extra caution over bruised or broken skin areas. The patient then should be rinsed with copious amounts of water.

The decontamination procedure should be carried out in a systematic fashion. To protect the airway, the head and face should be decontaminated first. Brush or blot visible contaminants away from the eyes, mouth, and nose; then soap and rinse in the same manner (Fig. 13-4). As soon as possible, the patient's airway should be isolated and protected with an oxygen mask, bag-valve mask, or self-contained breathing apparatus (SCBA). Areas of skin damage or gross contamination should be decontaminated next. Use care not to allow contamination into areas of tissue damage. Lightly covering damaged tissues after decontamination with a plastic cover or wrap will help prevent recontamination. The rest of the patient's body then can be decontaminated as necessary.

Ambulatory Patients

At major incidents, many ambulatory patients may need to be decontaminated. Ambulatory-patient decontamination procedures start with the patients exiting the contaminated area. Hoses or shower units should be available (Fig. 13-5). Some teams have made mass-casualty shower units from free-standing shelters or tarps, PVC pipes, and shower nozzles. If possible, set up two separate shower areas, one for females and one for males.

Have patients enter the shower area and assist them as necessary in quickly removing clothing, jewelry, and shoes. If possible, isolate these items in plastic bags. Have patients brush off any visible powder or blot away liquid contaminants. Have the patients rinse off, soap up, and rinse again. Warm water (85° F [29.4° C]) should be used, if possible. Mild liquid soap in small squeeze bottles can be made available for patient use. Special attention should be paid to areas of gross contamination, injured areas, hair, and opposing body surfaces such as the underarms and groin. As in the nonambulatory patient procedure, the medical providers assisting in this process should be trained to use PPE and should wear appropriate respiratory protection and protective clothing. In cases of extremely toxic agents, patients may need to be assessed with air monitoring equipment after exiting the decon area. Redressing areas (one for each gender) should also be established. Clean patients should be provided with blankets, sheets, or disposable clothing. After decontamination and redressing, all patients should be checked by EMS personnel and transported as necessary.

Runoff from the decontamination process (ambulatory or nonambulatory) should be contained, if possible. Children's wading pools, commercially manufactured units/tables, draft tanks, or makeshift plastic/frame units may be useful for runoff containment. The nonambulatory patient should be elevated out of the runoff in the bottom of the containment pool. Plastic sawhorses, stretcher stands, chairs, or wood blocks all can be utilized. Patient decontamination will be much easier if the patient is elevated to waist high on the decontamination

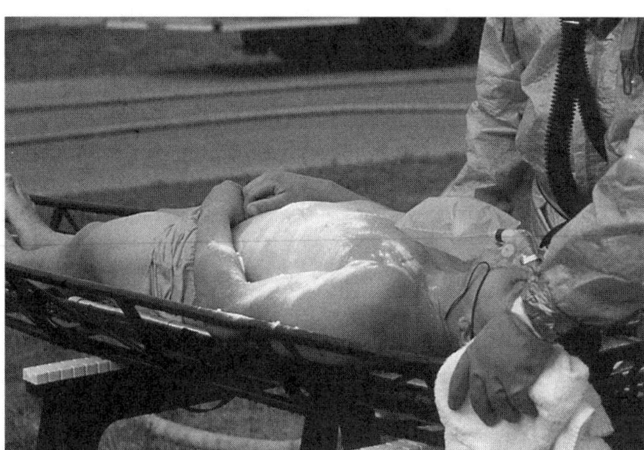

FIG. 13-4 Brush or blot visible contaminants away from the eyes, mouth, and nose first.

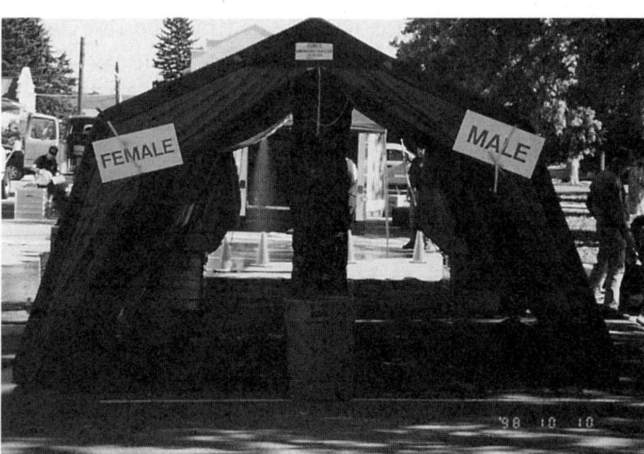

FIG. 13-5 Mass casualty shower system.

personnel. The ambulatory patient should also have something to stand on to elevate him or her out of the pooled runoff. The contaminated runoff can be pumped from the pools into barrels. Hand pumps or boat bilge pumps can be used. Some teams successfully pump the runoff into water bed mattresses instead of barrels. Patient decontamination should not be delayed to obtain containment pools. If no containment pools or tanks are immediately available, try to channel the runoff to a containment area. With mass casualties, runoff containment may not be feasible because of the volume of water that must be used. Remember to contact local authorities and water treatment plants if the runoff cannot be contained.

Patient decontamination procedures may need to be modified in cases of water- or air-reactive products that are embedded in the skin and in cases of radioactive contamination. If water-reactive products (i.e., lithium, magnesium, potassium) are embedded in the skin, no water should be applied. The embedded products should be covered with a light oil (mineral or cooking oil) and the patient rapidly transported for surgical debridement. If the products are not embedded, gently brush away the contaminant as much as possible and then flush with copious amounts of water to rapidly remove any residual product. Phosphorus is air reactive. It spontaneously ignites when in contact with air. If phosphorus particles are embedded in the skin, continuous water irrigation; water emersion; or sterile, water-soaked dressings should be applied during transport to the hospital for surgical debridement. Do not use oil for phosphorus exposure because it may promote dermal absorption.

Radioactive Decontamination

In transportation incidents in which radioactive materials are the only significant hazard, special decontamination procedures are required. Packages for large-quantity or high-level radioactive shipments are designed to withstand accident conditions and therefore are unlikely to release their contents when involved in an accident. Small-quantity radioactive shipments, such as a medical imaging isotope, are much more likely to be involved in a radiation release. Life-threatening conditions from the radioactive material released in these situations is unlikely. The trauma that the patient sustained is a much greater risk. Prolonged field decontamination of patients with life-threatening injuries may delay needed trauma care. In addition, alpha and beta particles may be difficult to remove from the skin. Effective, complete decontamination may require radiological monitoring equipment that may not be available in the field. Most important, improper decontamination methods may facilitate absorption (internalization) by transferring contamination to areas of tissue damage or by converting contaminants to a form that could be more readily absorbed through the skin.

Decontamination for victims of transportation accidents in which releases of small quantities of radioactive materials are the only significant hazard should be modified. When removed from the area of contamination, patients with electromagnetic radiation (gamma) exposure only will require no further decontamination. The clothing, jewelry, and shoes of patients with particle (alpha and beta) or liquid exposure should be removed quickly and isolated. The patient then should be packaged, using reverse isolation procedures such as specially designed patient transportation bags, plastic, or blankets. This will help prevent the spread of contamination during transport. EMS personnel should ensure adequate ambulance ventilation by using both intake and exhaust fans. PPE, such as air-purifying respirators (APRs) and outer protective garments, should be used if they are available and response personnel have received adequate training. Transportation should be to a receiving hospital that is capable of decontaminating a patient exposed to radioactive products. This should be established in preplanning. The hospital emergency department should be notified that a potentially contaminated patient is en route and supplied with all available information concerning the identity and nature of the contaminant. Complete decontamination of the patient should be carried out at the emergency department, guided by radiological monitoring devices and under the direction of a physician and/or health physicist. During decontamination, extreme care should be exercised to keep contaminants away from areas of tissue damage and body cavity openings. Assistance and advice on patient decontamination and management concerns may be obtained 24 hours a day from the Oak Ridge Radiation Emergency Assistance Center and Training Site by calling (615) 576-3131 or (615) 481-1000, ext. 1502 or beeper 241. In transportation incidents involving a large-quantity shipment in which the container has been breeched, or in a large release at a fixed facility, or if other chemical contaminants besides radioactive materials are suspected, standard field and emergency department decontamination guidelines should be followed.

Rapid Decontamination

In some cases, patients may need expedient decontamination before the HAZMAT team arrives. Patients may have made their way out of the contaminated area on their own or may have been rescued by firefighters wearing PPE. A rapid decontamination can be carried out by having them remove their clothes and rinsing with copious amounts of water from a partially opened fire nozzle. Be sure to keep the flow as gentle as possible. Try to keep runoff away from sensitive areas such as drains and bodies of water. Although this is not an optimal procedure, it may stop the action of the chemical on the patient and allow quicker medical intervention. The patient still may have some level of contamination after this rapid decontamination procedure. Personnel providing medical care for these patients should wear appropriate PPE (such as

SCBA and chemical-protective clothing [CPC] or firefighter protective clothing). The patient should undergo a more detailed decontamination procedure once the HAZMAT team arrives. If the HAZMAT team has an extended response time and the patient absolutely must be transported before their arrival, try to clean the patient as much as possible before transporting him or her. Isolate the patient for transport, using reverse isolation procedures. Ambulance intake and exhaust fans should be used to ensure adequate ventilation in the patient compartment. PPE should be used if available and if personnel have been adequately trained. The patient should undergo thorough decontamination on arrival at the receiving hospital.

Postdecontamination Procedures

After decontamination, patients should be transferred by a clean backboard (plastic backboards should be used whenever possible) or scoop stretcher to triage or a noncontaminated transport team in the cold zone. All articles that possibly are contaminated must be isolated for further decontamination, testing, and/or proper disposal according to federal, state, and local regulations. These items may include patient clothes or personal possessions, any contaminated patient-care equipment, and the responder's contaminated uniforms or PPE. The disposal of hazardous waste is strictly regulated. Contact the local or state health department for assistance. Any equipment that was used on the patient before decontamination must be considered contaminated and left in the warm zone until it can be decontaminated or disposed of properly.

Responder Decontamination

All responders who were contaminated at the scene also must be decontaminated (Fig. 13-6). The best protection for responders is to avoid contact with either the hazardous material or something that has been in contact with the material because then responder decontamination is unnecessary. In addition, standard operating procedures should be established that maximize worker protection. For example, proper procedures for donning and doffing PPE will minimize the potential for contaminants to bypass the protective clothing and escape decontamination. In general, all fasteners should be used (i.e., zippers fully closed, all buttons used, all snaps closed). Inner and outer gloves should be used. Disposable boot covers will help protect reusable boots. If responders are contaminated, they should follow a procedure that will ensure proper decontamination.

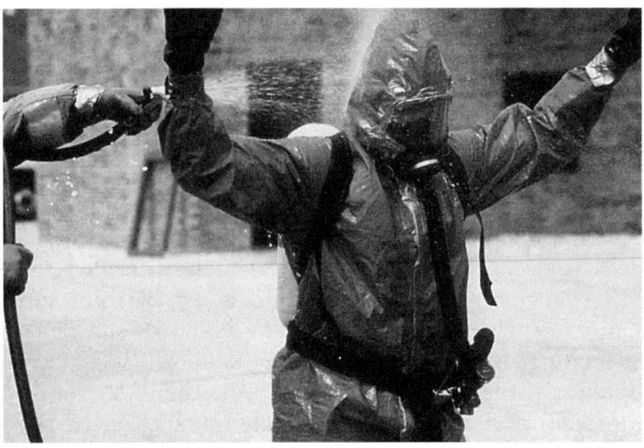

FIG. 13-6 All responders who become contaminated must undergo decontamination.

The original decontamination plan must be adapted to specific conditions found at each incident. The plan should be revised whenever the type of PPE or scene conditions change, or whenever the hazards are reassessed based on new information. Depending on numerous factors, these conditions may require more or less personnel decontamination than planned.

Determining the Extent of Decontamination

Contaminant properties

First, the extent of personnel decontamination will depend on the hazards associated with the material and its physical and chemical properties. If the material is suspected to be highly toxic or destructive to skin, full decontamination procedures for personnel who were contaminated should be followed. If permeable garments, such as firefighters gear, are contaminated with oxidizers or flammable liquids/vapors, detailed decontamination or disposal is essential. Solids and liquids will require more detailed decontamination than gas or vapor exposure. The substance's vapor pressure will significantly affect the extent of decontamination needed. If equipment is contaminated with a high-vapor–pressure liquid, then the majority of the product will evaporate, reducing the need for detailed decontamination.

Location

The location of the contamination is an important factor in determining the extent of decontamination. If contamination is isolated to glove and boot covers, gross decontamination can be accomplished by removing the contaminated items. If the entire suit is contaminated, more in-depth decontamination is called for.

PPE

The level of protection and type of protective clothing worn also are factors to be considered. Each level of protection incorporates different problems in decontamination and doffing of the equipment. For example, decontamination of the harness straps and backpack assembly of a SCBA is difficult. Encapsulated Level B or Level A suits will protect the SCBA from contamination. However, these suits will mandate almost complete suit decontamination when changing air tanks. If nonencapsulated Level B clothing is worn, a change of air tanks can be accomplished after the back and SCBA connections have been decontaminated. The type of protective clothing (limited use or multiuse) also will be a factor. For limited-use garments the decontamination must be adequate to remove the responder safely from the garment. The garment is then isolated and disposed of as hazardous waste. If multiuse garments are used, delayed permeation is a factor. Because these garments will be used again, decontamination must be complete.

Degree of exposure

The task that each responder performs determines the potential for contact with hazardous materials. If tasks do not bring the responder into contact with the hazardous substance, minimal, if any, decontamination is appropriate. Anybody with a potential of direct contact with the hazardous material will require more thorough decontamination.

The quantity of contaminants on equipment and protective clothing also will determine the extent of decontamination needed. If there is visible contamination or obvious discoloration/degradation of PPE, then decontamination is needed. The problem is that many contaminants are invisible to the eye. Therefore, the responder's work function and the type of release that has occurred must be assessed, and if it is possible that either responders or equipment may have had contact with the hazardous material, then thorough decontamination is required.

Finally, the reason for leaving the hot or warm zone also determines the need and extent of decontamination. A responder going to the edge of the contaminated area to pick up or drop off tools or instruments in a designated area and immediately returning to work may not require decontamination. A worker leaving to get a new SCBA cylinder will require some degree of decontamination. Individuals departing the hot or warm zone at the end of the response must be thoroughly decontaminated to prevent migration of the hazardous materials.

Decontamination Procedures

All personnel, clothing, and equipment leaving the hot or warm zone must be decontaminated to remove any harmful chemicals or infectious organisms that may have adhered to them. Decontamination methods accomplish one of the following:

- Physical removal of contaminants
- Inactivation of contaminants by chemical detoxification or disinfection/sterilization
- Removal of contaminants by a combination of both physical and chemical means

Removal methods

Dilution involves rinsing off the contaminant with water. Dilution often is used because water is readily available. However, this method has many disadvantages. Dilution does not change the hazards associated with the substance but does increase the volume of the substance. Containing the contaminated runoff also is a problem. This runoff is hazardous waste and must be disposed of properly. Also, many substances may not be readily removed by dilution.

Absorption is a process that usually is used for equipment, tools, and flat surfaces. In cases of gross contamination of protective clothing or equipment, absorbent pads or sheets may be used to physically remove as much contaminant as possible before another method is used. The disadvantages of absorption are that the absorbent must be picked up and the absorption process does not change the hazards of the chemical.

Hazardous contaminants sometimes can be removed by brushing or wiping away the substance. This is called *physical removal.* Special vacuums also may be used. The vacuums must have special high-efficiency filters on the exhaust. Physical removal may cause solid contaminants to become airborne as dusts and pose further threats of contamination and respiratory exposure.

Solidification is a process of turning a liquid into a solid. Solidifying liquid or gel contaminants can enhance their physical removal. Mechanisms of solidification include moisture removal through the use of adsorbents, chemical reactions via catalysts or chemical reagents, and freezing by using ice water or dry ice. Because of the associated hazards, these methods are restricted to tools and equipment. Technical assistance will be needed to determine the proper solidifying agent. The resulting product also must be considered hazardous waste and must be disposed of properly.

At times, equipment may not be able to be safely and completely decontaminated. Instead of trying to decontaminate these items, it may be better to isolate and dispose of them as hazardous waste. Porous items, such as fire hoses, ropes, and canvas stretchers, are extremely difficult to decontaminate. In some cases, limited-use protective clothing may be carefully stripped away, avoiding skin contact. Articles should be isolated and treated as hazardous waste.

Chemical disinfectants are a practical means of inactivating infectious agents on tools and equipment. Unfortunately, standard sterilization techniques generally are impractical for large equipment and for PPE.

Chemical neutralization or degradation may be used in the decontamination process. Chemical methods of decontamination require that the contaminant be identified. A decontamination chemical then is needed that will change the contaminant into a less harmful substance. Especially troublesome are unknown substances or mixtures from various known or unknown substances. Because of the potential hazards, using chemicals for decontamination should be done only by experienced personnel and only if recommended by an experienced chemist, industrial hygienist, or other qualified health professional. Chemical removal of surface contaminants sometimes can be accomplished by dissolving them in a solvent. The solvent must be chemically compatible with the equipment being cleaned. In addition, care must be taken in selecting, using, and disposing of any organic solvents that may be flammable or potentially toxic. Surfactants can be used to reduce adhesion forces between contaminants and the surface being cleaned. Household detergents are among the most common surfactants. Neutralization may be used to reduce the hazard potential of specific hazardous substances (acids and alkalis). This process may reduce the chemical hazard but may cause an exothermic reaction, toxic gas production, and suit degradation.

Chemical decontamination will require the use of decontamination solutions (Box 13-2). The solutions usually comprise water and chemical compounds that are designed to react with specific contaminants. Standard solutions are used for decontaminating PPE and equipment.

Decontamination solutions should be used for equipment only. Only in extremely rare circumstances (e.g., very dilute solution B (0.5%) for nerve agent or biological agent exposure, and solution D for last-resort radionuclide contamination) should they ever be applied to skin surfaces. Using chemical decontamination on skin may result in skin damage, thermal burns from the exothermic neutralization reaction, or increased absorption from the solvent. Unless specifically advised by a knowledgeable physician, the only thing that should be used for skin decontamination is mild soap and copious amounts of water. The chemical manufacturer or the Agency for Toxic Substances and Disease Registry (ATSDR) or CHEMTREC (see Chapter 6) may be consulted for specific recommendations on equipment decontamination.

The appropriate procedure will depend on the contaminant and its physical properties. Thorough research of the chemical involved, its properties, and expert consultation are necessary to make appropriate decontamination decisions. Many factors, such as cost, availability, and ease of implementation, influence the selection of a decontamination method. Care must be taken to ensure that decontamination methods do not introduce new hazards into the situation. Additionally, the residues of the decontamination process must be treated as hazardous wastes. From a health and safety standpoint, two key questions must be addressed:

- Is the decontamination method effective for the specific substances present?
- Does the method itself pose any health or safety hazards?

BOX 13-2

Equipment Decontamination Solutions

DECON SOLUTION A—5% SODIUM CARBONATE AND 5% TRISODIUM PHOSPHATE

Useful for:

Inorganic acids, metal processing wastes, heavy metals, solvents, polychlorinated biphenyls

To prepare:

Add 4 pounds of sodium carbonate (soda lime) and 4 pounds of trisodium phosphate to 10 gallons of water. Stir until evenly mixed.

DECON SOLUTION B—10% CALCIUM HYPOCHLORITE

Useful for:

Pesticides (especially organophosphates), fungicides, chlorinated phenols, phencyclidine (PCP), cyanides, ammonia

To prepare:

Add 8 pounds of calcium hypochlorite to 10 gallons of water. Stir with plastic or wooden stirrer until evenly mixed.

DECON SOLUTION C—5% TRISODIUM PHOSPHATE

Useful for:

Solvents, other lipid-soluble organic compounds

To prepare:

Add 4 pounds of trisodium phosphate to 10 gallons of water. Stir until evenly mixed.

DECON SOLUTION D—DILUTED HYDROCHLORIC ACID

Useful for:

Oily, greasy, unspecified substances, alkali and caustic substances

To prepare:

Add 1 pint of concentrated hydrochloric acid to 10 gallons of water. Stir with a plastic or wooden stirrer until evenly mixed.

DECON SOLUTION E—A CONCENTRATED SOLUTION OF LAUNDRY DETERGENT AND WATER

Useful for:

Radioactive substances and adhesive chemicals

To prepare:

Mix into a paste and scrub with a brush. Rinse with water.

Decontamination line

Decontamination procedures must provide an organized process by which levels of contamination are reduced. The decontamination process should consist of a series of procedures performed in a specific sequence. For example, outer, more heavily contaminated items (e.g., outer boots and gloves) should be decontaminated and removed first, followed by decontamination and removal of inner, less contaminated items (e.g., jackets and pants). Each procedure should be performed at a separate station to prevent cross-contamination (Fig. 13-7). The sequence of stations is called the *decontamination line* (Fig. 13-8). The responder decontamination line usually is set up in the same general area but separately from the patient decontamination area. Stations in the decontamination line should be separated physically to prevent cross-contamination and should be arranged in order of decreasing contamination, preferably in a straight line. Entry and exit points should be well marked.

The EPA has established suggested decontamination setups. They range from a maximum layout of 19 stations to a minimum layout of 7 stations. The number of stations will depend on the extent of decontamination required.

SAMPLE DECONTAMINATION SETUP. A typical emergency response decontamination setup for responders in Level B protection might include:

1. **Equipment drop.** A tarp or plastic sheet should be placed just inside the hot zone at the exit point to the warm zone. Equipment that will be needed again should be left at the equipment drop.
2. **Primary decontamination.** This step may actually entail many intermediate steps. Personnel should undergo water rinsing and soap or solution washes as necessary to remove as much contaminant as possible.
3. **Secondary decontamination.** The number of washes will depend on the nature of the contaminant. If the worker will be returning to the hot zone and only needs an air bottle change, primary decontamination can be done at this time.
4. **Removal and isolation of chemical-protective clothing.** Outer protective clothing, including outer gloves and overboots, are removed at this station.
5. **Removal and isolation of respiratory-protective equipment.** The SCBA harness should be removed, but the mask should remain connected and in place on the worker's face. The protective clothing then can be removed, using special care to reduce the risk of contaminating the worker. Once the outer clothing is removed, the SCBA mask can be removed. Inner gloves are the last piece of PPE to be removed.
6. **Removal of personal clothing.** With extremely hazardous substances, removal and isolation of the responder's personal clothing may be necessary. All clothing should be isolated for later cleaning or disposal.
7. **Field wash/personnel shower.** Personnel should wash their face and hands. To ensure complete decontamination, all personnel should shower as soon as possible. In cases of PPE failure or ex-

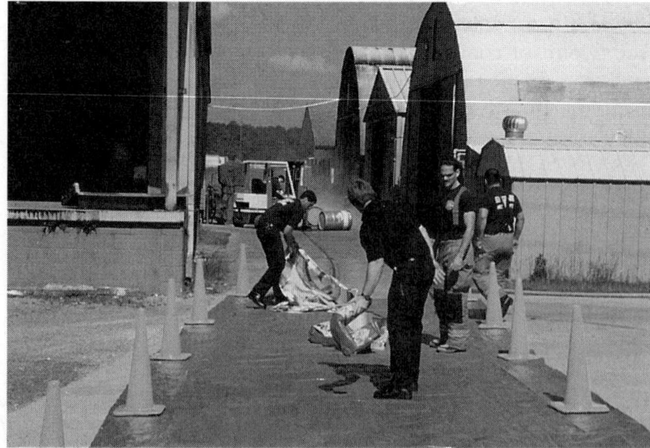

FIG. 13-7 Responders setting up a decontamination line in the warm zone.

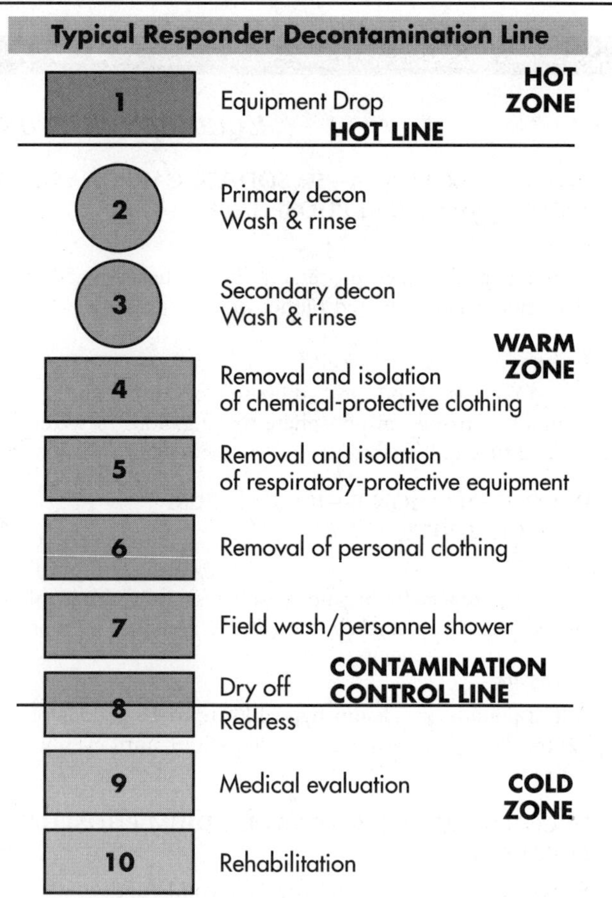

FIG. 13-8 Responder decontamination line.

posure without PPE, this shower should be conducted in the field.

8. **Drying off and redress.** Disposable towels should be used for drying. Clean clothes then can be donned. Many teams use disposable coveralls or hospital scrubs.
9. **Medical evaluation.** All personnel involved in mitigation activities must undergo a medical evaluation. Entry personnel should have received a preentry baseline examination. Vital signs, indications of exposure, and signs of heat stress all should be evaluated.
10. **Rehabilitation.** A clean area in the cold zone should be established as a rehabilitation area. Food and liquid supplements should be provided in this area. The welfare of response personnel is a vital step and should not be overlooked.

Personnel will work their way through the decontamination corridor, becoming cleaner as they progress. The object is to be absolutely clean by the time they leave the contamination reduction corridor.

DRY DECONTAMINATION. The trend is toward dry decontamination (Box 13-3) in cases where contamination is minimal. Dry decontamination involves using disposable clothing and systematically removing these garments in a manner that precludes contact with the contaminant.

BOX 13-3

RESPONDER DRY DECONTAMINATION PROCEDURE

1. Remove the tape securing the gloves to the suit.
2. Remove the outer gloves, turning them inside-out as they are removed.
3. Remove the suit, turning it inside-out. Avoid shaking it.
4. Remove the plastic shoe cover from one foot, and step over the "clean line." Remove the other shoe cover, and put that foot over the line.
5. Remove the mask. The last staff member to remove his or her mask may want to wash all masks with soapy water before removing his or her suit and gloves. Place the masks in a plastic bag, and hand the bag over the clean line and into a second bag being held by another staff member. Send the masks for further decontamination and proper inspection or disposal.
6. Remove the inner gloves and discard them in a drum or bag inside the dirty area.
7. Close off the dirty area until the level of contamination is established and the area is properly cleaned.
8. Personnel then should move to a shower area, remove their uniform, and place it in a plastic bag.
9. Shower and redress in clean attire.

Dry decontamination will probably be the method of choice for EMS personnel who transported patients to the hospital.

Equipment Decontamination

In selecting equipment, consider whether the equipment itself can be decontaminated for reuse or can be disposed of easily. For example, canvas stretchers are extremely difficult to decontaminate. Wooden handles cannot be decontaminated. Plastic-handled tools are a better choice, but some substances may degrade or decompose the plastic. Painted and bare metal surfaces usually can be decontaminated by solutions or steam cleaning. Structural firefighters protective clothing (bunker gear) must be carefully decontaminated. Never use an oxidizer solution such as calcium hypochlorite. Oxidizers will severely reduce the strength of the bunker gear fabric. Use only soap and water or contact the clothing manufacturer for specific recommendations. Leather cannot be decontaminated and therefore items including bunker gear with leather trim, gloves, boots, belts, watchbands, and wallets must be disposed of properly. SCBA straps and harnesses may be difficult to decontaminate. Refer to the manufacturer for specific advice.

Heavy Equipment

Heavy equipment and ambulances used at the scene may come into contact with hazardous substances. If so, decontamination must be carried out before the equipment is removed from the scene. Accessible areas on the equipment can be washed with water and decontamination solutions. All runoff must be contained as hazardous waste. Pay close attention to tires, wheel wells, and exposed surfaces. In extreme cases, steam cleaning or sand blasting may be needed. The ambulance used for transport may have a contaminated patient compartment. Returning the unit to service prematurely will prolong the exposure to EMS personnel and create a hazard for other patients. The unit should be isolated until it can be decontaminated. This includes a thorough decontamination of the patient compartment as well as mechanical and exterior decontamination as necessary. Tests should be carried out to verify proper decontamination. In most cases, soap and water are adequate for vehicle decontamination. CHEMTREC, ATSDR, and the local health department can assist with decision making. This is another reason to ensure adequate decontamination occurs before transport. If the patient is clean, then the ambulance and everything that he or she touches also will be clean. If the substance was released as an airborne contaminant, then air filters and vehicle interiors may need to be decontaminated.

Equipment Used for Decontamination

All equipment used for decontamination also must be decontaminated or disposed of properly. Buckets, brushes, clothing, tools, and other contaminated equipment should be collected, placed in containers, and labeled. Also, all spent solutions and wash water should be collected and disposed of properly. The local health and environmental regulatory agencies should be contacted for advice. In some cases, decontamination water may be disposed of by discharging it into a sanitary sewer. Approval from the local regulatory agencies and wastewater treatment facility is mandatory. In other cases, the water must be placed in containers and disposed of as hazardous waste. Clothing that is not completely decontaminated should be placed in plastic bags, pending further decontamination and/or proper disposal.

Decontamination Personnel

Decontamination workers who come in contact with personnel, victims, and equipment leaving the hot zone will require protection from contaminants. Generally, decontamination personnel may be sufficiently protected by wearing protective clothing that is one level lower than that of responders in the hot zone (e.g., decontamination personnel wear Level B protective clothing when responders in the hot zone are wearing Level A protective clothing). Supplied-air respirators (air lines) can increase the efficiency of the decontamination team by allowing them an extended time period in protective equipment. Air-purifying respirators (APRs) may be used if the contaminant has been identified, its concentration is known, and all requirements for the use of such equipment are met. Even decontamination workers assisting in removing protective clothing that has been decontaminated should take precautions by using a minimum of chemical-protective gloves and protective eyewear.

All decontamination workers are in a contaminated area and must themselves be decontaminated before entering the cold zone. The extent of their decontamination should be determined by the types of contaminants they may have contacted and the type of work they performed. Generally, the decontamination worker closest to the hot zone should progress through the other stations, following the station that they were staffing, to be decontaminated. They are followed by the next closest person and so on down the decontamination line. The last person (closest to the cold zone) decontaminates himself or herself at the last station.

Testing the Effectiveness of Decontamination Procedures

Decontamination methods vary in their effectiveness for removing different substances. The effectiveness of any decontamination method should be assessed throughout the response. If contamination is not being removed or if it is penetrating protective clothing, the decontamination plan must be revised. The problem is that no reliable test exists to determine immediately how effective decontamination is. In some cases, effectiveness can be estimated by visual observation. Discolorations, stains, corrosive effects, visible products, or alterations in the fabric of protective clothing may indicate that contaminants have not been removed. However, not all contaminants leave visible traces. Certain contaminants fluoresce and can be detected visually when exposed to ultraviolet light. Exposure to ultraviolet light may be harmful, and appropriate safety precautions must be followed. If an air monitoring device is available that will detect the presence of the contaminant, it may be useful to determine if gross contamination still is present. Wipe testing provides after-the-fact information on the effectiveness of decontamination. In this procedure, a dry or wet cloth, glass fiber filter paper, or swab is wiped over the surface of the potentially contaminated object and then analyzed in a laboratory. Both the inner and outer surfaces of protective clothing should be tested. Skin also may be tested, using wipe samples. Another way to test the effectiveness of decontamination procedures is to analyze for contaminants left in the cleaning solutions. Elevated levels of contaminants in the final rinse solution may suggest that additional cleaning and rinsing are needed. Reusable PPE also may be tested for permeation. Testing for the presence of permeated chemical contaminants requires that pieces of the protective garments be sent to a laboratory for analysis.

Summary

Decontamination procedures will help protect responders from hazardous substances that may contaminate victims, PPE, tools, vehicles, and other equipment used at the scene. Because decontamination stops the chemical action on the victim, it also is a valuable part of patient treatment. Decontamination protects personnel by minimizing the transfer of harmful materials into clean areas. Decontamination also will help protect the community by preventing uncontrolled migration of contamination away from the scene.

CHAPTER REVIEW QUESTIONS

1. At a hazardous materials emergency, when should the decontamination process be established?
2. What are the negative aspects of using off-site facilities, such as firehouses, garages, or indoor car washes, during inclement weather?
3. Why should patient decontamination be carried out before transport?
4. List at least three factors that should be considered when deciding if patient decontamination is necessary.
5. What is secondary contamination, and how does it happen?
6. What should take place if patients need immediate decontamination and no runoff containment pools are available?

7. Describe the patient decontamination process.
8. How should the standard patient decontamination process be modified for a trauma patient with low-level radiation contamination?
9. Why shouldn't chemical neutralization routinely be used for skin decontamination?
10. Why is a strict decontamination process or decontamination line necessary?

BIBLIOGRAPHY

Agency for Toxic Substances and Disease Registry: *Managing hazardous materials incidents, emergency medical services: a planning guide for the management of contaminated patients,* Atlanta, Ga, 1992, US-DHHS.

Andrews LP, editor: *Emergency responder training manual for the hazardous materials technician,* New York, 1992, Van Nostrand Reinhold.

Bowen JE: *Emergency management of hazardous materials incidents,* Quincy, Mass, 1995, National Fire Protection Association.

Bronstein AC, Currance PL: Module 4: emergency medical operations. In Ayers S, Christopher J, editors: *Medical response to chemical emergencies,* Washington, DC, 1994, Chemical Manufacturers Association.

California EMS Authority: *Hazardous materials medical management protocols,* 1991.

Carroll TR: *Contamination and decontamination of turnout clothing,* Emmitsburg, Md, 1993, Federal Emergency Management Agency, US Fire Administration.

Currance PL: *Hazmat for EMS,* St Louis, 1995, Mosby (videotape and guidebook).

EPA: *EPA standard safety operating guidelines,* Washington, DC, 1984, US Government Printing Office.

Goldfrank LR et al: *Goldfrank's toxicological emergencies,* ed 4, Norwalk, Conn, 1990, Appleton & Lange.

Gosselin RE, Smith RP, Hodge HC: *Clinical toxicology of commercial products,* ed 5, Baltimore, 1994, Williams & Wilkins.

Guidelines for public sector hazardous materials training. 1998 ed, HMEP Curriculum Guidelines, Emmitsburg, Md, 1998, National Emergency Training Center.

Hazardous materials response training program, New Jersey/New York, 1988, Hazardous Materials Worker/Training Program.

National Fire Protection Association: *NFPA 471, Recommended practice for responding to hazardous materials incidents.* Quincy, Mass, 1992, The Association.

NIOSH/OSHA/USCG/EPA: *Occupational safety and health guidance manual for hazardous waste site activities,* Washington, DC, 1985, DHHS (NIOSH) Publication No 85-115, US Government Printing Office.

Noll GG, Hildebrand MS, Yvorra JG: *Hazardous materials: managing the incident,* ed 2, Stillwater, Okla, 1995, Fire Protection Publications.

Olson KR, editor: *Poisoning & drug overdose,* ed 2, East Norwalk, Conn, 1994, Appleton & Lange.

OSHA: 29 CFR 1910.120, Hazardous waste operations and emergency response; Final rule, March 6, 1989; Washington, DC: US Government Printing Office.

Ricks RC, Leonard RB: *Hospital emergency department of radiation accidents,* Washington, DC, 1984, Emergency Management Institute, National Emergency Training Center.

Strong CB, Irvin TR: *Emergency response and hazardous chemical management: principles and practices,* Delray Beach, Fla, 1996, St. Lucie Press.

Tokle G, editor: *Hazardous materials response handbook,* ed 2, Quincy, Mass, 1993, National Fire Protection Association.

Varela J, editor: *Hazardous materials handbook for emergency responders,* New York, 1996, Van Nostrand Reinhold.

SECTION THREE

Management of the Exposed Patient

14

Body System Response to Poisons

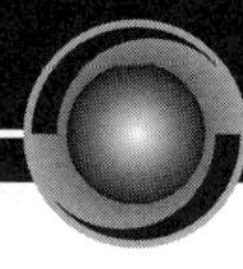

Alvin C. Bronstein, M.D., FACEP

CHAPTER OBJECTIVES

At the conclusion of this chapter the student will be able to:

- Describe the mechanisms of pulmonary toxicity.
- Name three chemicals that cause pulmonary toxicity.
- Discuss the different types of shock states produced by hazardous materials poisoning.
- Name three chemicals that cause cardiac toxicity.
- Describe the general medical approach to a hazardous materials exposure victim.

CASE STUDY

The location is a chemical plant near New York Harbor. At 11 AM, a 34-year-old chemical engineer was checking documents on a loading dock when a tanker truck exploded. The blast knocked him off the dock and onto the concrete pad below. He experienced transient loss of consciousness and sustained a fracture dislocation of his left ankle. Paramedics arrived within 10 minutes and transferred him to a hospital. No other individuals were injured. The rescue workers noted a strong, chlorinelike chemical odor. On arrival in the emergency department, the engineer was noted to be slightly short of breath. Radiographs of the chest and ankle were ordered. The shortness of breath was attributed to the patient's anxiety and pain from the ankle fracture. Pulse oximetry on 2 liters of nasal oxygen was 85%. The chest radiograph was interpreted as normal; the ankle film showed the fracture. Orthopedics was called and as it was lunch time, the emergency department attending physician went to the hospital cafeteria. The orthopedist arrived 15 minutes later. The patient received 100 mg of Demerol intravenously, and the orthopedist reduced the ankle fracture. At 1:30 PM, the patient was admitted to the orthopedic floor. At 2:30 PM, his nurse noted that he was experiencing increasingly severe shortness of breath. On chest auscultation, diffuse rales and rhonchi were heard. He was transferred to the intensive care unit, where he expired at 6:30 PM.

- What hazardous material did the victim most likely encounter in the explosion?
- What is the patient's major injury and life threat?
- Hazardous materials poisoning victims usually have what associated medical problem?
- What information should have been given in the paramedic report to the emergency department physician?
- What does the pulse oximeter reading of 85% at a near sea-level elevation mean?

How do health care providers learn to look for diagnostic clues in cases of hazardous materials poisoning? It is impossible to know the health effects of every hazardous material in use. However, it is possible to acquire a basic understanding of hazardous materials toxicology (e.g., knowledge of general chemical families and associated typical organ system toxicity manifestations). Although the information they contain is limited, material safety data sheets (MSDS) are a way that health care providers can learn about chemicals. Another way is for them to learn about body system responses to various hazardous materials so that they can be alert for the life-threatening symptoms most likely to result from exposure to a particular chemical. With this information, proper diagnostic and treatment decisions can be made.

Body Systems Response

Using a body systems approach is helpful in studying an individual's response to hazardous materials or chemical exposure. It is impossible to have detailed knowledge of all chemical poisoning symptoms, but a general understanding of life threats to body systems helps to focus the health management of a patient potentially poisoned by hazardous materials. This chapter will examine various body systems and provide examples of the adverse health effects that can be encountered.

Eyes

Chemicals may cause direct or indirect damage to the optic system. Agents such as chlorine, acids, alkalis, or isocyanates can cause ocular irritation to the conjuctiva and sclera surrounding the globe, leading to conjunctivitis. Severe cases of inflammation secondary to the chemical's inflammatory properties may lead to corneal scarring. Exposure to a strong caustic substance can cause rupture of the globe itself. In general, any chemical that causes skin or mucous membrane irritation can cause ocular damage through a similar mechanism. Drugs and chemicals or their metabolites can damage the retina directly. Although the mechanism is not understood, quinine acts on the retina itself to cause blindness. Ocular symptoms can be delayed for hours. Methyl alcohol is metabolized to formaldehyde and formic acid, which causes retinal damage, resulting in blurred vision, photophobia, and blindness. Methanol-poisoned patients report their vision to be like that of being in a snowfield. Pupils become fixed and dilated. Examination of the retina shows edema and optic disc hyperemia, which leads to blindness.

Ears, Nose, and Throat

The external ear (pinna) is vulnerable to direct toxicity from chemicals that cause mucous membrane irritation or burns. Acids or caustics can cause permanent disfiguration of the pinna. Direct auditory nerve toxicity is unlikely unless there is massive central nervous system (CNS) toxicity. Hazardous agents, including propylene glycol, ethyl alcohol, and mercury, have been reported to cause auditory nerve toxicity.

Skin and mucous membrane irritants can cause burns to nasal and pharyngeal mucosa. Examples of these agents are chlorine, ammonia, and other caustic compounds. Depending on the water solubility of the compound, nasal irritation or burns may or may not signal damage farther down the respiratory tree. Although less water soluble than chlorine, phosgene and sulfur dioxide, depending on the concentration and duration of exposure, can cause pharyngeal irritation. In severe cases, glottal swelling can lead to the development of stridor, which, in turn, can lead to hypoxia and, in severe cases, death.

Respiratory System

Because inhalation is the primary exposure route for most occupational and hazardous materials exposures, it is not surprising that damage to the respiratory system is the major life threat for hazardous materials poisoning victims (see Chapter 5). Respiratory symptoms may be viewed as a spectrum, with less severe damage, such as respiratory system mucosal irritation, on the left side of the spectrum and noncardiac pulmonary edema (NCPE), on the right side.

Various factors influence the effects that exposure to hazardous materials will have on the respiratory system (Box 14-1). Knowledge of a chemical's solubility can help predict its site of action in the respiratory tree. Understanding this also can help predict the probability of the patient developing NCPE, which, as we have seen from the case study, can lead to death.

Most hazardous materials exposures are by the respiratory route. The five major life threats possible from inhalation exposure are as follows:

- ◆ Hypoxia and asphyxiation
- ◆ Direct respiratory system injury
- ◆ Cardiovascular collapse
- ◆ Central nervous system toxicity
- ◆ Systemic poisoning

Examples of respiratory system hazardous materials exposure include chlorine gas, which can cause direct pulmonary injury and subsequent NCPE. Depending on the dose, inhalation of hydrogen cyanide gas can result in rapid loss of consciousness, leading to respiratory depression and cardiovascular collapse. Trichloroethylene inha-

BOX 14-1

FACTORS THAT INFLUENCE PULMONARY EFFECTS OF HAZARDOUS MATERIALS EXPOSURE

Chemical properties
Dose
Particle size
Water solubility
Patient's medical status

lation induces CNS depression and/or cardiac arrhythmias. Liver toxicity may be a late complication.

Water solubility of the hazardous material largely will influence where damage will occur in the respiratory tract and also the time of symptom onset. Highly water-soluble compounds, such as chlorine, easily react with water in the upper airway to produce rapid symptom onset. Symptoms with a rapid onset include ocular, nasal, and pharyngeal irritation. Scleral irritation with red, watery eyes usually is observed. Upper airway signs are manifested by nasal and throat irritation. Coughing, shortness of breath, chest tightness, and discomfort or pain may be present. Alternatively, phosgene has a much lower water solubility, which allows it to reach deeper into the respiratory tract before it reacts with respiratory tract mucosal water to produce irritation and possible NCPE.

Water solubility is only one exposure parameter to be considered when predicting respiratory system health effects. Air concentration, particle size, and duration of exposure before victim decontamination and hospital transport also must be considered. Prolonged exposure to even relatively water-soluble substances may produce pulmonary edema; conversely, exposure to low water-soluble compounds may cause upper airway signs and symptoms as well.

The size of the inhaled particles also plays a key role in pulmonary toxicity and in predicting the site of respiratory system injury (Box 14-2). Respirable particles measuring between 5 and 30 μm usually are deposited in the upper airway (see Chapter 5). To reach the lower airways, particles must be in the 1- to 5-μm range. For lung parencyhma and/or alveoli deposition, respirable particles must measure no more than 1 μm in diameter. Particle size must be coupled with the agent's water solubility when evaluating where damage may occur in the respiratory tract and also time of symptom onset.

Poisoning as a result of fire and explosions presents a special case. In addition to concerns regarding local or systemic health threats from the products of combustion of hazardous materials, victims of these types of events also experience life threats from carbon monoxide (CO) and/or cyanide poisoning. Many plastics release cyanide when they burn. CO always is associated with fire. Both CO and cyanide poisoning should be considered in the differential diagnosis of a fire or explosion victim. The classical symptoms sometimes reported with CO or cyanide poisoning may not be evident. Empirical use of the cyanide antidote kit for people severely injured in fires is controversial. Such use of this kit should be discussed with the local medical control physician. Prompt initiation of oxygen therapy will help reverse the effects of both cyanide and CO poisoning until specific diagnoses can be made.

Cardiovascular System

Many hazardous materials may cause cardiovascular system toxicity (Box 14-3). These substances range from heavy metals to a wide variety of hydrocarbon solvents. Cardiovascular effects can result from any exposure route. Once again the pulmonary exposure route is the most rapid way to cause cardiac toxicity.

Cardiac arrhythmias may be encountered with inhalation of most hydrocarbon solvents. Cardiac toxicity is common with the impaired oxygen (O_2) delivery encountered in severe CO poisoning. Because cardiac tissue has high O_2 requirements, cardiac arrhythmias frequently are generated by CO poisoning. The same mechanism applies to poisoning with simple asphyxiants, which also deprive the coronary circulation of required O_2. Victims with preexisting cardiovascular disease are particularly vulnerable to the decreased O_2 levels experienced in cases of poisoning by simple or chemical asphyxiants. The effects of simple and chemical asphyxiants are compounded by the fact that the relative hypoxia induced by these agents shifts the O_2-hemoglobin (Hgb) dissociation curve to the left, further compromising the body's ability to receive O_2 still bound to Hgb.

Shock and Related Hypoperfusion States

Various types of shock also may be observed after hazardous materials poisoning. These shock states include hypovolemic, cardiogenic, anaphylactic, and vasogenic shock.

BOX 14-2

Relationship Between Particle Size and Site of Pulmonary Deposition/Action

Upper airway

5 to 30 μm

Lower airway

Bronchiolar region
 1 to 5 μm
Alveolar region
 ≤1 μm

BOX 14-3

Effects of Cardiovascular System Toxicity

Arrhythmias
Shock
Cardiovascular collapse

Hypovolemic shock

Hypovolemic shock is secondary to a chemical exposure that causes increased permeability of the blood vessel walls. Leakage of plasma across cell membranes out of the vascular system and into the interstitial or cellular space occurs. Thus a relative state of hypovolemia is produced. Trauma, which often is associated with hazardous materials incidents, also may cause hemorrhage, which, if untreated, will produce hypovolemic shock.

Hypovolemic shock usually is manifested by increased heart rate and decreased blood pressure. Usually the pulse rate is greater than 120 beats per minute (bpm). The pulse pressure is weak. Depending on the clinical situation, bradycardia or a normal rate may be observed. Blood pressure usually will be less than 90 mm Hg systolic, and jugular venous pressure is decreased. Positive orthostatic changes usually are present (a pulse rate increase of 20 or more, or a blood pressure decrease of 20 mm Hg or more, or a combination of 20 or more when the patient is moved from the supine to the standing position). The respiratory rate will be increased, and respirations will be shallow. The patient may experience anxiety, restlessness, confusion, decreased level of consciousness, and coma. The skin will most likely be pale, diaphoretic, and cool. In cases of dehydration, the skin may be warm and dry.

Cardiogenic shock

Chemical agents, such as chlorinated hydrocarbon solvents, may produce direct cardiac toxicity, leading to reduced blood pressure and tissue perfusion. Cardiogenic shock may result. Many types of cardiac problems, including electrical conduction deficits and loss of contractility, may be seen. Signs and symptoms include substernal chest pain or a heavy pressure sensation in the chest. The blood pressure usually will be less than 90 mm Hg systolic. The pulse rate may be normal, fast, or slow and may be irregular. Jugular venous pressure is increased but may be normal initially. Associated respiratory system changes may include increased respiratory rate with shallow respirations. Signs of pulmonary edema may be present. The skin may be cyanotic, cool, and diaphoretic. The patient may exhibit signs of anxiety, restlessness, confusion, decreased level of consciousness, and coma.

Anaphylactic and anaphylactoid reactions

True anaphylactic shock or anaphylactoid reactions may be seen in some types of chemical exposure. In severe allergic reactions to chemicals such as metabisulfite, the body reacts to a foreign substance by releasing histamine and other chemical mediators of anaphylaxis. This Type 1 allergic reaction requires previous sensitization to the substance. Anaphylactoid reactions, which are indistinguishable from anaphylactic reactions, also may be seen. An anaphylactoid response is a dose-dependent, nonimmunological reaction caused by chemical drug-induced histamine release from mast cells and basophils. The reaction is independent of antigen-antibody reactions. An anaphylactoid reaction may occur on a patient's first exposure to a chemical. Both of these reactions cause bronchial spasm and wheezing, dilation of peripheral blood vessels, and alterations in capillary permeability. Capillary cell membranes become leaky, allowing fluid to move from the vascular space and into the interstitial space. This results in a relative hypovolemic shock and noncardiogenic pulmonary edema. Signs and symptoms of anaphylactic or anaphylactoid reactions usually include an increased pulse rate with blood pressure less than 90 mm Hg systolic. A tight feeling may be present in the chest. Respiratory symptoms may include cough and stridor, indicating upper airway obstruction secondary to mucosal swelling. Dyspnea and diffuse wheezing may be present. The patient may complain of headache, anxiety, shortness of breath, and restlessness. Decreased level of consciousness or coma may rapidly ensue. The skin may be flushed and edematous. Rash, redness, and itching may be present. It must be emphasized that the symptom progression in anaphylactic and anaphylactoid reactions is usually rapid and without prompt treatment may result in death.

Vasogenic shock

Hazardous materials exposure may cause vasogenic shock. Chemical agents may interfere with smooth muscle function in blood vessel walls, causing relaxation and vasodilation. Widespread vasodilation without primary loss of volume causes hypotension. Nitrates and nitrites are capable of this phenomenon. Clinical signs usually include a weak, rapid heart rate (pulse rate greater than 120 bpm). Bradycardia or a normal pulse rate may be encountered. Blood pressure typically is less than 90 mg Hg systolic, and jugular venous pressure is decreased. Positive orthostatic changes most likely are present. Respiratory rate will be increased, and respirations will be shallow. The skin may be warm, dry, and flushed. Anxiety, restlessness, confusion, decreased level of consciousness, and coma may occur.

Gastrointestinal System

Occasionally, hazardous materials exposure will occur orally. Many times these exposures are intentional ingestions. Poisoning also may result from smoking in industrial areas or as a result of poor decontamination. Ingestion of hazardous materials may result in the following six major, acute, life-threatening poisoning possibilities:

- Cardiovascular collapse
- Pulmonary toxicity
- CNS toxicity
- Gastrointestinal (GI) tract injury
- Metabolic poisoning effects
- Systemic toxicity

Examples of agents that act on the GI system include sodium hydroxide, which when ingested causes GI hemorrhage and ulceration. Esophageal stricture formation may be a late complication. The absence of oral burns does not correlate with the presence or absence of burns in the esophagus or stomach. Potassium cyanide, a solid form of cyanide, produces cardiovascular collapse on ingestion. Ethylene glycol and diethylene glycol ingestion cause CNS depression. A hallmark of ethylene glycol poisoning is the development of an anion gap metabolic acidosis. Left untreated, renal failure follows. Symptoms may be delayed depending on the rate of absorption and the presence of any coingestants, such as ethanol, which slows the metabolic conversion of ethylene glycol to oxalic/glycolic acids (i.e., oxalate/glyoxalate). Poisoning from ethylene glycol is another example of lethal synthesis in which the parent compound has limited toxicity. The primary toxicity stems from the calcium oxalate metabolism products.

In general, GI signs and symptoms of hazardous materials poisoning may include nausea, vomiting, drooling, intestinal obstruction, abdominal pain, hemorrhage, ulceration, perforation, diarrhea, and melena. Once absorbed, the agent may produce systemic toxicity.

Genitourinary System

The genitourinary (GU) system also is at risk from hazardous materials insult. Chemicals such as benzidine may cause bladder cancer. Cadmium has been linked to the development of both prostate cancer and renal disease.

Problems with reproduction can result from hazardous materials exposure. Human malformations have many causes, ranging from genetic defects and maternal infections to drug and toxin exposure. To accurately assess the potential effects of chemicals on reproduction, one must thoroughly understand the male and female reproductive systems. A knowledge of fetal development is necessary. Although these discussions are beyond the scope of this text, some generalizations can be made. Agents such as the metals arsenic, beryllium, cadmium, lead, or mercury can adversely affect the female reproductive cycle and fetal development. Deleterious effects also may be seen on the male reproductive system. For example, lead can cause abnormal or decreased sperm counts, leading to infertility or birth defects.

Skin

Next to inhalation the second most common route of exposure to hazardous materials is the dermal or ocular route. Dermal exposures have the following three major, acute, life-threatening poisoning possibilities:

- Spectrum of local skin irritation to burns
- CNS toxicity after systemic absorption
- Cardiac toxicity after systemic absorption

Local skin symptoms may include blistering, chemical burns, irritant dermatitis, allergic dermatitis, and allergic reactions. Absorption of agents such as toluene may produce systemic toxicity. Cardiovascular collapse, pulmonary toxicity, and metabolic acidosis may be observed. Seizures, altered level of consciousness, and coma will be seen with CNS toxicity.

Examples of dermal injury resulting from hazardous materials exposure range from superficial redness (erythema) to full-thickness chemical burns. Hydrofluoric acid causes local burns ranging from skin irritation to erythema, vesicle formation, and partial or full-thickness burns. Hydrofluoric acid penetrates tissues down to and including bone. Large areas of skin exposure and/or concentrated hydrofluoric acid solutions can produce systemic fluoride toxicity. Life-threatening hypocalcemia and hypomagnesemia may result. Hypocalcemia may be refractory to even the most aggressive calcium replacement treatment. Dermal exposure to organophosphate insecticides or nerve agents may produce cardiovascular collapse and death.

Abraded skin or open, soft-tissue traumatic injuries promote surface absorption of poisons. Remember that the concentration of the chemical, duration of exposure, and skin surface disruption will influence the rate of absorption and magnitude and expression of the symptoms.

CNS

Various hazardous materials may directly or indirectly affect the CNS. Seizures, including status epilepticus, altered level of consciousness, and coma will be seen with CNS toxicity. Many metabolic disturbances, such as hypocapnia, cerebral anoxia, water intoxication, electrolyte disturbances, and hypoglycemia, may result from hazardous materials exposure. Seizures may result from direct CNS effects or any of the metabolic abnormalities just mentioned.

Certain compounds, such as strychnine, picrotoxin, pentylenetetrazol, camphor, DDT, chlorinated insecticides, parathion and other organophosphates, nerve agents, and fluoroacetates, may cause seizures. Aliphatic and aromatic hydrocarbon solvent inhalation can result in CNS poisoning. Toluene, a common aromatic solvent found in gasoline and glues, has been shown not only to cause behavioral changes in acute and chronic exposures but also white matter degeneration on magnetic resonance imaging scans of the brain. The solvents n-hexane and methyl-n-butyl ketone (2-hexanone) not only are capable of causing CNS depression but also their common primary metabolite 2,5 hexanedione produces a sensorimotor polyneuropathy.

Summary

The foregoing discussion has touched briefly on each body system and a few of the many toxic responses each system may experience as a result of exposure to hazardous materials. Although it is impossible to know the effects of all chemicals, a general awareness of the possible body system responses likely to be encountered is extremely helpful in providing proper patient care.

CHAPTER REVIEW QUESTIONS

1. What is noncardiogenic pulmonary edema?
2. Name three chemicals that can cause skin irritation.
3. Name the five major life threats from hazardous materials exposure by inhalation.
4. Compare the onset of action of poorly water-soluble and highly water-soluble compounds in the respiratory tract.
5. What is the primary cardiovascular toxicity of hydrocarbon solvents?
6. Name the six major life threats from exposure by oral ingestion.
7. Name two metals that can affect the reproductive system.
8. What factors influence the health effects of a dermal exposure?
9. Describe the effects of toluene on the central nervous system.
10. Name three substances that can cause seizures.

BIBLIOGRAPHY

Bronstein AC, Currance PL: *Emergency care for hazardous materials exposure,* ed 2, 1994, St. Louis, Mosby.

Hessler R: Cardiovascular principles. In Goldfrank LR et al, editors: *Goldfrank's toxicologic emergencies,* 1994, Norwalk, Conn, Appleton & Lange.

National Institute for Occupational Safety and Health. Current intelligence bulletin 48: *Organic solvent neurotoxicity,* 1987, Cincinnati, NIOSH.

Newman LS: Pulmonary toxicology. In Sullivan JB, Krieger GR, editors: *Hazardous material toxicology,* 1991, Baltimore, Williams & Wilkins.

Snyder R, Andrews LS: Toxic effect of solvents and vapors. In Klaassen CD et al, editors: *Casarett and Doull's Toxicology: the basic science of poisons,* ed 5, 1996, New York, McGraw-Hill.

USDHHS: *ATSDR case studies in environmental medicine: tetrachloroethylene toxicity,* Monograph 9, June 1990.

USDHHS: *ATSDR case studies in environmental medicine: trichloroethylene toxicity,* Monograph 6, January 1992.

USDHHS: *ATSDR case studies in environmental medicine: benzene toxicity,* Monograph 11, October 1992.

USDHHS: *ATSDR case studies in environmental medicine: gasoline toxicity,* Monograph 31, September 1993.

15

Triage and Chemical Exposure Syndromes

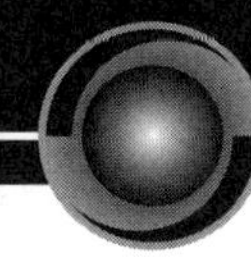

Alvin C. Bronstein, M.D., FACEP

CHAPTER OBJECTIVES

At the conclusion of this chapter the student will be able to:

- Describe special triage problems presented by hazardous materials accidents.
- Discuss why trauma frequently is associated with hazardous materials poisoning.
- Define a toxidrome.
- Describe three poisoning symptom complexes.
- Discuss basic emergency department laboratory studies.

CASE STUDY

Paramedics are dispatched to a small house. It is a warm summer day. There they find a young mother in the back yard kneeling near her young son. She is crying hysterically. The child is lying quietly on the ground and is sweating profusely. Occasional muscle twitches in the extremities are noted. He is responsive to deep pain only. Vomitus that has a strong chemical odor is noted on his shirt. Nearby is a half-full, gallon plastic milk container. The mother states that the boy was playing outside. She states that she thinks he was thirsty and drank from the milk container. The woman reports that she is beginning to get light-headed from the odor coming from the child's shirt.

- Describe the toxic syndrome or toxidrome the child is exhibiting.
- What is most likely in the milk container?
- Describe the initial treatment plan for the child.
- What should be done for the mother?

As has been discussed in previous chapters, Emergency Medical Services (EMS) providers must be familiar with decontamination procedures and poison-specific treatment modalities in order to decrease morbidity and mortality. Because many chemical incidents involve multiple patients, triage techniques need to be reviewed and modified for hazardous materials incidents. Triage procedures also must address the additional decontamination and medical treatment needs of hazardous materials poisoning victims. In addition, to protect health care providers, strict adherence to the Centers for Disease Control and Prevention (CDC) Standard Precautions (formerly Universal Precautions) is required.

The assessment and treatment of patients exposed to hazardous materials require specialized diagnostic skills. Many poisons cause multiple symptom complexes. Many authors have used the term *toxidrome* to refer to these poisoning symptom constellations. Understanding common toxidromes helps the prehospital provider to focus field treatment plans.

Triage

Patients exposed to hazardous materials present special triage problems. Hazardous materials incidents often involve multiple patients. Some of these patients may have received only minor, low-risk exposures. However, others may have received high-risk exposures and experience serious immediate or delayed symptoms. Hazardous materials poisoning victims also may have traumatic injuries.

Hazardous Materials Exposure

Hazardous materials exposure influences triage decisions in numerous ways. Access to patients and provision of emergency treatment may be delayed because of scene conditions and patient decontamination requirements. Additions to scene time because of patient decontamination may stall definitive patient care. Chemicals may modify the physiological response to trauma by amplifying signs and symptoms or decreasing the efficiency of various protective mechanisms. For example, nitrates, nitrites, or hydrocarbon solvents can cause or augment hypotension, compromising an individual's response to hypovolemic and other forms of shock.

Many chemicals may not produce immediate symptoms. The ability of hazardous materials exposure to postpone or delay poisoning symptoms must be considered to make appropriate triage decisions. For example, oral ingestion of a fat-soluble substance, such as an organophosphate insecticide, can result in delayed symptom onset because of the time it takes for absorption and redistribution of the organophosphate throughout the body. Conversely, even a drop of an organophosphate such as Sarin (GB) deposited on the skin can result in unconsciousness, seizures, and death in a matter of minutes.

Warning Properties

Victims at the periphery of the hazardous materials release may experience a very minor exposure. Some chemicals have warning properties that are detectable far below the harmful level. The Occupational Safety and Health Administration (OSHA) has determined that the 8-hour permissible exposure limit–time weighted average (PEL–TWA) for toluene is 200 ppm. The odor threshold for toluene is only 160 parts per billion (ppb) and only 40 ppb for taste when dissolved in water. Thus the human nose can detect toluene at a level approximately 500 times less than the PEL. The sense of taste for this chemical is obviously more precise than the odor detection level. Thus the human senses of smell and taste often can detect a chemical's presence far below the posted toxic level. This ability is a double-edged sword. Simply detecting the odor of a chemical does not always equate to a high-risk exposure. These facts, coupled with the emotional impact of being involved in a hazardous materials release, can cause many people to react to the warning properties just as if they had been exposed to a dangerous chemical air level. This situation accounts for some of the cases of so-called mass hysteria associated with hazardous materials incidents. EMS providers must be able to evaluate the scene for real vs. imagined risk and toxicity.

Relying on detection of a chemical's warning properties to determine if a scene is safe from exposure to hazardous materials is fraught with problems. The chief difficulty is that an individual's odor-sensing ability for a particular chemical rapidly diminishes with prolonged exposure. Thus a chemical may still be present but a responder may fail to sense its presence. Also, for many chemicals, the health effects of continued inhalation, even at low levels, may be unknown. In addition, many chemicals have no perceptible warning properties. Some chemicals may not be able to be detected until the exposure limit is well above their immediately dangerous to life and health (IDLH) value. Furthermore, the ability to detect a chemical's warning properties may vary among individuals. For example, cyanide's warning property is that it smells like bitter almonds. However, it is estimated that up to 50% of the population is unable to detect this odor.

Hazardous materials exposure can present multiple hazards. The chemical compounds may be toxic, corrosive, reactive, and/or flammable, adding to the exposure threat. All possible dangers from a particular exposure incident must be considered. In addition, the chemical's state of matter (i.e., solid, liquid, or gas) during the release must be considered in assessing risk. Gases and vapors present the greatest risk for respiratory system or skin toxicity because they spread the fastest and farthest.

Remember that chemical incidents are commonly caused by some type of accident. The hazardous materials incident may involve the release of both kinetic and chemical energy. Therefore, as just stated, trauma and chemical exposure may coexist. Triage decisions must take the associated risks of trauma into account.

Exposure Timeline Development

Patient symptoms at the time of the exposure and at the time of triage assessment should be taken into consideration. Develop a patient timeline exposure history. It is important to note the time and chart the direction of a patient's clinical course. Irritant or corrosive chemicals that are highly water soluble will present immediate upper-airway symptoms. Many compounds may have a delayed symptom onset and unlike toluene and other hydrocarbon solvents have no detectable warning signs. Patients exposed to chemicals with the potential to cause delayed symptoms warrant further observation. Providers should ascertain the ability of the chemical in question to cause delayed symptoms.

Immediate vs. Delayed Symptoms

A major challenge to effective triage is that many chemical exposures do not result in immediate symptoms but rather in symptoms that may be delayed for hours or days, or result in long-term sequelae. Substances may cause both immediate and delayed symptoms, depending on level of exposure and an individual's response. Toxic decomposition and metabolic products may cause delayed problems. The thermal decomposition products of many chemicals may produce more poisonous products than the parent compound. Alternatively, some compounds undergo a metabolic process of lethal synthesis. Each exposure must be evaluated for its individual toxicity and symptom pattern.

Population Modifiers of Chemical Exposure

Certain population groups may experience more problems from chemical exposure than others (Fig. 15-1, *A* and *B*). These groups include patients with preexisting medical conditions such as cardiovascular or respiratory tract disease. These individuals are more sensitive to exposures that cause respiratory, cardiovascular, and/or neurological compromise.

The pregnant patient presents a special risk. The fetus not only is at risk from teratogenic agents but is more sensitive to poisons such as carbon monoxide (CO) and other chemical asphyxiants. CO binds tighter to fetal hemoglobin (Hgb) than it does to adult Hgb. Additionally, CO shifts the oxyhemoglobin dissociation curve to the left, thus further slowing oxygen delivery to fetal tissue from the oxygen still bound to Hgb. Other chemicals, such as chlorinated hydrocarbon solvents, that depress cardiac function may also increase fetal hypoxia.

Pediatric patients are at greater risk from hazardous materials poisoning than are adults. Toxic responses generally result from exposure to doses that are lower than in adults. Similarly, geriatric patients are at higher risk for morbidity and mortality than young, presumably healthy adult patients. Preexisting medical conditions, decreased pulmonary/cardiovascular reserve, and decreased immune system function limit physiological reserve in the elderly. Knowledge of the patient's medical history in any age group is important because many preexisting medical conditions may be aggravated by chemical exposure.

A

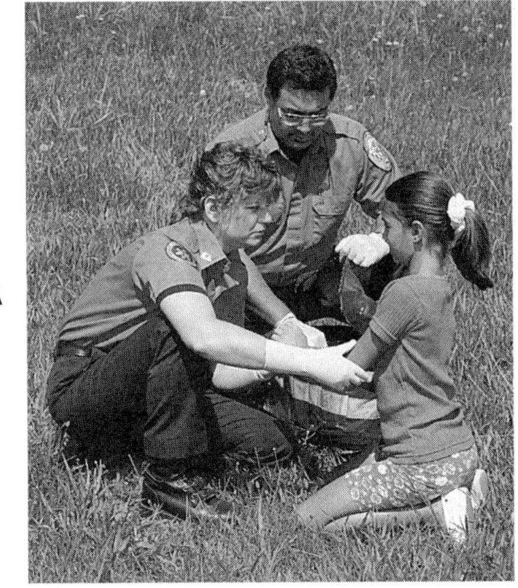

B

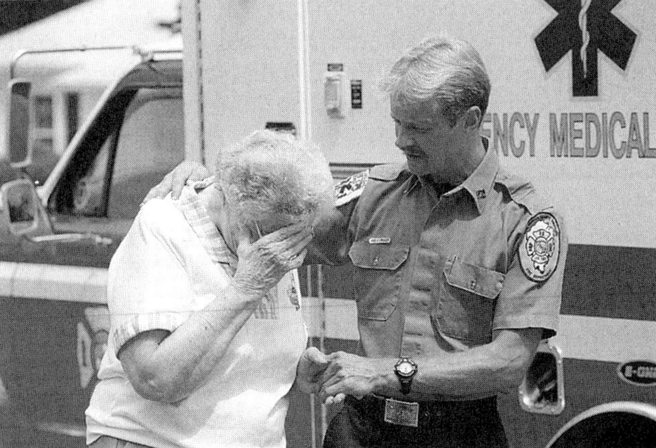

FIG. 15-1 Pediatric **(A)** and elderly **(B)** patients may be more sensitive to chemical exposure.

Standard Precautions

It is necessary that the EMS provider not only consider all of the issues just discussed when making triage decisions but also that he or she operates in an environment that follows standard precautions (body substance isolation). Not all hazardous materials accidents are chemical spills. Incidents involving biological contamination may be encountered. Accidental or intentional biological problems may arise. Patients may have preexisting infectious processes that will require implementation of standard precautions and/or other special handling techniques to prevent disease transmission (Box 15-1).

Formerly called Universal Precautions, *Standard Precautions,* or *body substance isolation guidelines,* were designed to prevent disease transmission to health care providers. The first published recommendations for isolation precautions in the United States appeared as early as 1877, when a hospital handbook recommended that pa-

BOX 15-1

Disease Transmission Prevention Techniques

Standard precautions
Airborne precautions
Droplet precautions
Contact precautions
Laboratory biosafety levels

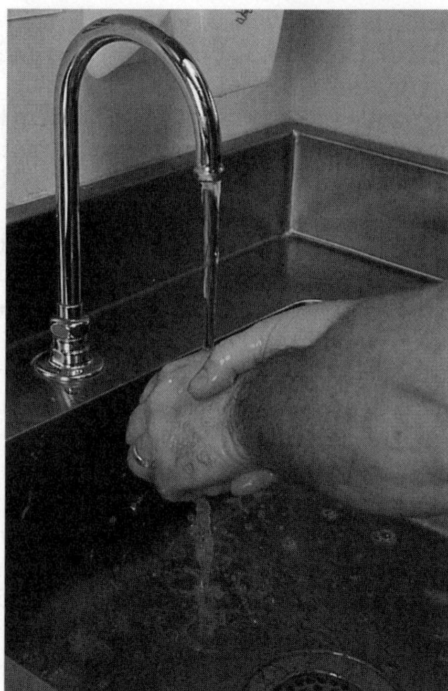

FIG. 15-2 Handwashing must be done according to strict protocols.

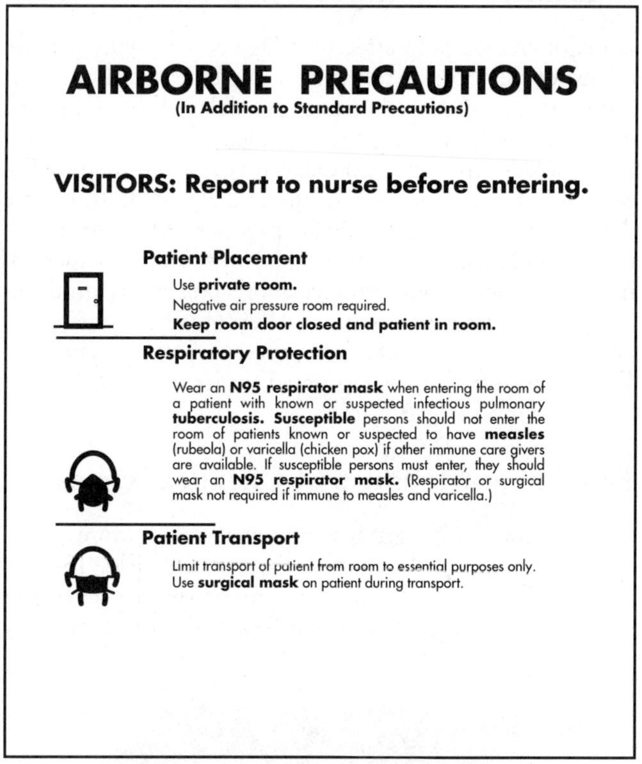

tients with infectious diseases be placed in separate facilities, which ultimately became known as infectious disease hospitals. Infection practices have been evolving ever since.

The fundamentals of standard precautions include handwashing, personal protective equipment (PPE) designed for infection control, resuscitation equipment, and safe disposal of needles and sharps. Handwashing (probably one of the most important ways to prevent the spread of infection) requires adherence to known defined protocols (Fig. 15-2). PPE includes gloves, splash-resistant and fluid-impervious gowns and protective clothing, and facial protection (surgical masks, goggles, and face shields). Use of resuscitation equipment is required to prevent direct oral contact during cardiopulmonary resuscitation. Safe procedures should be followed for the use and disposal of needles and sharps in appropriate containers to prevent exposure to human immunodeficiency virus (HIV), hepatitis B, hepatitis C, and other bloodborne pathogens.

In addition to the procedures just outlined, standard precautions can be modified for specific modes of infectious disease transmission. There are three types of specific transmission precautions: airborne, droplet, and contact.

Airborne Precautions

Airborne precautions should be used in addition to standard precautions in cases of patients known or suspected to be infected with microorganisms transmitted by airborne droplet nuclei (5 μm or smaller) (Fig. 15-3).

AIRBORNE PRECAUTIONS

(In Addition to Standard Precautions)

VISITORS: Report to nurse before entering.

Patient Placement

Use **private room.**

Negative air pressure room required.

Keep room door closed and patient in room.

Respiratory Protection

Wear an **N95 respirator mask** when entering the room of a patient with known or suspected infectious pulmonary **tuberculosis. Susceptible** persons should not enter the room of patients known or suspected to have **measles** (rubeola) or varicella (chicken pox) if other immune care givers are available. If susceptible persons must enter, they should wear an **N95 respirator mask.** (Respirator or surgical mask not required if immune to measles and varicella.)

Patient Transport

Limit transport of patient from room to essential purposes only.

Use **surgical mask** on patient during transport.

FIG. 15-3 Airborne precaution placard.

Examples of infectious diseases requiring airborne precautions include tuberculosis, measles, and varicella (including disseminated zoster).

Droplet Precautions

Standard precautions are further modified for microorganisms transmitted by droplets larger than 5 μm that can be disseminated by coughing, sneezing, talking, or while suctioning patients (Fig. 15-4). Microorganisms and diseases that can be transmitted by droplets include: *Neisseria meningitidis* (meningitis, pneumonia, and sepsis), multidrug-resistant streptococcal pneumonia, diphtheria, pertussis (whooping cough), streptococcal pharyngitis, influenza, *Mycoplasma* pneumonia, mumps, rubella, and invasive *Haemophilus influenzae* Type b, which can cause meningitis, pneumonia, epiglottitis, and sepsis. Other serious bacterial respiratory infections spread by droplet transmission include pneumonic plague streptococcal (group A) pharyngitis, pneumonia, or scarlet fever in infants and young children. Serious viral infections spread by droplet transmission include adenovirus, influenza, mumps, parvovirus B-19, and rubella.

Contact Precautions

Standard precautions may be further modified by the use contact precautions for patients known or suspected to

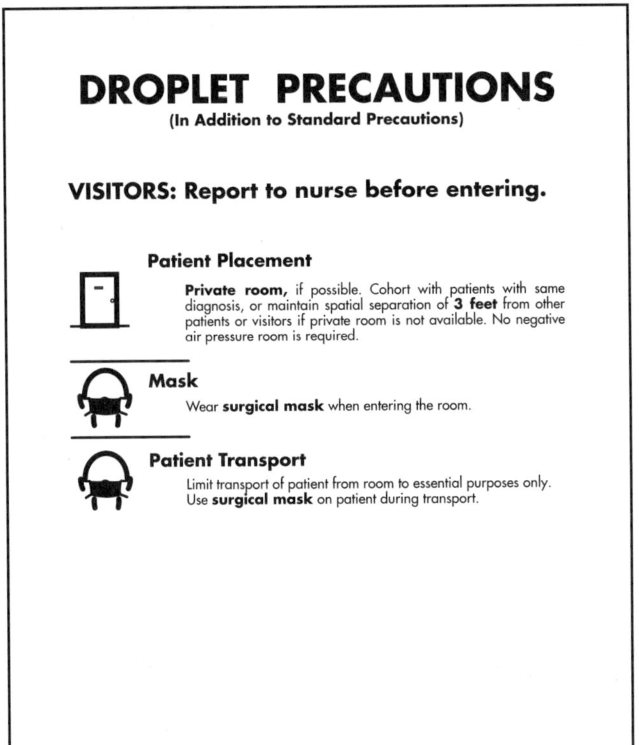

FIG. 15-4 Droplet precaution placard.

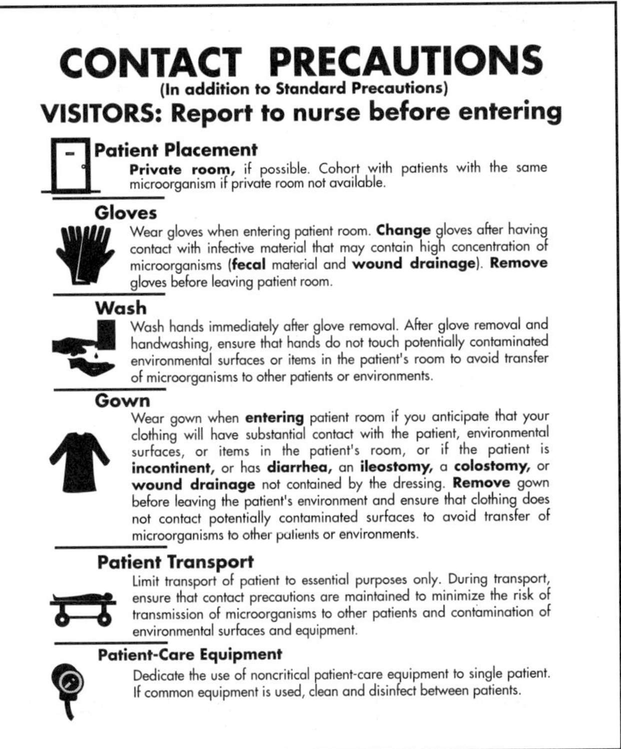

FIG. 15-5 Contact precaution placard.

have serious illnesses easily transmitted by direct patient contact (skin to skin) or by contact with items in the patient's environment (Fig. 15-5). Examples of organisms transmitted by direct contact include scabies; staphylococcal skin infections; zoster (disseminated or in the immunocompromised host); viral/hemorrhagic conjunctivitis; impetigo; enteric infections with a low infectious dose or prolonged environmental survival such as *Clostridium difficile, Escherichia coli,* and respiratory syncytial virus (RSV); parainfluenza virus; or enteroviruses. Patients with gastrointestinal, respiratory, skin, or wound infections with multidrug-resistant bacteria may present increased risk. For diapered or incontinent patients, enterohemorrhagic *Escherichia coli* O157:H7, *Shigella,* hepatitis A, or rotavirus present an infection risk.

Biological Laboratories

Four biosafety levels (BSL) are in use for microbiological and biomedical laboratories to provide increasing levels of personnel and environmental protection. BSL-1 is appropriate for working with microorganisms that are not known to cause disease in healthy humans (examples include *Bacillus subtilis* and infectious canine hepatitis virus). BSL-2 applies to agents with moderate risk to personnel and the environment. Examples of these agents include measles virus or hepatitis B virus. BSL-3 is designated for laboratories working with infectious agents that may cause serious or potentially lethal diseases as a result of inhalation exposure. BSL-3 agents include research with *Mycobacterium tuberculosis* or St. Louis encephalitis virus.

It is unlikely that you will ever encounter BSL-4 maximum containment facility biothreat agents (Boxes 15-2 to 15-4). These are the most toxic biological agents known and require the highest level of biosafety containment. These are dangerous or exotic agents that pose a high risk of life-threatening disease. They may be aerosol-transmitted laboratory infections or related agents with an unknown risk of transmission.

Consult your local medical control physician for more information on the indications and application of standard precautions, airborne, droplet, and contact precautions in your response area.

Toxidromes

A *sign* is defined as any objective evidence or manifestation of an illness or disordered body function. Signs are usually definitive, objective, and obvious. They are distinguished from the patient's impressions and complaints, which are termed *symptoms.* In contrast to signs, symptoms are usually defined as being subjective in nature. A syndrome is defined as a group of symptoms and signs of disordered function related to one another by means of some anatomical, physiological, or biochemical abnor-

BOX 15-2

Examples of Biosafety Level 4 Viral Agents

Crimean-Congo haemorrhagic fever virus
Eastern equine encephalitis virus
Ebola virus
Equine morbillivirus
Lassa fever virus
Marburg virus
Rift Valley fever virus
South American haemorrhagic fever viruses (Junin, Machupo, Sabia, Flexal, Guanarito)
Tick-borne encephalitis complex viruses
Variola major virus (smallpox virus)
Venezuelan equine encephalitis virus
Viruses causing hantavirus pulmonary syndrome
Yellow fever virus

BOX 15-3

Examples of Biosafety Level 4 Bacterial Strains

Bacillus anthracis (anthrax)
Brucella abortus, B. melitensis, B. suis
Burkholderia (Pseudomonas) mallei
Burkholderia (Pseudomonas) pseudomallei
Clostridium botulinum
Francisella tularensis
Yersinia pestis

mality. This definition does not include a precise cause of an illness but rather a reference framework for investigating the syndrome. Poisoning syndromes have come to be known as *toxicological syndromes,* or *toxidromes.* Knowledge of these poisoning symptom complexes can be helpful for the hazardous materials responder. Understanding these toxidromes can facilitate patient diagnosis and treatment. As in medical illness symptom groups, patients may not demonstrate all of the signs and symptoms of a certain hazardous materials poisoning or toxidrome at any one time. Symptoms and signs may change, with the resolution of some and the appearance of others. Diagnosis by toxidrome can be difficult because of the patient's constantly changing clinical picture. (Therefore diagnosis by toxidrome is not universally supported by all medical toxicologists.) To understand the toxidrome concept we will look at some of the more common hazardous materials toxidromes.

BOX 15-4

Examples of Biosafety Level 4 Toxins

Abrin
Aflatoxins
Botulinum toxins
Clostridium perfringens epsilon toxin
Coccidioides immitis
Conotoxins
Diacetoxyscirpenol
Ricin
Saxitoxin
Shiga toxin
Staphylococcal enterotoxins
Tetrodotoxin
T-2 toxin

BOX 15-5

SLUDGE Syndrome

*S*alivation
*L*acrimation
*U*rination
*D*efecation
*G*astrointestinal symptoms
*E*mesis

Cholinergic Poisoning (Nerve Agent Poisoning)

The cholinergic toxidrome comprises signs and symptoms that usually result from exposure to substances that cause an oversupply of the neurotransmitter acetylcholine (ACh). Nerve agents and the organophosphate and carbamate insecticides are causative agents. Based on neuroreceptor physiology, this toxidrome can be divided into muscarinic, nicotinic, and central nervous system (CNS) effects. Muscarinic effects of this toxidrome usually are remembered by the mnemonic SLUDGE (Box 15-5).

Dermal muscarinic effects usually are manifested by diaphoresis (profuse sweating). Ocular signs include small pupils (miosis), lacrimation, and blurry vision. Cardiovascular signs encompass bradycardia, hypotension, or hypertension. Pulmonary toxicity is manifested by wheezing, rales, rhonchi, and increased pulmonary secretions culminating in noncardiogenic pulmonary edema. Gastrointestinal (GI) signs and symptoms are salivation, cramps, nausea, emesis, diarrhea, involuntary defecation, and muscle spasms. Incontinence usually is observed as a sign of genitourinary effect.

Nicotinic cholinergic symptoms include muscle fasciculations, muscle cramps, weakness, muscle twitching, and paralysis of respiratory muscles (diaphragm). Excess ACh release at sympathetic ganglia include tachycardia and hypertension.

CNS effects are manifested by anxiety, restlessness, confusion, ataxia, seizures, and coma.

Anticholinergic Poisoning

The opposite of cholinergic poisoning is anticholinergic poisoning. It usually is caused by anticholinergic drugs such as the overadministration of atropine. This toxidrome also can be caused by mushroom ingestion, antihistamines, jimsonweed, phenothiazines, scopolamine, and tricyclic antidepressants. Individuals with anticholinergic poisoning usually have flushed, dry skin and dry mucous membranes. Pupils are dilated (mydriasis). CNS effects include altered mental status, psychosis, hallucinations, ataxia, and seizures. Cardiovascular system signs include tachycardia, hypertension, and cardiovascular collapse. Decreased GI motility is observed. Urinary retention also is common.

Solvent Poisoning

Hydrocarbon solvent poisonings usually present as CNS and cardiovascular toxicity. Signs of CNS toxicity include dizziness, giddiness, and euphoria. Concentration deficits, attention deficits, and altered mental status may be seen. In cases of severe exposure, CNS depression and seizures may result.

Cardiovascular signs and symptoms, including cardiac arrhythmias and sudden death resulting from nonperfusing dysrhythmias, can occur. Solvents can irritate the respiratory tract. Liver dysfunction is manifested by elevation in hepatic transaminases. Jaundice may occur. Blood coagulation problems, evidenced by elevations in prothrombin time and international normalized ratio (INR), may be present. Liver enzyme and coagulation problems usually are not seen initially but become evident after the acute presentation.

Radiation Poisoning

Radiation poisoning symptoms depend on the dose of radiation absorbed, dose rate, and individual susceptibility. The acute radiation toxidrome begins with GI signs of nausea, vomiting, intestinal cramps, diarrhea, salivation, and dehydration. CNS effects include apathy and fatigue. Cardiovascular signs include hypotension. Depending on the absorbed dose, these initial signs and symptoms may be followed by a variable latent period. The next phase focuses on the hematopoetic system, with decreases in all blood cell types. Because of GI tract poisoning, dehydration, electrolyte abnormalities, and hypovolemic shock may develop.

Biological Poisoning

Poisonings by biological agents rarely have acutely demonstrable signs or symptoms. Furthermore, signs and symptoms are almost always delayed. Once apparent, symptoms run the gamut of those seen in any infectious disease. Depending on the biological agent, signs and symptoms may include fever, cough, respiratory difficulties, fatigue, skin rash, and bleeding abnormalities. The patient with botulism may present with slow respirations and normal mental status. Usually there is a history of GI upset. The patient may complain of dry mouth and dysphagia (difficulty swallowing). Blurred vision and paralysis of eye movements, especially to the outside (abducens palsy), are highly suggestive of botulism. Eye muscle paralysis usually presents first, followed by paralysis of the extremities and respiratory muscles.

Cyanide Poisoning

Cyanide is a complex cellular poison. CNS signs include agitation, anxiety, seizures, and alterations in mental status. The respiratory rate usually is rapid initially (tachypnea), followed by apnea. Cardiovascular signs include tachycardia initially, followed by various dysrhythmais. Sinus arrhythmias may be seen. The so-called T-on-R phenomenon (progressive shortening of the ST segment until the T wave appears to originate on the R wave) also has been described.

The groups of signs and symptoms just discussed are a few examples of toxidromes. Remember that patients usually do not present with complete symptom patterns for a particular chemical agent. Sometimes a patient may have only one sign of the several that compose a toxidrome. To enhance your hazardous materials poisoning diagnostic skills, learn to categorize signs and symptoms of poisoning. The toxidrome concept may be useful as you expand your toxicological database.

Summary

The assessment and management of patients exposed to or contaminated by hazardous materials can be complicated. The materials involved, onset of symptoms, and possible clinical outcomes can present numerous variables. Standard triage and treatment procedures may need modification. Always observe standard precautions, and use the highest level of specific disease transmission prevention techniques required. Grouping signs and symptoms of poisoning from hazardous materials into toxidromes may be a useful diagnostic tool.

CHAPTER REVIEW QUESTIONS

1. Why may access to patients and treatment be delayed at a hazardous materials accident?
2. Why is it important to develop an exposure timeline for patient symptoms?

3. Is the use of a chemical's warning properties a good way to monitor scene safety?
4. Compare and contrast immediate and delayed symptoms resulting from hazardous materials poisoning.
5. Name two population modifiers of chemical exposure.
6. Define standard precautions (body substance isolation).
7. When should standard precautions be instituted?
8. Name three agents that are spread by droplet contamination.
9. Describe the organophosphate insecticide-induced toxidrome.
10. Why is trauma usually associated with hazardous materials exposure injuries?

BIBLIOGRAPHY

Aaron CK: Cyanide antidotes. In Goldfrank LR et al, editors: *Goldfrank's toxicologic emergencies,* Norwalk, Conn, 1994, Appleton & Lange.

Bronstein AC, Currance PL: *Emergency care for hazardous materials exposure,* ed 2, St. Louis, 1994, Mosby.

Ecobichon DJ: Toxic effect of pesticides. In Klaassen CD, Amdur MO, Doull J, editors: *Casarett and Doull's Toxicology: the basic science of poisons,* ed 5, New York, 1996, McGraw-Hill.

Howland MA, Aaron CK: Pralidoxime. In Goldfrank LR et al, editors: *Goldfrank's toxicologic emergencies,* Norwalk, Conn, 1994, Appleton & Lange.

Howland MA: Ethanol. In Goldfrank LR et al, editors: *Goldfrank's toxicologic emergencies,* Norwalk, Conn, 1994, Appleton & Lange.

Smith EA, Oehme FW: A review of selected herbicides and their toxicities, *Vet Hum Toxicol* 33:596-608, 1991.

16

Treatment of Hazardous Materials Poisoning

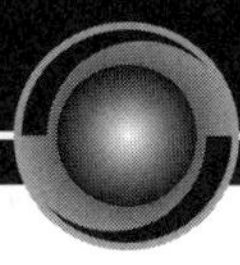

Alvin C. Bronstein, M.D., FACEP

CHAPTER OBJECTIVES

At the conclusion of this chapter the student will be able to:

- Discuss the treatment approach to hazardous materials poisoning victims.
- Discuss cardiac treatment protocols for hazardous materials exposure victims.
- Describe the mechanism of injury of pulmonary edema.
- Describe the treatment for hypovolemic shock.
- Describe the signs and symptoms of noncardiogenic pulmonary edema.

CASE STUDY

A 42-year-old male truck driver is brought to the emergency department by ambulance. He was driving a chemical tanker truck, which slid off the interstate. The truck was leaking a liquid material, and the paramedics reported a strong gasoline-like odor at the scene. The patient was not decontaminated. An intravenous line of normal saline was started at a rate of 50 cc/hour. Oxygen via nasal cannula had been started in the field. No signs of trauma were found. His pulse was 100 by palpation and irregular. An electrocardiogram (ECG) rhythm strip revealed a sinus tachycardia with multifocal premature ventricular contractions (PVCs).

- ◆ What is the most likely cause of the driver's PVCs?
- ◆ What is the most appropriate treatment for the PVCs?
- ◆ What other injuries should be considered?
- ◆ What is the potential for delayed health effects?

This case illustrates a hazardous materials poisoning victim with cardiac effects secondary to hydrocarbon exposure. Other than decontamination, which was not done in the field, basic cardiac care protocols are followed. Most cardiac problems are treated by following current Advanced Cardiac Life Support (ACLS) protocols. However, knowledge of the toxic agent is necessary because special conditions may apply to exposure from certain poisons, possibly changing normal care patterns. For example, most texts advise not using epinephrine for patients exposed to hydrocarbon solvents.

Most hazardous materials poisoning victims require standard supportive care measures. Sometimes these protocols must be adjusted for the specific toxic agent. This chapter outlines major treatment approaches. These approaches may need to be modified to fit your community standards. Baseline emergency laboratory studies also are presented.

Cardiac Treatment Protocols/ACLS Algorithms

The new ACLS algorithms are reprinted in Appendix 1 of this textbook to guide cardiac management decisions. Specific information for chemically induced pulmonary edema and shock conditions should be established by your local medical control physician.

Pulmonary Edema

Mechanism of Injury

Pulmonary edema is caused by fluid leaking into the alveoli from the pulmonary capillaries. It can be caused by various mechanisms, including circulatory overload, cardiac failure, and toxic inhalation. Toxic inhalation can cause either cardiac failure or direct damage to the alveolar basement membranes (noncardiogenic pulmonary edema [NCPE]). It is important to distinguish between cardiac and NCPE to be able to determine proper treatment. The lungs normally contain 20% water by weight. With acute pulmonary edema, fluid content can reach 1000 times normal. Acute pulmonary edema usually has a rapid onset. Toxic exposures may exhibit a delayed onset, from hours to 3 days, of pulmonary edema.

Cardiovascular signs and symptoms may include increased heart rate and jugular venous distention. Respiratory examination may reveal dyspnea; cough; Cheyne-Stokes respirations; orthopnea; moist breath sounds (rales and rhonchi); and in severe cases, pink, blood-tinged, frothy sputum. Central nervous system (CNS) findings include anxiety, decreased level of consciousness, and coma.

Basic treatment starts with ensuring an open airway, with suctioning as necessary. Respiratory support is vital. Administer oxygen by nonrebreather mask at 10 to 15 L/min. If possible, place the patient in a sitting position to increase gas exchange. Place arms and legs in a dependent position, if possible.

Advanced treatment may involve orotracheal or nasotracheal intubation for airway control. Positive end-expiratory pressure (PEEP) ventilation may be necessary to overcome increased pulmonary resistance. Cardiac rhythm should be monitored. Treat arrhythmias as necessary according to appropriate ACLS protocol. In some cases, furosemide (Lasix) to decrease fluid preload may be used. Inhaled metaproterenol sulfate (Alupent) or intravenous aminophylline may be used to decrease reversible bronchospasm if wheezes are present. Morphine sulfate is not indicated in cases of NCPE. Administration of corticosteroids for NCPE is controversial. Recent studies have demonstrated increased benefit from early steroid administration. Specific field treatment guidelines should be developed by your medical control director.

Shock

Acute poisoning can cause four different types of shock states: hypovolemic, cardiogenic, vasogenic, and anaphylactic or anaphylactoid reactions. Hypovolemic and cardiogenic shock are the most frequent types encountered after toxic exposures. It is helpful to differentiate among these shock types so that optimal treatment can be achieved.

Hypovolemic

Mechanism of injury

Chemical exposure may cause increased permeability of the blood vessel walls, with leakage of plasma (water) out of the vascular system and across cell membranes, resulting in hypovolemia. Hemorrhagic shock from trauma may be an associated finding.

Cardiovascular signs and symptoms include tachycardia (usually the heart rate is greater than 120 beats/minute [bpm]). The pulse usually is weak. Occasionally, bradycardia or a normal pulse rate may be observed. Blood pressure typically is less than 90 mm Hg systolic, with decreased jugular venous pressure. Positive orthostatic changes are present (pulse rate increase of 20 or more, or a blood pressure decrease of 20 mm Hg or more, or a combination of 20 or more when the patient is moved from the supine to the standing position). Respiratory findings usually will show an increased rate, with shallow respirations. CNS findings of anxiety, restlessness, or confusion may be observed. These findings may lead to a decreased level of consciousness, progressing to coma. The skin will be pale, diaphoretic, and cool or, in cases of dehydration, warm and dry.

Basic treatment involves establishing airway control. Maintain an open airway and support ventilation as necessary. Administer oxygen by nonrebreather mask at 10 to 15 L/min. Control any external bleeding. Elevate the legs 10 to 12 inches. Splint any obvious fractures. Maintain body temperature. Monitor and record vital signs every 5 minutes.

Advanced treatment may involve orotracheal or nasotracheal intubation for adequate airway control. Start an intravenous (IV) line of either lactated Ringer's (LR) or normal saline (NS). Administer a fluid bolus of 250 to 500 mL in the adult patient (20 mL/kg in the pediatric patient). Fluid boluses may be repeated up to three times in the field unless otherwise directed by medical control. Titrate the IV infusion rate to maintain an adequate blood pressure.

Special considerations

The use of the pneumatic antishock garment (PASG) is controversial. Application of the PASG may be useful in certain circumstances. Indications for use should be developed in consultation with your local medical advisor. Hypotension is a late sign. Be prepared to institute treatment before the blood pressure falls. After IV fluids are started during initial resuscitation efforts, watch for signs of fluid overload and cerebral and/or pulmonary edema. Elderly patients and patients with chronic hypertension may be hypovolemic, with vital signs that appear normal. Cardiac tamponade and tension pneumothorax may coexist with hypovolemic shock, especially with trauma. Rapid transport to an appropriate treatment center is essential. Do not waste time at the scene.

Cardiogenic

Mechanism of injury

Chemical agents can impair the cardiovascular system by direct cardiotoxicity, reducing cardiac output. Many types of cardiac problems, including electrical conduction deficits and loss of contractility, may be seen.

Cardiovascular signs and symptoms may include chest pain or a heavy pressure sensation in the chest. The systolic blood pressure will be less than 90 mm Hg. The pulse rate may be normal, fast, or slow, and may be irregular. Jugular venous pressure is increased but may be normal initially. The respiratory rate will be increased, with shallow respirations. Signs of pulmonary edema may be present. As in hypovolemic shock, CNS findings of anxiety, restlessness, confusion, decreased level of consciousness, and/or coma may be present. The skin may be cyanotic, cool, and diaphoretic.

Basic treatment starts with ensuring an open airway. Support ventilation as necessary. Administer oxygen by nonrebreather mask at 10 to 15 L/min. Keep the patient as quiet as possible. Position for comfort as necessary.

Advanced treatment may involve orotracheal or nasotracheal intubation for airway control. Monitor the cardiac rhythm, and treat arrhythmias as necessary according to appropriate ACLS protocol. Start an IV infusion of 5% dextrose in water (D_5W) at a keep-open rate. Vasopressors may be necessary. Norepinephrine (Levophed) or dopamine (Intropin) are two commonly used vasopressors. The adult dosage for norepinephrine infusion is 0.5 to 30 μg/min. Dopamine is administered at an adult dosage of 2.5 to 20 μg/kg/min. Titrate the agent chosen to a systolic blood pressure of 90 to 100 mm Hg. Vasopressor use should be governed by your local medical control physician. Treat symptoms of pulmonary edema as necessary. If signs of hypovolemia are present, use a cautious fluid challenge of 250 mL NS or LR.

Anaphylaxis and Anaphylactoid Reactions

Mechanism of injury

In severe allergic reactions to a foreign substance, the body releases histamine and other chemical mediators of anaphylaxis. These are termed *Type 1 allergic reactions* and require that the individual first be sensitized to the hazardous material from a previous exposure. An anaphylactic reaction may manifest by bronchial spasm, dilation of peripheral blood vessels, and alterations in the permeability of the cell membranes, allowing fluid to leak from the vascular space into the interstitial spaces.

Anaphylactoid reactions have identical clinical presentations but differ in that no prior exposure or sensitization to the offending agent is required to produce the allergic-type phenomenon. Sulfite exposure is a classic example of an agent that can cause an anaphylactoid reaction.

Cardiovascular signs and symptoms usually include an increased pulse rate, with a systolic blood pressure of less than 90 mm Hg systolic. The patient may complain of a tight feeling in the chest. Respiratory findings of dyspnea and diffuse wheezing usually will be present. Cough and stridor, which indicate an upper airway obstruction caused by soft tissue swelling, may be observed. The patient usually will experience CNS involvement, including headache, anxiety, and restlessness. Because of the potential for rapid respiratory compromise, be alert for a rapidly decreasing level of consciousness, leading to coma. Facial edema and a flushed appearance with a hivelike rash, redness, and itching may be seen.

Basic treatment starts with maintaining an open airway. Support ventilation as necessary. Administer oxygen by nonrebreather mask at 10 to 15 L/min.

Advanced treatment may involve orotracheal or nasotracheal intubation for airway control. Be alert for signs of airway obstruction. Intubation may be necessary. Monitor the cardiac rhythm, and treat arrhythmias according to ACLS protocols. Start an IV infusion of LR or NS at a keep-open rate. Epinephrine is the drug of choice. The adult dosage is 0.3 mg of a 1:1000 dilution subcutaneously (SQ). If symptoms are severe, give 0.1 to 0.5 mg (usually 0.3 mg in the adult) of 1:10,000 dilution IV push. This should be done under direct physician order or standing order protocol. Consider the use of inhaled metaproterenol sulfate (Alupent) to decrease reversible bronchospasm. The adult dosage is one unit-dose vial of 0.6% via nebulizer by direct physician order. Corticosteroids such as hydrocortisone, Benadryl (diphenhydramine), cimetidine, and/or aminophylline may be used to reverse the anaphylaxis or anaphylactoid symptoms.

Special considerations

Rapid transport is essential. Use epinephrine with caution in children and elderly patients.

Vasogenic

Mechanism of injury

Chemical agents may cause a defect in the responsiveness of vascular smooth muscles to neural or hormonal stimuli, or depress vasomotor center activity in the brainstem. In either case, widespread vasodilation without primary loss of volume causes hypotension.

Cardiovascular signs and symptoms usually include a pulse rate that is greater than 120 bpm and weak. Bradycardia or a normal pulse rate also is possible. The blood pressure may be greater than 90 mm Hg systolic, and jugular venous pressure is decreased. Positive orthostatic changes usually are present. The respiratory rate usually will be increased. Respirations usually will be shallow. CNS findings of anxiety, restlessness, confusion, decreased level of consciousness, and rapid progression to coma may be observed. The skin will be warm and dry. Sometimes, flushing (redness) will be present. Hives (urticaria) also may be seen.

Basic treatment starts with ensuring an open airway. Support ventilation as necessary. Administer oxygen by nonrebreather mask at 10 to 15 L/min. Elevate the legs 6 to 12 inches.

Advanced treatment may involve orotracheal or nasotracheal intubation for airway control. Start an IV infusion of NS or LR at a keep-open rate. If a vasopressor is indicated, administer dopamine or norepinephrine. Dopamine is administered at an adult dosage of 2.5 to 20 μg/kg/min. Norepinephrine is administered at an adult dosage of 0.5 to 30 μg/min. Titrate to a systolic blood pressure of 90 to 100 mm Hg.

Special considerations

Rapid transportation to a medical facility is essential. Do not delay at the scene.

Seizures

Mechanism of Injury

Many metabolic disturbances may result from toxic exposures. These derangements may include hypocapnia, cerebral anoxia, water intoxication, and hypoglycemia. Seizures may result from any of these abnormalities. Certain compounds, such as hydrocarbon solvents, picrotoxin, pentylenetetrazol, camphor, DDT, chlorinated insecticides, parathion and other organophosphates, and fluoroacetates may cause seizures.

Any type of seizure presentation is possible; focal or grand mal seizures and/or status epilepticus are possible. Seizure activity may be associated with increased temperature, fractures, or dislocations. Trauma to the tongue and incontinence of urine and stool may occur.

Basic treatment starts with ensuring an open airway. Support ventilation as necessary. Administer oxygen by nonrebreather mask at 10 to 15 L/min. Do not force anything between the teeth. Protect the patient from injury. Do not restrain or attempt to mechanically stop seizure motor activity. Time the duration of the seizure. Be alert for repeat seizure activity. Reassess the patient after the seizure has ended.

Advanced treatment may involve orotracheal or nasotracheal intubation for airway control in the unconscious patient or patient with status epilepticus (continuous seizure activity). Monitor the cardiac rhythm, and treat arrhythmias according to ACLS protocol. Start an IV infusion of LR or NS at a keep-open rate. Blood may be drawn for later laboratory analysis. Monitor for signs of hypoglycemia (decreased level of consciousness, tachycardia, pallor, dilated pupils, and diaphoresis). If available, perform a dextrose stick analysis. If signs of hypoglycemia and/or low blood glucose (<50 mg/dL) are found, administer 50% dextrose, if necessary. Obtain a blood sample for glucose determination before dextrose administration. The adult dosage for dextrose is 25 g IV push. In the adult patient, if he or she is actively convulsing, administer diazepam (Valium) 2 to 10 mg in 2-mg increments by slow IV push, or lorazepam (Ativan) 4 to 8 mg in 2-mg increments by slow IV push.

Special Considerations

Diazepam and lorazepam may depress respiratory drive; therefore, be prepared to assist respirations. Reduce external stimuli as much as possible.

Chemical Burns

Mechanism of Injury

Various chemicals and corrosives (acids and alkalis) can cause tissue damage ranging from skin irritation to severe burns. Depending on concentration and other factors, the liquefaction necrosis effect of alkalis generally produces more tissue damage than do acids. Hydrofluoric (HF) acid is an exception.

Dermal signs and symptoms of exposure include irritation, redness, and vesicle formation. Partial or full-thickness burns may result. Some chemicals (e.g., HF acid) may penetrate into deep tissues. Soft-tissue damage, down to and including bone, may occur with severe exposures.

Basic treatment starts with ensuring that the patient is properly decontaminated. All clothing, shoes, and jewelry should be removed. The patient should have been decontaminated with soap and water. Ensure an open airway, and support respirations as necessary. Check for singed nasal hair, the presence of carbon particles, or oral burns. Administer oxygen at 10 to 15 L/min. by nonrebreather mask. Assess and treat any other injuries.

An estimation of the extent of burned body surface area is necessary to provide appropriate fluid resuscitation. Two systems in use provide a way to quickly estimate the extent of the burned area. These systems are as follows:

- Rule of Nines: The body surface is divided into 11 areas, each containing 9% or multiples of 9%. The perineum is counted as 1% (Fig. 16-1).
- Lund-Browder Classification: The body surface is mapped, and percentages are attached to the various areas. The body surface map corrects for the patient's age (Fig. 16-2).

Burned areas should be covered with dry, sterile dressings. Maintain body temperature with blankets. Do not apply external heat. Evaluate for possible systemic toxicity caused by absorption of the hazardous material.

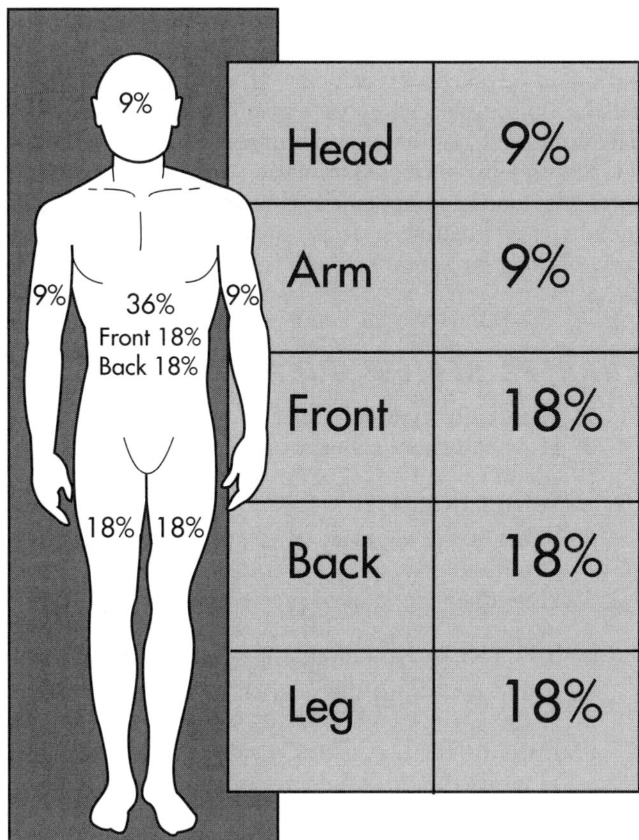

FIG. 16-1 Rule of Nines.

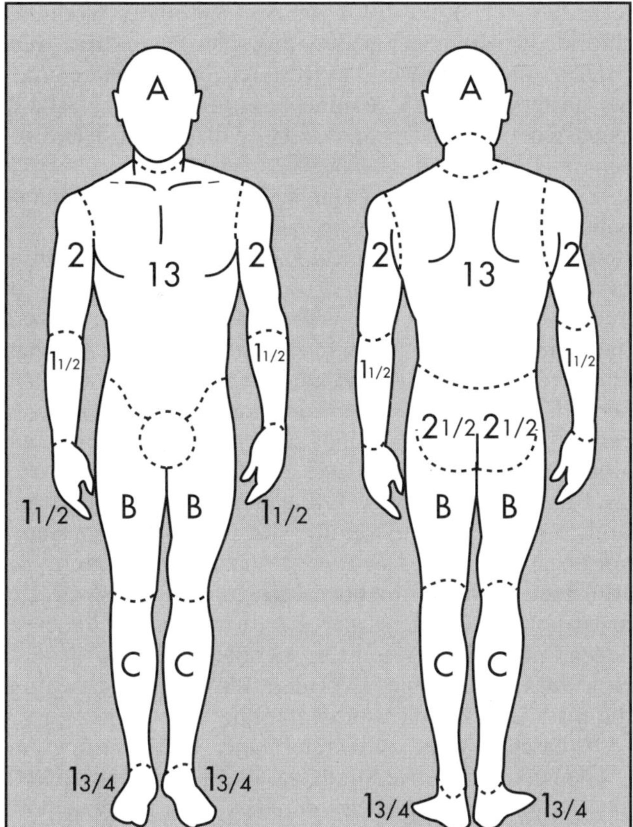

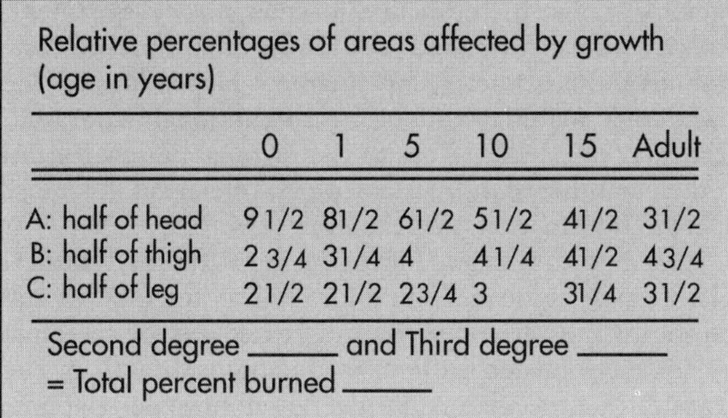

Relative percentages of areas affected by growth (age in years)

	0	1	5	10	15	Adult
A: half of head	9 1/2	8 1/2	6 1/2	5 1/2	4 1/2	3 1/2
B: half of thigh	2 3/4	3 1/4	4	4 1/4	4 1/2	4 3/4
C: half of leg	2 1/2	2 1/2	2 3/4	3	3 1/4	3 1/2

Second degree _____ and Third degree _____
= Total percent burned _____

FIG. 16-2 Lund-Brower Classification.

Advanced treatment may involve orotracheal or nasotracheal intubation at the first indication of stridor or respiratory distress. Start an IV infusion of LR or NS initially at a keep-open rate. Depending on the surface area, size of the burn, and hemodynamic state of the patient, administer fluids according to the Parkland formula (4 mL/kg/% body surface burn) according to medical control direction. Typically, half of the total fluid requirement is replaced in the first 8 hours. One fourth is given over the next 8 hours, and the final fourth is given in the third 8-hour period. Of course, when possible, fluid replacement is guided by urine output and other clinical parameters.

If no respiratory distress or trauma is present, then consider the administration of morphine sulfate as an analgesic. The adult dosage for morphine sulfate is 2 to 5 mg slow IV push and titrate to symptom improvement. Administer this drug with a direct physician order only.

Special Considerations

Use calcium gluconate gel to treat minor HF acid burns. Embedded fragments of water-reactive metals, such as sodium, lithium, or magnesium, may be covered by a light cooking oil to help reduce possible tissue reaction. Embedded fragments of phosphorus should be immersed in water or covered with moist, sterile dressings during transport. Do not use any topical antibiotic or anesthetic ointments on the burned area. The routine use of prophylactic antibiotics is not recommended.

Emergency Department Initial Laboratory Considerations

Once the patient arrives in the emergency department, baseline laboratory studies should be obtained. It is not possible to get all necessary laboratory tests, but a basic panel merits consideration. These studies include a complete blood count (CBC); serum electrolytes (sodium, chloride, bicarbonate, potassium); blood urea nitrogen (BUN); blood glucose; the liver enzymes aspartate aminotransferase (AST), alanine aminotransferase (ALT), gama-glutamyl transpeptidase (GGT), lactate dehydrogenase (LDH), and alkaline phosphatase (AP).

The anion gap is a useful measure in cases of metabolic acidosis and should be calculated based on the serum electrolytes. The osmolal gap (useful in ethylene glycol and methanol poisoning) also may be computed, if indicated. A urinalysis should be obtained. Depending on the patient's clinical presentation, other blood tests, such as arterial blood gases and carboxyhemoglobin, may be needed. In cases of suspected organophosphate or carbamate pesticide poisoning, determination of the red blood cell cholinesterase level and plasma cholinesterase level usually is necessary. Other useful tests include coagulation studies and serum calcium and magnesium. Poison-specific blood or urine tests are rarely helpful or available in a timely manner. Exceptions to this rule are methanol and ethylene glycol measurements. However, depending on local resources, these tests may not have a rapid turnaround time. Treatment must still be based on the history and clinical presentation.

A baseline chest radiograph and electrocardiogram (ECG) usually are needed. Serial ECGs may be required in cases of cardiac toxicity or chest trauma. Peak flow measurements can be a useful adjunct in assessing pulmonary status. In the field and emergency department, the patient can be placed on a cardiac monitor and continuous pulse oximetry implemented. Depending on the hazardous material in question, additional laboratory tests may be needed. Consult the regional poison control center or other standard toxicology references for more specific information on laboratory testing.

Laboratory tests only reveal part of the total clinical picture and are no substitute for clinical judgment. Each poisoning must be evaluated and treated case by case. Just as not all poisoned patients will demonstrate all of the features of a specific toxidrome, not all poisoned patients will require every laboratory test just listed.

Summary

Victims of hazardous materials poisoning may require basic and advanced life support procedures. Depending on the poison, special considerations may be necessary. Treatment of cardiac arrhythmias follows standard ACLS guidelines. Decontamination and treatment measures may need to happen simultaneously. Above all, remember that treatment decisions are based on the history, clinical presentation, and specific toxicity of the poison.

CHAPTER REVIEW QUESTIONS

1. Name four types of shock.
2. How can chemical exposure cause pulmonary edema?
3. What is NCPE?
4. What is the mainstay of treatment for most hazardous materials poisoning victims?
5. How does the clinical presentation of an anaphylactoid reaction differ from anaphylaxis?
6. Name three compounds that cause seizures.
7. Name two drugs that can be used to treat seizures.
8. Describe the use of the Lund-Browder chart.
9. What is the drug therapy for minor HF acid burns?
10. Name three symptoms of acute pulmonary edema.

BIBLIOGRAPHY

Bronstein AC, Currance PL: *Emergency care for hazardous materials exposure,* ed 2, St. Louis, 1994, Mosby.

Meduri GU et al: Effect of prolonged methylprednisolone therapy in unresolving acute respiratory distress syndrome: a randomized controlled trial, *JAMA* 280:159-165, 1998.

Sanchez MR: Dermatologic principles. In Goldfrank LR et al, editors: *Goldfrank's toxicologic emergencies,* Norwalk, Conn, 1994, Appleton & Lange.

Witschi HR, Last JA: Toxic responses of the respiratory system. In Klaassen CD, Amdur MO, Doull J, editors: *Casarett and Doull's Toxicology: the basic science of poisons,* ed 5, New York, 1996, McGraw-Hill.

17

Antidotes for Hazardous Materials Poisoning

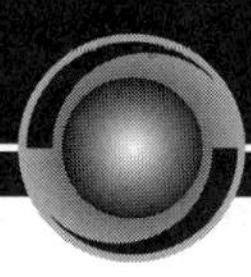

Alvin C. Bronstein, M.D., FACEP

CHAPTER OBJECTIVES

At the conclusion of this chapter the student will be able to:

- List the major antidotes used for hazardous materials poisoning.
- Describe the treatment for organophosphate poisoning.
- Discuss the use of methylene blue for the treatment of methemoglobinemia.
- Describe the treatment for cyanide poisoning.
- Discuss the use of activated charcoal.

CASE STUDY

The emergency department of a hospital in a small Kentucky town receives a call from the state patrol. Four employees have been injured in an explosion at a local extermination company. They are covered in an unpleasant-smelling hydrocarbon-like fluid. One employee is unconscious after having a seizure. Although he is given 2 mg of intravenous atropine, he experiences a respiratory arrest. The other three employees are disoriented and sweating profusely. The trooper reads the label from a spilled container. It states, "Parathion." Additional Emergency Medical Services (EMS) personnel arrive and administer 4 mg of atropine to the unconscious victim, exhausting the second unit's supply.

- ◆ Would your hospital have the proper antidotes to treat these patients?
- ◆ Would your hospital have enough of the needed antidotes?
- ◆ What antidotes are valuable for field use?
- ◆ What are adequate antidote inventories?

A quick check of the hospital pharmacy reveals only 16 0.4-mg doses of atropine and no multidose atropine vials in stock. Six 1-gram vials of pralidoxime (2PAM) are available.

The organophosphate poisoning victim with mild to moderate symptoms will require a minimum of 2 mg of atropine intravenously initially and approximately 25 mg over a 24-hour period. This patient also will need at least 6 g of pralidoxime over the first 24 hours. Studies show that hospitals have limited stockpiles of these physiological antagonists. In one study of 16 hospitals in the metropolitan Denver area, sufficient atropine was available to treat 343 patients but only enough pralidoxime for 11 patients. To mount a credible hazardous materials response, adequate antidote stockpiles must be available.

Treating patients who develop toxicity from exposure to hazardous materials presents a continuing challenge. Very few specific antidotes or physiological antagonists are available. The cornerstone of treatment is prompt supportive care. The case just presented reminds us that even though the appropriate antidote (atropine) was used, unless respiratory support is achieved, adverse events can occur. Remember that atropine will stop pulmonary secretions but not prevent fatigue of the diaphragm and respiratory arrest. Reliance on antidotes alone is not enough to treat the patient. Adequate supportive care dictated by clinical signs and symptoms is necessary.

Keeping an adequate inventory of the antidotes needed for mass disasters is a major problem for all hospitals, regardless of size. Several studies have shown that no one hospital has enough of any one antidote to treat large numbers of victims or enough for a few severely poisoned patients. This chapter reviews the major antidotes for hazardous materials and summarize their actions and uses.

We will begin with the drugs atropine and pralidoxime, which are used for insecticides, such as organophosphates and carbamates, and the cholinergic nerve agents tabun (GA), sarin (GB), soman (GD), and VX. These poisons work by inhibiting acetylcholinesterase (AChE). This enzyme is ubiquitous throughout the body. It is found at the nerve endings to exocrine glands and smooth and cardiac muscle. Poisoning by these compounds results in the accumulation of acetylcholine (ACh) at muscarinic, nicotinic, and central nervous system (CNS) synapses. Antidotal therapy uses drugs that can reverse this ACh accumulation.

ATROPINE

Major Actions

Atropine is an antimuscarinic agent, which blocks parasympathetic muscarinic receptor sites and inhibits ACh at postganglionic cholinergic sites. It blocks cholinergic-mediated neuromuscular junctions. Atropine competitively antagonizes ACh at postsynaptic parasympathetic sites.

Major cardiac effects of atropine are that it increases heart rate by blocking vagal stimulation and increases conduction through the atrioventricular (AV) node. It reduces tone and motility of the gastrointestinal (GI) tract. Atropine inhibits exocrine gland secretion (salivary, bronchial, and sweat), and it dilates pupils (mydriasis).

Indications

Atropine is used to treat sinus bradycardia or ventricular rates with concomitant hypotension. Additional indications include asystole and high-degree atrioventricular (AV) blocks with slow ventricular rates. Atropine also is a specific physiological antagonist for poisoning from toxic exposures to organophosphates, carbamates, and nerve agents.

Adult Dosage

Cardiac arrhythmias: 0.5 to 1 mg slow IV push, repeat every 3 to 5 minutes as needed, up to a maximum of 0.03 to 0.04 mg/kg. A total dose of 3 mg (0.04 mg/kg) results in full vagal blockade (cardiac) in humans. In asystole, a 1-mg bolus should be given initially and repeated in 3 to 5 minutes.

Pediatric Dosage

Cardiac arrhythmias: 0.02 mg/kg slow IV push, with a minimum dose of 0.1 mg and a maximum single dose of 0.5 mg in a child and 1 mg in an adolescent. The dose may be repeated in 5 minutes, to a maximum total dose of 1 mg in a child and 2 mg in an adolescent.

Adult Dosage

Symptomatic toxic exposure to organophosphates, carbamates, or acetylcholinesterase poisoning from nerve agents (GA, GB, GD, and VX): Administer an initial dose of 2 mg slow IV push. Repeat this dose every 3 to 5 minutes as needed. Atropine should be given until the lungs are clear to auscultation.

Pediatric Dosage

Symptomatic toxic exposure to organophosphates, carbamates, or similar-acting nerve agents: Administer an initial dose of 0.05 mg/kg slow IV push up to a maximum of 2 mg. Repeat this dose (0.05 mg/kg, maximum of 2 mg) every 3 to 5 minutes as needed. Atropine should be given until the lungs are clear to auscultation.

NOTE: The initial atropine dose may be given intramuscularly (IM) or via endotracheal (ET) tube followed by 3 to 4 rapid ventilations to disperse the drug, since the required dose may be very large; switch to the IV route as soon as possible.

For severely poisoned patients, a continuous infusion at 0.02 to 0.08 mg/kg/hour may be required.

Precautions

Severely poisoned patients are relatively atropine resistant. They do not respond to the drug as do patients with cardiac instability. *Massive amounts may be necessary.* Adequate oxygenation and ventilation should be assessed before atropine administration. Smaller doses of atropine may produce paradoxical bradycardia.

Do not treat bradycardia (heart rate <60) unless signs of inadequate perfusion (hypotension) are present. In acute myocardial infarction, infarct size may be enlarged by increasing myocardial oxygen demand.

Atropine increases intraocular pressure and dilates the pupil. Its use therefore is contraindicated in individuals who demonstrate increased intraocular pressure.

Use with caution in patients with hepatic or renal insufficiency. In children younger than 2 years and the elderly, atropine's half-life is prolonged. If large doses are necessary, preservative-free preparations should be used to prevent benzyl alcohol or chlorobutanol poisoning.

How Supplied

Atropine sulfate

- 1 mg/10 mL preloaded syringes (0.1 mg/mL)
- 0.5 mg/5 mL preloaded syringes (0.1 mg/mL)
- 1 mg/1 mL ampule (1 mg/mL)
- Multidose vials of 8 mg/20 mL (0.4 mg/mL)
- Autoinjector of 2 mg for IM use. Adult use only.

Pharmacy Stocking Recommendations

For each 70-kg patient: 20 mg

PRALIDOXIME CHLORIDE (PROTOPAM CHLORIDE, 2PAM CHLORIDE, 2-PYRIDINE ALDOXIME METHOCHLORIDE)

Major Actions

Pralidoxime is a quaternary ammonium oxime acting as a cholinesterase reactivator. It binds with the organophosphate (OP) bound to the acetylcholinesterase, removing it from the enzyme and thus restoring cholinesterase function. Unlike atropine, which only acts to block muscarinic receptor sites, pralidoxime acts at nicotinic *and* muscarinic cholinergic receptor sites. Pralidoxime is synergistic with atropine. Regeneration of nicotinic sites at the diaphragm stops paralysis of the respiratory muscles. Optimally, pralidoxime should be administered as soon as possible preferably within the first 24 hours, after cholinesterase poisoning. After 24 hours of exposure, the enzyme-OP complex undergoes covalent bonding, or "aging." In cases of nerve agent exposure this "aging" process may occur in minutes. Once covalent bonding occurs, the cholinesterase moiety is irreversibly inactivated by the OP. In symptomatic patients, consider pralidoxime administration even 48 hours or longer after exposure. Because it is relatively slow acting, pralidoxime must be used in conjunction with atropine.

Indications

Pralidoxime is indicated for the treatment of poisoning caused by pesticides and chemicals of the organophosphate class that have anticholinesterase activity. Organophosphate insecticides are thought to cause irreversible inactivation of acetylcholinesterase enzymes, whereas insecticides of the carbamate class cause reversible enzyme binding. For this reason, use of pralidoxime in carbamate poisoning is debated. Often quoted is pralidoxime's controversial use for poisoning with carbaryl (Sevin), a carbamate insecticide. Most authorities agree that regardless of the theoretical considerations, if symptoms are severe from carbamate poisoning, pralidoxime may be indicated. Pralidoxime is administered by direct physician order only.

Adult Dosage

Administer 1 to 2 g of pralidoxime chloride IV drip in 100 mL of normal saline (NS) over 15 to 30 minutes. The dose may be repeated in 1 hour if symptoms are still present. The dose can then be repeated every 6 to 8 hours as necessary for 24 to 48 hours. Symptomatic patients may require extended treatment after 48 hours.

Pediatric Dosage

The dose is 20 to 40 mg/kg to a maximum dose of 1 g of pralidoxime chloride IV drip in a 5% solution of NS over 15 to 30 minutes. The dose may be repeated in 1 hour if symptoms are still present. The dose can then be repeated every 6 to 8 hours as necessary for 24 to 48 hours. Symptomatic patients may require extended treatment after 48 hours.

If nicotinic effects persist, a continuous infusion of 2.5% pralidoxime in NS may be used. The adult dose is 500 mg/hr. The pediatric dose is 9 to 19 mg/kg/hr (do not exceed 500 mg/hr). Continuous infusion may be more beneficial than repetitive, single-dose therapy. The clinical response determines the treatment end point.

Precautions

Tachycardia, laryngospasm, and muscle rigidity have been reported from a too-rapid infusion rate. Dizziness, blurred vision, diplopia, headache, drowsiness, nausea, hyperventilation, and muscle weakness also have been observed. Give cautiously to patients with impaired renal function. Use pralidoxime chloride with caution when treating organophosphate overdose in cases of myasthenia gravis because it may precipitate a myasthenic crisis.

Atropine and pralidoxime chloride are synergistic and should be used together. With concomitant use of 2PAM, the signs of atropinization may occur earlier than might be expected when atropine is used alone.

Pralidoxime chloride is not effective in the treatment of poisoning caused by phosphorus, inorganic phosphates, or organophosphates not having anticholinesterase activity. Pralidoxime chloride generally is not recommended for treatment of intoxication from the carbamate class of insecticides, especially carbaryl, unless poisoning symptoms are severe. The carbamate/cholinesterase bond is not permanent and will allow the cholinesterase to reactivate spontaneously.

How Supplied

- ◆ 20-mL vial containing 1 g of sterile pralidoxime chloride (white to off-white porous cake) and one 20-mL ampule of sterile water for injection to be used as a diluent
- ◆ Autoinjector of 600 mg for IM use. Adult use only

Stocking Recommendations

For each 70-kg patient: 6 g

ATROPINE AND PRALIDOXIME AUTOINJECTORS

Both atropine and pralidoxime are issued to military personnel in autoinjector form (Fig. 17-1). The atropine device delivers 2 mg of atropine. The pralidoxime injector delivers 600 mg of 2PAM. Both injectors deliver the medication deep IM. Armed forces personnel receive three of each injector type. One 10-mg diazepam injector also is issued. If exposure to a nerve agent occurs, one atropine and one pralidoxime injector is used. If symptoms continue, then another atropine and pralidoxime injector

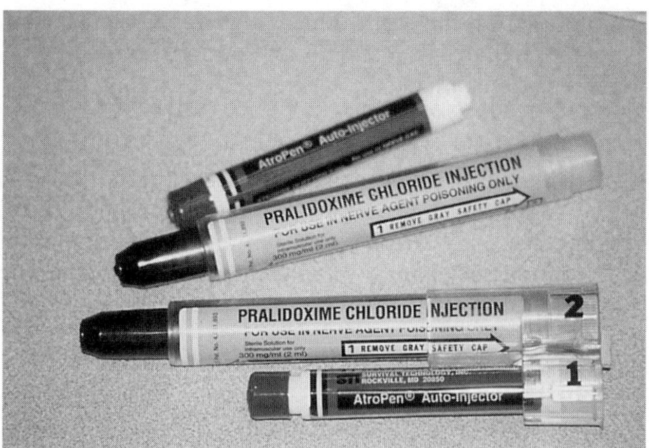

FIG. 17-1 Military Mark I Kit with self-injectable atropine and 2PAM.

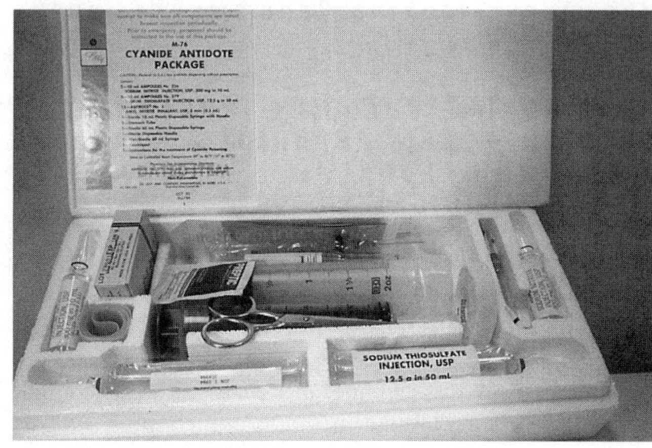

FIG. 17-2 Cyanide antidote kit.

are given. Severe symptoms may require that all three sets be used. After the victim has received all six injectors, then the diazepam injector is administered. It is thought that the diazepam potentiates the action of the 2PAM and atropine in the case of nerve agent exposure and also acts to prevent seizures. Autoinjectors for use in mass casualty situations may be available to EMS responders through your state health department. The injectors provide a convenient way to administer atropine and pralidoxime for mass casualties in both the field and emergency departments.

CYANIDE ANTIDOTE KIT

Major Actions

The cyanide kit consists of three drugs: amyl nitrite (AN), sodium nitrite ($NaNO_2$), and sodium thiosulfate ($Na_2S_2O_3$) (Fig. 17-2). AN reacts with hemoglobin (HB) to form an approximate 5% methemoglobinemia (MHB). $NaNO_2$ reacts with HB to form an approximate 20% to 30% methemoglobinemia. Theoretically, methemoglobin attracts cyanide (CN) ions bound to the cytochrome oxidase system in the mitochondria, forming cyanmethemoglobin (CNMHB). Sodium thiosulfate converts cyanmethemoglobin to thiocyanate (HSCN), which is excreted in the urine by the kidneys. This scenario can be described by the following chemical reactions:

$$AN + HB = MHB$$

$$NaNO_2 + HB = MHB$$

$$CN + MHB = CNMHB$$

$$Na_2\,S_2O_3 + CNMHB + O_2 = HSCN$$

Amyl nitrite, sodium nitrite, and sodium thiosulfate are administered in the above order. This combination of drugs is the only therapy against cyanide and hydrocyanic acid poisoning currently approved by the Food and Drug Administration (FDA).

Indications

The cyanide antidote kit is used to treat victims of cyanide poisoning and exposure to hazardous materials that are metabolized to cyanide. Amyl nitrite and sodium nitrite without sodium thiosulfate is used for hydrogen sulfide poisoning.

Adult Dosage

1. Aspirols of amyl nitrite should be broken and held, one at a time, in front of the patient's nose. They should be left in place for 15 seconds, then followed with a 15-second rest, and repeated until sodium nitrite can be administered. This produces an approximate 5% methemoglobin. The use of amyl nitrite should not delay prompt respiratory support. In case of respiratory arrest, place an aspirol inside the bag/valve/mask and ventilate (remove after 15 seconds, ventilate for 15 seconds, and repeat) until sodium nitrite can be administered.
2. Stop amyl nitrite administration and administer 300 mg of sodium nitrite (10 mL of 3% solution) by IV push over 5 minutes. This will produce a theoretical 20% to 30% methemoglobin.
3. Immediately follow sodium nitrite with 12.5 g of sodium thiosulfate (50 mL of a 25% solution) IV push over 5 minutes.
4. If toxic signs reappear, repeat both sodium nitrite and sodium thiosulfate at half the original dose.

Pediatric Dosage

1. Aspirols of amyl nitrite should be broken and held, one at a time, in front of the patient's nose. They should be left in place for 15 seconds, then followed with a 15-second rest, and repeated until sodium nitrite can be administered. This produces an approximate 5% methemoglobin. The use of amyl nitrite should not delay prompt respiratory support. In case of respiratory arrest,

place an aspirol inside the bag/valve/mask and ventilate (remove after 15 seconds, ventilate for 15 seconds, and repeat) until sodium nitrite can be administered.

2. The sodium nitrite dose is based on one of three dosing parameters: (1) the child's hemoglobin concentration, (2) body surface area (BSA) estimation, or (3) weight in kilograms. Although the hemoglobin concentration dosing regimen method is preferred, in most cases, the child's hemoglobin concentration will not be readily available. *Failure to dose according to one of these dosing parameters may lead to a fatal overdose of sodium nitrite by causing development of life-threatening methemoglobinemia.*

a. Sodium nitrite dose based on hemoglobin concentration:

HEMOGLOBIN IN GRAMS	INITIAL IV DOSE
8	0.22 mL (6.6 mg)/kg
10	0.27 mL (8.3 mg)/kg
12	0.33 mL (10 mg)/kg
14	0.39 mL (11.6 mg)/kg

Do not exceed 10 mL or 300 mg.

b. Sodium nitrite dose based on BSA: Administer 6 to 8 mL/m^2 or approximately 0.2 mL/kg IV. Do not exceed 10 mL or 300 mg.

c. Sodium nitrite dose based on body weight estimation: If a child weighs less than 25 kg and it is not possible to obtain a hemoglobin determination rapidly, then administer 10 mg/kg (0.33 mL/kg). Do not exceed 10 mL or 300 mg.

3. The sodium thiosulfate dose also is based on one of three dosing parameters: (1) the child's hemoglobin concentration, (2) BSA estimation, or (3) weight in kilograms. Calculate the correct dose, using either the measured hemoglobin concentration, BSA, or child's weight.

a. Sodium thiosulfate dose based on hemoglobin concentration:

HEMOGLOBIN IN GRAMS	INITIAL IV DOSE
8	1.1 mL/kg
10	1.35 mL/kg
12	1.65 mL/kg
14	1.95 mL/kg

Do not exceed 12.5 g.

b. Sodium thiosulfate IV dose based on BSA: Administer 7 g/m^2. Do not exceed 12.5 g.

c. Sodium thiosulfate IV dose based on body weight: If a child weighs less than 25 kg and it is not possible to obtain a hemoglobin determination rapidly, then administer 1.65 mL/kg of the 25% solution. Do not exceed 12.5 g.

4. If toxic signs reappear, repeat both sodium nitrite and sodium thiosulfate at half the original dose.

Precautions

Administration of 1% methylene blue is controversial if signs of methemoglobinemia occur (i.e., severe cyanosis, vomiting, coma, and shock), because bound cyanide may be released. Give only under the *direct verbal order of the medical control physician.* Both sodium nitrite and amyl nitrite in excessive doses can induce a dangerous methemoglobinemia in children or adults and can be fatal. Sodium nitrite can cause hypotension. Drug therapy should be in addition to ventilation, oxygen therapy, and rapid transport to a medical facility.

How Supplied

Cyanide antidote package

Special Considerations

Other countries have approved different cyanide antidote treatments. 4-DMAP (4-dimethylaminophenol) is used in Europe. 4-DMAP is an extremely potent methemoglobin-forming agent and can generate methemoglobin levels as high as 25% to 35% in the adult after one intravenous dose. Its use is followed by the standard dosing regimen of sodium thiosulfate. Hydroxocobalamin (vitamin B_{12a}) is widely used in Europe and is under investigation in the United States. Hydroxocobalamin works by reacting with cyanide to form cyanocobalamin (vitamin B_{12}), which is excreted in the urine. Dicobalt EDTA (Kelocyanor) currently is used in Europe. It acts by chelating cyanide to form stable cobalt-cyanide, which is excreted in the urine.

Hyperbaric oxygen therapy is a useful adjuctive therapy and may increase the efficiency of the cyanide antidote kit.

Stocking Recommendations

For each 70-kg patient: One kit

METHYLENE BLUE 1%

Major Actions

Methylene blue is a thiazine dye (Fig. 17-3). Methylene blue has two opposite actions on hemoglobin. At low doses, methylene blue reduces methemoglobin to hemoglobin. This reaction can go both ways and at high doses methylene blue will oxidize hemoglobin iron in the ferrous state (Fe^{+2}) to ferric iron (Fe^{+3}), forming methemoglobin. Only iron in the ferrous state can bind with oxygen. Methylene blue functions as an electron donor for the reversible reduction of methemoglobin to hemoglobin by methemoglobin reductase.

Indications

Methylene blue is indicated for hazardous materials poisoning that results in an absolute methemoglobinemia

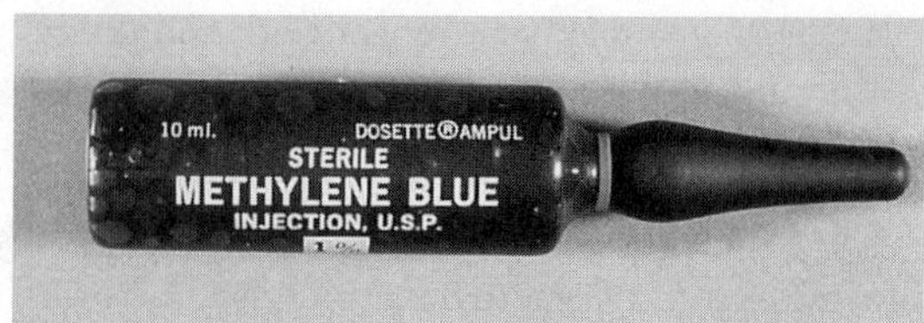

FIG. 17-3 Methylene blue.

level greater than 30% or for a methemoglobinemia patient with signs and symptoms of hypoxia.

Dosage

For adults administer 1 to 2 mg/kg (0.1 to 0.2 mL/kg) of a 1% solution slow IV push over 5 minutes. Repeat as necessary up to a total dose of 7 mg/kg. The pediatric dose is the same as the adult dose.

Precautions

Methylene blue is for IV use only. It must be injected slowly over a period of 5 minutes to prevent local high concentration of the compound from producing additional methemoglobin. Do not exceed the recommended dose. Large doses may produce nausea, chest and abdominal pain, dizziness, headache, profuse sweating, mental confusion, and the formation of methemoglobin. Tissue infiltration may cause necrotic abscesses. Methylene blue is contraindicated in patients with glucose-6-phosphate deficiency (G6PD). Methylene blue gives urine, feces, and glandular secretions a blue-green color. Explain this fact to the patient. It may also stain skin. Do not use for patients with renal failure.

How Supplied

- 10 mg/1 mL ampule

Stocking Recommendations

For each 70-kg patient: 30 to 40 mL (3 to 4 vials)

NALOXONE (NARCAN)

Major Actions

Naloxone is a pure narcotic (opiate) antagonist. It has a rapid onset of action, with a short half-life (approximately 20 minutes after intravenous injection).

Indications

Naloxone is used to reverse narcotic effects, especially respiratory depression. It may be a diagnostic tool in coma or seizures without a reliable history.

Dosage

The adult dose is 0.1 to 2 mg slow IV. The pediatric dose is 0.01 mg/kg slow IV.

NOTE: Naloxone may be repeated at 2- to 3-minute intervals, if necessary. It may be given via ET or IM routes if IV access is delayed.

Precautions

Naloxone may precipitate opiate withdrawal symptoms. Withdrawal can be violent; try to titrate the dose to reverse respiratory depression only. Naloxone use may cause hypertension and tachycardia. If no response is observed in an adult after a total dose of 10 mg, continued administration probably is of no value. Because the half-life of naloxone is shorter than many narcotics, symptoms may recur. Repeat administration based on clinical symptoms may be necessary.

How Supplied

- 0.4 mg/1 mL ampule, preloaded syringe (0.4 mg/mL)
- 1 mg/1 mL ampule, preloaded syringe (1 mg/mL)
- 2 mg/2 mL ampule, preloaded syringe (1 mg/mL)
- 0.04 mg/2 mL ampule (0.02 mg/mL) neonatal

Stocking Recommendations

For each 70-kg patient: 10 mg

ETHANOL (ETHYL ALCOHOL)

Major Actions

Hepatic alcohol dehydrogenase has preferential affinity for ethanol. Administration of ethanol saturates alcohol dehydrogenase and blocks the metabolism of either methanol or ethylene glycol to toxic byproducts. Methanol or ethylene glycol therefore is excreted unchanged in the urine. Use of ethanol in these patients buys time until hemodialysis can be started to definitively remove the ethylene glycol or methanol.

Indications

Ethanol is used for poisoning from methanol or ethylene glycol.

Dosage

Adult: IV loading dose of 0.7-0.8 g/kg. Administer 10 mL/kg of a 10% ethanol solution (0.75 g/10 mL). A maintenance dose of 0.1 g/kg/hr (1.4 mL/kg/hr of 10% ethanol) should be established to maintain a serum ethanol concentration of 100 to 125 mg/dL.

Pediatric: The dose is the same as for an adult. Monitor the blood glucose level because hypoglycemia is common in children.

Precautions

Because a 10% solution is the highest concentration that can be safely administered intravenously, a large amount of solution may be needed. An 80-kg patient requires an 800-mL loading dose. Monitor for pulmonary edema during administration.

The maintenance dose will need to be adjusted in patients with chronic alcoholism and during dialysis to maintain a serum alcohol level of 100 to 125 mg/dL.

Maintenance therapy should be guided by determination of serum ethanol concentrations. Ethanol is difficult to dose to achieve optimal blood concentration to block alcohol dehydrogenase. Reloading and maintenance infusion adjustment are required along with frequent blood alcohol levels.

Ethanol may cause CNS depression, respiratory depression, hypothermia, hypotension, nausea, and vomiting. Hypoglycemia, especially in children, may occur. Hourly glucose monitoring is required. Therapy should be started as soon as possible after exposure.

Ethanol therapy is of limited value because it may take several days to excrete the methanol or ethylene glycol. Definitive treatment is hemodialysis. Ethanol treatment is therefore used to block alcohol dehydrogenase metabolism while preparations are made for hemodialysis. Pyridoxine (vitamin B_6) and thiamine also are used in ethylene glycol poisonings to promote the formation of nontoxic metabolites. Folic acid is administered to methanol victims for the same reason.

How Supplied

- Absolute ethanol (95%) must be diluted to 10% vol/vol for IV administration.
- 10% ethanol and 5% dextrose for injection
- 5% ethanol and 5% dextrose for injection

Stocking Recommendations

For each 70-kg patient: Ethanol 15 g—first 4 hours

FOMEPIZOLE (ANTIZOLE, 4-METHYLPYRAZOLE [4-MP])

Major Actions

Fomepizole recently was approved by the FDA as an antidote for ethylene glycol poisoning. Fomepizole effectively blocks alcohol dehydrogenase, inhibiting ethylene glycol and methanol metabolism. It is a more effective inhibitor of alcohol dehydrogenase than ethanol. Because it is easy to use and dose and does not present the logistical problems of keeping the patient intoxicated, fomepizole most likely will replace ethanol as the antidote of choice for ethylene glycol and methanol poisonings.

Indications

Fomepizole is used as an antidote for methanol or ethylene glycol poisoning. It may be given to patients with a history of toxic alcohol ingestion with increased anion gap metabolic acidosis or increased osmolar gap. Fomepizole is indicated if ethylene glycol or methanol blood levels are greater than 20 mg/dL. Consider using fomepizole in suspected ingestion when hemodialysis will be delayed.

Dosage

Loading dose for both adult and pediatric: 15 mg/kg IV

Maintenance dose for both adult and pediatric: 10 mg/kg IV every 12 hours × four doses. Additional doses during hemodialysis may be necessary.

Precautions

Flushing has been observed with infusion. Overall, fomepizole has fewer complications than does ethanol.

Stocking Recommendations

For each 70-kg patient: 1.5 g (one vial)—first 4 hours

ACTIVATED CHARCOAL

Major Actions

Activated charcoal is a nonspecific adsorbent for various chemicals and drugs. By definition, commercial preparations (1 g) must adsorb 100 mg of strychnine in 50 mL of water to meet USP standards. Activated charcoal does not adsorb cyanide, ethanol, methanol, ferrous sulfate, caustics, lithium, mineral acids, or hydrocarbon solvents.

Indications

Activated charcoal is used to treat poisonings with chemicals or drugs adsorbable by activated charcoal. Multiple-dose activated charcoal (MDAC) may be used to adsorb drugs that exhibit enterohepatic recirculation. MDAC has proved useful for phenobarbital, theophylline, carbamazepine, and digoxin poisonings.

Dosage

Oral or orogastric tube

Adult: 30 to 100 g

Pediatric: 30 to 50 g or 1 g/kg

Sorbitol

Activated charcoal usually is given with the osmotic laxative agent sorbitol to decrease GI transit time. Use with caution in cases of GI obstruction.

Adult: 100 g (150 mL of 70% solution)

Pediatric: 1 to 2 mL/kg of 70% solution

Precautions

Activated charcoal is contraindicated in caustic ingestions. Use with caution if decreased bowel activity or intestinal obstruction is present. The adsorbed chemical/drug may be released into the GI tract for reabsorption. Administration of activated charcoal followed by GI tract perforation and charcoal peritoneum has been occasionally reported.

How Supplied

Powder for suspension:

- 30 g Acta-Char
- 50 g Acta-Char

Suspension:

- 0.625 g/5 mL (15 or 30 g) Acta-Char, Insta-Char in aqueous or sorbitol solution
- 0.7 g/mL (50 g) Acta-Char liquid in sorbitol solution

- 1 g/5 mL (12.5, 25, 30, 40, 50 g) in 70% sorbitol solution: Actidose, Charcoaid
- Also in aqueous solution: Actidose-Aqua, Activated Charcoal Liquid, Insta-Char, Liqui-Char

Stocking Recommendations

For each 70-kg patient: 100 g

CALCIUM GLUCONATE

Major Actions

Calcium gluconate is used to treat hydrofluoric acid (HF) burns and fluoride toxicity. The calcium in the calcium gluconate binds to the fluoride ion, preventing tissue and systemic injury. Depending on the type and extent of exposure, calcium gluconate may be administered via several routes. Calcium gluconate gel may be administered topically. Subcutaneous (SQ) injections or intraarterial (IA) infusion of calcium gluconate may be used for definitive treatment of local injuries. Intravenous therapy may be needed for systemic signs and symptoms. For local injury, the end point of therapy is the elimination of pain. For systemic poisoning, therapy should be guided by clinical presentation and laboratory values (calcium, magnesium, and potassium).

Calcium Gluconate Gel

Indications

Calcium gluconate gel is indicated for mild to moderate skin burns resulting from exposure to HF acid (Fig. 17-4).

Dosage

To make 2.5% wt/vol gel, mix 3.5 g of USP calcium gluconate powder in 5 oz of water-soluble lubricant (KY or Surgilube) and apply over painful areas. Cover with sterile dressings. The product must be mixed. Calcium gluconate gel is not available for sale in the United States. Over the counter 2.5% calcium gluconate gel and jelly (H-F Antidote Gel) preparations are available from Pharmascience, Inc., Montreal, Quebec, Canada. Commercial H-F Antidote Gels also are available from Moore & Company, Ltd., in Essex, England, and Industrial Pharmaceutical Service, Ltd., in London, England.

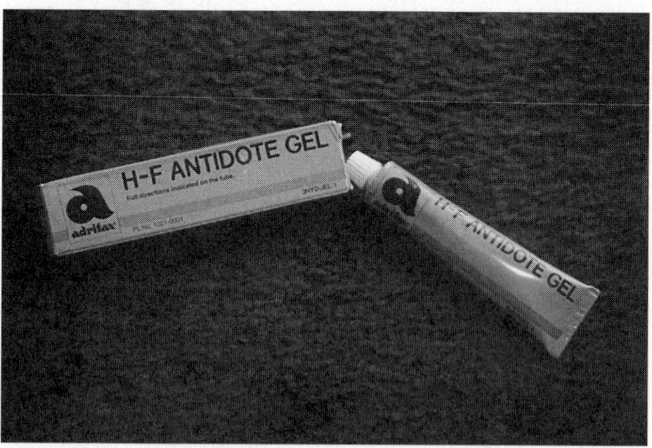

FIG. 17-4 Calcium gluconate gel.

Precautions

The exposed skin surface may look normal. Beware, however, that the burn is in the lower skin layers and, other than for pain, symptoms may not be readily apparent. The HF acid may penetrate to the bone, seeking the large supply of calcium there. Severe burns may require SQ or IA injections. Rapid transport to a medical facility is essential. Watch for systemic poisoning signs and symptoms.

Subcutaneous Injections

Indications

SQ injection is indicated for moderate to severe local tissue damage resulting from exposure to HF acid. Patients with no significant pain relief after 45 minutes of topical treatment may be candidates for SQ injection.

Dosage

Using a 30-gauge needle, calcium gluconate 10% is infiltrated into the subcutaneous tissue. The injected volume should not exceed 0.5 mL/cm^2. Some texts advocate nail removal. Some evidence suggests that nail removal may not be necessary if the patient was exposed to an HF acid solution of less than 10%.

Precautions

Small surface area exposure to dilute solutions of HF acid may not require SQ injections. This can be an extremely painful procedure. Local anesthesia should not be used because the therapeutic end point is pain reduction. Because of the potential for tissue vascular compromise from the SQ calcium injection, only physicians experienced in this treatment method should perform it. Calcium chloride is irritating to the tissues and should not be used. Excessive administration may result in vascular compromise. Burn symptoms may be delayed for several hours. Treatment should be guided by history and clinical presentation. Watch for signs and symptoms of systemic poisoning.

Intraarterial Injections

Indications

IA injection is used for moderate to severe extremity tissue damage resulting from exposure to HF acid. Patients with no significant pain relief after 45 minutes of topical treatment may be considered for IA treatment.

Dosage

Perform an arteriogram to determine which artery supplies the affected tissue. Mix 10 mL of calcium gluconate with 50 mL of 5% dextrose solution and administer over a 4-hour period intraarterially using a parenteral infusion pump. Repeat if pain recurs. If the patient does not experience pain relief, repeat the arteriogram to ensure correct artery selection.

Precautions

Small surface area exposure to dilute solutions of HF acid may not require IA injections. This is an invasive procedure, requiring hospital administration. IA calcium gluconate administration should be performed by a physician experienced in IA use of calcium gluconate. Ensure adequate tissue perfusion during the procedure. Burn signs and symptoms may be delayed for several hours. Treatment should be guided by history and clinical presentation. Watch for signs and symptoms of systemic hypocalcemia poisoning.

Intravenous Injection

Indications

IV calcium gluconate is indicated for systemic poisoning resulting in severe hypocalcemia secondary to HF acid exposure. If a serum calcium concentration is not readily available, dosing is guided by the history of HF acid exposure, symptoms, and ECG changes consistent with hypocalcemia (i.e., prolonged QT interval).

Dosage

Administer 0.1 to 0.2 mL/kg IV up to 10 mL. Repeat the dose as necessary. Larger than usual doses may be necessary. Therapy should be guided by serum calcium and serum potassium determinations.

Precautions

Closely monitor the ECG and serum calcium and potassium concentrations during therapy. Hypotension, bradycardia, and arrhythmias may occur. Calcium gluconate is contraindicated in patients with digitalis toxicity.

Stocking Recommendations

For each 70-kg patient: 1 g

Field Use of Antidotes

In certain instances, paramedic administration of specific physiological antagonists (antidotes) may be appropriate in the field under medical supervision. In all cases, antidote therapy is not without its own potential toxicity. Strict medical supervision must be established and followed for protocols involving antidote therapy. Specific treatment for various chemical exposures can be found in standard reference texts such as Mosby's *Emergency Care for Hazardous Materials Exposure.* All treatment modalities must be carried out under protocol and be approved by local medical control.

Oxygen

Oxygen is the most often administered prehospital therapeutic agent. Although it is used for many patient conditions, it is a valuable treatment modality for many toxic exposures. Oxygen administration elevates arterial oxygen tension, increases arterial oxygen content, and improves tissue oxygenation. Remember that there is a difference between oxygenation and ventilation. The patient's respiratory rate and depth must be supported by ventilation as well as oxygenation. Dose and delivery devices will depend on the specific problem.

Cyanide Antidote Kit

Under special conditions, the cyanide antidote kit can be a valuable antidote for field use. Indications for administration of the kit include treatment of cyanide poisoning and poisoning from cyanide metabolites. The use of amyl nitrite and sodium nitrite (without sodium thiosulfate) is a controversial but accepted treatment for hydrogen sulfide poisoning. The cyanide antidote kit supplied as the Taylor Cyanide Antidote Package consists of three drugs—amyl nitrite, sodium nitrite, and sodium thiosulfate. Amyl nitrite and sodium nitrite react with hemoglobin to form methemoglobin. Methemoglobin attracts cyanide ions from tissue and binds with them to become cyanmethemoglobin. Sodium thiosulfate converts cyanmethemoglobin to thiocyanate, which is excreted by the kidneys. Amyl nitrite, sodium nitrite, and sodium thiosulfate, administered in that order, is the only therapy against cyanide and hydrocyanic acid poisoning currently approved by the FDA. Both sodium nitrite and amyl nitrite in excessive doses can induce a dangerous methemoglobinemia, which can be fatal. Sodium nitrite can cause hypotension. Drug therapy should be in addition to ventilation, oxygen therapy, and rapid transport. Hyperbaric therapy may increase the efficacy of the cyanide antidote kit.

Atropine Sulfate

Atropine sulfate is a useful antidote for nerve agent and certain insecticide exposures. Atropine acts as an antimuscarinic, inhibiting acetylcholine and the parasympathetic nervous system; increasing heart rate and conduction through the AV node; reducing the tone and motility of the GI tract; inhibiting salivary, bronchial, and sweat gland secretions; and dilating the pupils (mydriasis). In cases of organophosphate or carbamate exposure, the amount of atropine sulfate needed may exceed the usual dose suggested by Advanced Cardiac Life Support (ACLS) protocol for cardiac arrhythmias. The end point of administration should be adequate breath sounds. The initial atropine dose may be given IM or via ET tube. Because the required dose may be very large, switch to the IV route as soon as possible. Adequate oxygenation and ventilation should be assessed before atropine administration. Smaller doses of atropine may produce paradoxical bradycardia. If large doses are necessary, preservative-free preparations should be used.

Pralidoxime Chloride (Protopam Chloride, 2PAM Chloride, 2-pyridine Aldoxime Methochloride)

Pralidoxime chloride is used as an adjunct to atropine for treating exposure to nerve agents and certain insecticides. It is used to treat poisoning caused by organophosphate pesticides that have anticholinesterase activity. Pralidoxime chloride generally is not recommended for treatment of intoxication from the carbamate class of insecticides, especially carbaryl. However, it may be used in severe poisonings. The carbamate/cholinesterase bond is not permanent and will allow the cholinesterase to reactivate spontaneously. Pralidoxime chloride binds with organophosphate (OP), removing it from the cholinesterase enzyme, so that cholinesterase function is restored. Its actions are synergistic with atropine and will assist in reversing paralysis of respiratory muscles. In most cases, except for nerve gas exposure, pralidoxime chloride can be administered after arrival at the hospital emergency department. It should be administered as soon as possible, preferably within the first 24 hours, after cholinesterase poisoning, before the enzyme-OP complex "ages" (covalently bonds). Once covalent bonding occurs, the cholinesterase-OP bond is irreversibly established. Pralidoxime chloride must be used with atropine because it is relatively slow acting. It is administered in an IV drip over 15 to 30 minutes.

Methylene Blue 1%

Methylene blue is a thiazine dye used to treat poisoning from nitrates, nitrites, amines, and other agents that cause methemoglobinemia greater than 30%, when accompanied by signs and symptoms of hypoxia. It has two opposite actions on hemoglobin: low doses of methylene blue will reduce methemoglobin to hemoglobin, and high doses will create additional methemoglobin. Hemoglobin is ferrous iron, and methemoglobin is ferric iron. Only iron in the ferrous state can bind with oxygen. It is administered via slow IV push.

Calcium Gluconate

Calcium gluconate is used to treat HF acid and fluoride toxicity. It binds the fluoride ion, preventing tissue and systemic injury. Depending on the type and extent of exposure, calcium gluconate may be administered via several routes. Calcium gluconate gel may be administered topically. SQ injections or IA infusion may be used in the hospital setting for definitive treatment of severe local injuries. Intravenous therapy may be needed for systemic signs and symptoms of fluoride poisoning. For local injury, the end point of therapy is the elimination of pain. For systemic poisoning, therapy should be guided by clinical presentation and laboratory values.

In cases of HF acid burns, the skin surface may look normal; however, the burn is in the lower skin layers and bone tissue may be involved. Severe burns may require SQ or IA injections, so rapid transport to a medical facility is essential. Watch for systemic poisoning leading to signs and symptoms of hypocalcemia, hypomagnesemia, and hyperkalemia.

Summary

Antidotal therapy is an important aspect of hazardous materials poisoning treatment. Unfortunately, most hazardous materials poisonings do not have a specific antidote. Antidotes are no substitute for supportive care. For those poisonings that do require specific antidotes, adequate field and hospital stocking is essential. Work with your local EMS and medical control to survey the antidote stocking inventories of area hospitals. All antidotes have the potential for adverse reactions. Knowledge of the correct use of these compounds is essential to ensure proper patient care.

CHAPTER REVIEW QUESTIONS

1. Name three uses of atropine.
2. Why should pralidoxime always be used with atropine?
3. Describe the mechanism of pralidoxime.
4. What is activated charcoal?
5. What three drugs are in the cyanide antidote kit?
6. How is sodium nitrite dosed in children?
7. What is methylene blue?
8. Describe how to mix calcium gluconate gel.
9. Name three ways calcium gluconate can be administered.
10. What is the indication for Narcan?

BIBLIOGRAPHY

Aaron CK: Cyanide antidotes. In Goldfrank LR et al, editors: *Goldfrank's toxicologic emergencies,* Norwalk, Conn, 1994, Appleton & Lange.

Bronstein AC, Currance PL: *Emergency care for hazardous materials exposure,* ed 2, St. Louis, 1994, Mosby.

Chyka PA, Conner HG. Availability of antidotes in rural and urban hospitals in Tennessee, *Am J Hosp Pharm* 51:1346-1348, 1994.

Dart RC et al: Insufficient stocking of poisoning antidotes in hospital pharmacies, *JAMA* 276:1508-1510, 1966.

Ecobichon DJ: Toxic effect of pesticides. In Klaassen CD, Amdur MO, Doull J, editors: *Casarett and Doull's Toxicology: the basic science of poisons,* ed 5, New York, 1996, McGraw-Hill.

Howland MA, Aaron CK: Pralidoxime. In Goldfrank LR et al, editors: *Goldfrank's toxicologic emergencies,* Norwalk, Conn, 1994, Appleton & Lange.

Howland MA: Activated charcoal. In Goldfrank LR et al, editors: *Goldfrank's toxicologic emergencies,* Norwalk, Conn, 1994, Appleton & Lange.

Howland MA: Calcium. In Goldfrank LR et al, editors: *Goldfrank's toxicologic emergencies,* Norwalk, Conn, 1994, Appleton & Lange.

Howland MA: Ethanol. In Goldfrank LR et al, editors: *Goldfrank's toxicologic emergencies,* Norwalk, Conn, 1994, Appleton & Lange.

Smith EA, Oehme FW: A review of selected herbicides and their toxicities, *Vet Hum Toxicol* 33:596-608, 1991.
USDHHS: ATSDR case studies in environmental medicine: nitrate/nitrite toxicity, Monograph 16, October 1991.
USDHHS: ATSDR case studies in environmental medicine: methanol toxicity, Monograph 20, July 1992.
USDHHS: ATSDR case studies in environmental medicine: ethylene/propylene glycol toxicity, Monograph 30, September 1992.
Weisman R: Naloxone. In Goldfrank LR et al, editors: *Goldfrank's toxicologic emergencies,* Norwalk, Conn, 1994, Appleton & Lange.

18

Patient Transportation

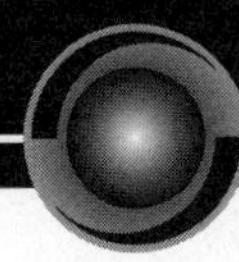

Phil Currance

CHAPTER OBJECTIVES

At the conclusion of this chapter the student will be able to:

- Discuss the need for early hospital notification during hazardous materials incidents.
- Identify the information that should be relayed to the hospital emergency department.
- Discuss how the regional poison center can assist as a contact in hazardous materials emergencies.
- Explain how to ensure that chemical information is relayed accurately.
- Identify conditions under which field decontamination may be less than complete.
- Discuss why adequate ventilation in the patient care compartment is important.
- Identify ways to reduce secondary exposure risk during transportation.
- Explain how reverse isolation procedures are carried out and their hazards.
- Discuss the need for personal protective equipment (PPE) during transportation of contaminated patients.
- Identify the risks in using air transport for patients at a hazardous materials emergency.

CASE STUDY

While chemicals are being mixed at a plant site, a reaction takes place, resulting in the exposure of numerous workers and visitors. In addition, the vapor cloud that has formed as a result of the reaction has drifted over a highway that runs near the plant, possibly exposing more people. Workers at the plant have been decontaminated as effectively as possible given the number of patients involved. The local Emergency Medical Services (EMS) agency is preparing for patient transport.

- ◆ Are special protective precautions necessary during transport?
- ◆ What kind of information is necessary to adequately prepare the receiving emergency department?
- ◆ Is air transport a safe alternative?

Hazardous materials events may involve numerous victims. They may be either ambulatory or nonambulatory. Ambulatory victims will often scatter 360 degrees from the incident. In large incidents, those victims may have already exited the area and may be on their way to the hospital before emergency responders have time to arrive and set up at the scene. Once the news media broadcast the details of the incident, patients who were on the periphery of the incident may think they were exposed and will be calling local hospitals for advice. Early in the incident, hospital emergency departments will be swamped with potentially contaminated patients and requests for information. Obviously, they have a need for information, and they need it as quickly as they can get it. Patients with known hazardous materials contamination will require decontamination for proper and safe treatment. Unfortunately, there is no effective way in the field to determine if the patient is completely decontaminated.

Special precautions should be taken to ensure that the patient and crew are protected during transport.

Early Communication

When responding to a possible hazardous materials incident, early notification and communication with the local hospital's emergency department is essential. Even if no patients are initially involved in the incident, early communication will provide the emergency department with the time needed to carry out research on the chemical(s) and obtain needed equipment and expertise. Remember that many people may be contacting the local hospital for information and advice. Early communication to the hospital should include the type of chemical, any known characteristics of the chemical, and the direction of chemical movement, if known. All hospitals in the area should be contacted, if possible. Your base hospital may be able to make the contacts to the other hospitals.

Poison Center

Many communities are using the regional poison center as an information resource. Most poison center staffs have the experience, expertise, and resources to obtain and communicate toxicology information. Many emergency response agencies and local hospitals have established a system in which the field personnel make first contact to the regional poison center. The center then will start gathering information on the chemical, contact the local hospitals and clinics, and work with the news media to get information to the public.

Hospital Emergency Department

If patients are involved or expected, the receiving emergency department staff need information. They will need to know the number of patients expected. The nature of the chemical and expected threats must be communicated. For example, if a flammable liquid has been released, patients may have burns as well as toxic exposure. The substance's identity is vital information for proper patient care. Make sure to accurately communicate the name of the chemical. A good way to ensure this is to spell the chemical name to the person on the other end of the radio or telephone and have that person spell it back to you for confirmation.

The expected route and possible duration of exposure are vital pieces of information for determining population groups at risk of exposure. Many hazardous materials exposures occur because of vehicle or industrial accidents. Any associated trauma must be reported. As with any patient, the examination findings and vital signs should be reported. Because many toxic substances have a delayed onset of symptoms, the symptom trend is important. Both the initial and current signs and symptoms should be noted and reported. The level of decontamination is important. Has the patient been decontaminated? Do you think that the patient will need any further decontamination on arrival? The report should also contain the estimated time of arrival. Remember that it is extremely important to make this contact as soon as possible. Patients who have been exposed to hazardous materials may present special treatment concerns. Because hazardous materials injuries may be complex in nature and require a multidisciplinary approach to treatment, the receiving hospital will need as much time and information as possible to prepare adequately (Box 18-1).

Contamination Hazards

Obviously an exposure potential exists if contaminated patients are transported before decontamination. Therefore, except in very specific instances, decontamination should always be carried out before transport (Fig. 18-1). As discussed in Chapter 13, cases of low-level particulate

BOX 18-1

INFORMATION TO BE COMMUNICATED TO RECEIVING HOSPITALS

Number of patients and potential additional patients
Nature of accident
Substance(s) involved
Route(s) of exposure
Duration of exposure
Associated trauma
Victim examination findings and vital signs
Initial signs and symptoms
Treatment administered
Current signs and symptoms
Decontamination carried out?
Need for further decontamination?
Estimated time of arrival

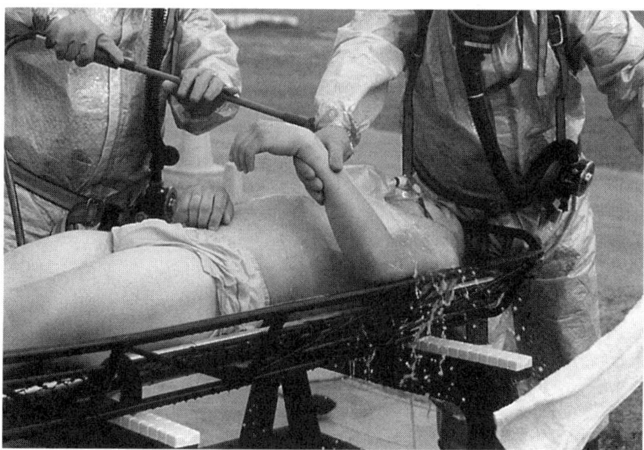

FIG. 18-1 Decontamination should always be carried out before transport.

radiation exposure or embedded air- or water-reactive products may need to be isolated and transported before decontamination for proper patient management. Even when patients are decontaminated, a small risk of secondary contamination may still exist. Field decontamination is carried out in less than ideal conditions. The material that the patient was exposed to may not be very water soluble. Weather conditions, patient numbers, and patient condition may all necessitate a quick field decontamination. Residual contamination may still exist on the patient.

Secondary Contamination

Because of the risk of secondary contamination of EMS responders when transporting patients who may have been contaminated, certain precautions should be taken. The best way to reduce this risk is adequate patient decontamination before transport. Because inhalation is the quickest and most vulnerable route of exposure, adequate ventilation in the ambulance is a must. A study conducted at the Solar Energy Research Institute (now the National Renewable Energy Laboratory) in Colorado showed that ambulances manufactured before 1993 have a relatively poor air-exchange rate, with a resulting increased risk of secondary exposure to EMS personnel. Newer ambulance units meeting KKK-A-1822 C 3.13.6 standards are required to have a complete air exchange every 2 minutes. Both intake and exhaust fans should always be used to ensure maximum ventilation in the patient care compartment. Some authorities suggest opening all of the windows in the ambulance. Many ambulances do not have windows in the patient compartment, but even with those that do, protection may be inadequate. Windows are bidirectional, allowing some contamination to come back into the ambulance. This may result in inadequate ventilation and an exposure risk. In addition, opening of rear windows may allow exhaust fumes, including carbon monoxide, into the ambulance. Another suggestion, given in many protocols, is to completely cover the walls and ceiling of the entire ambulance patient compartment in plastic. Unless time is taken though to cut holes for ventilation units and adequately tape down the plastic so there are no flaps, ventilation in the patient compartment will be radically decreased, resulting in an increase of the secondary inhalation hazard

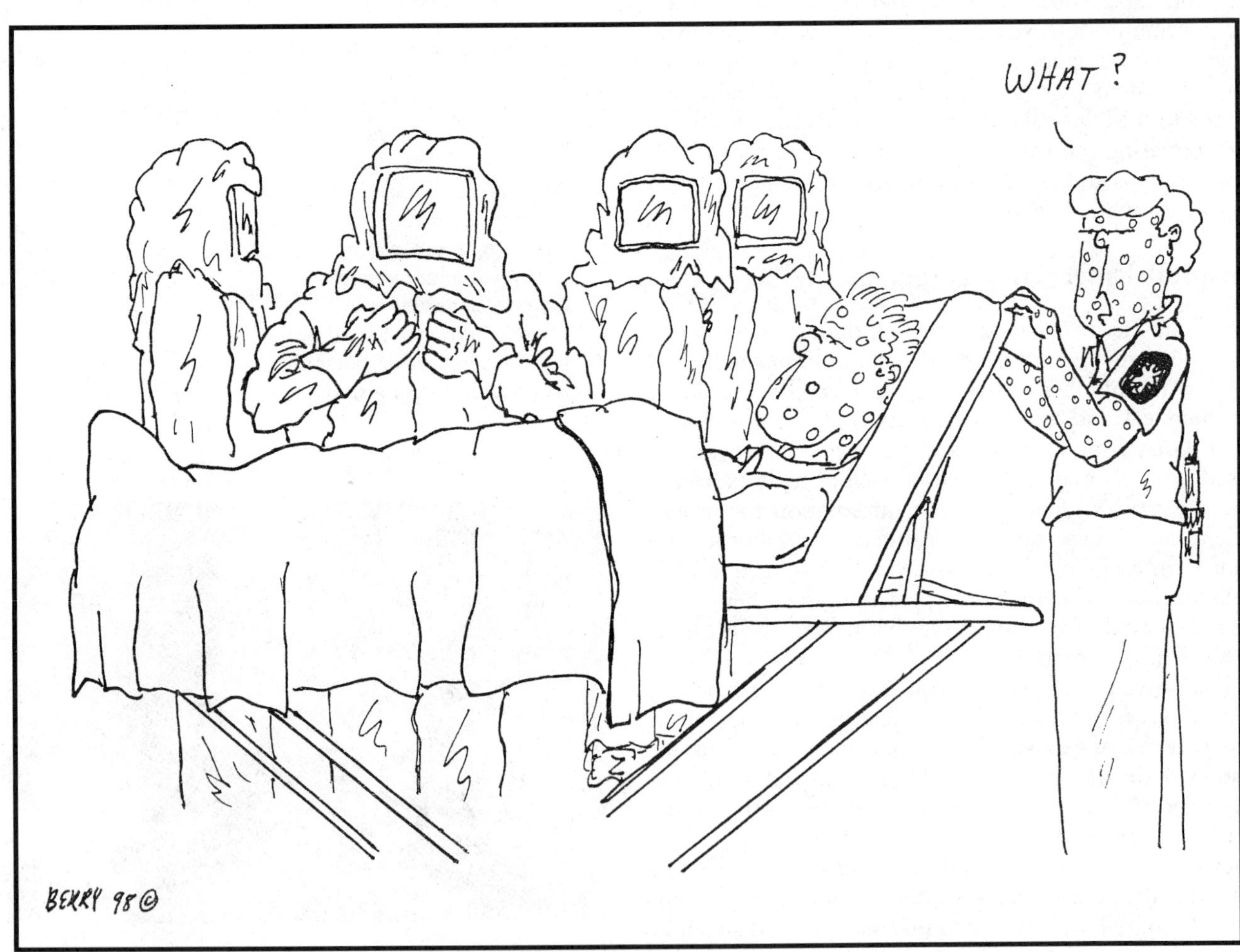

Reprinted with permission from Steve Berry's *I'm Not an Ambulance Driver* cartoon book series.

to patients and EMS responders. Plastic is useful on the stretcher, floor, and bench to reduce contact exposure from patients who are wet with decontamination water (Fig. 18-2). Pre-cut pieces are useful in reducing excess plastic that may result in a tripping hazard. Any water on the plastic also will create a slip hazard.

Reverse Isolation

Another method that sometimes is recommended is reverse isolation (Fig. 18-3). These procedures include postdecontamination isolation of the patient in specially designed contaminated-patient transportation bags, plastic, sheets, blankets, or zip-front body bags. Although this process will reduce the risk of secondary contamination of EMS responders, it may increase the risk of further contamination to the patient. When wrapped up, especially in plastic or a body bag, the temperature will increase, resulting in sweating, open pores, and dilated peripheral blood vessels. If the patient has not been adequately decontaminated, skin absorption may be increased, which, in turn, increases the patient's chemical exposure risk. It has been argued that if adequate patient decontamination has been carried out, there is no need for reverse isolation procedures. Because it is almost impossible to determine if the patient has been adequately decontaminated in the field, a combination of good decontamination and reverse isolation procedures may be useful. Check with your medical control physician and follow his or her recommendations.

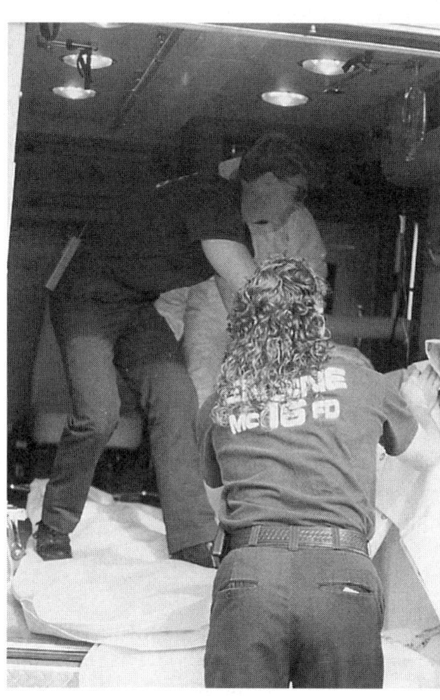

FIG. 18-2 Plastic can be useful in reducing contact exposure.

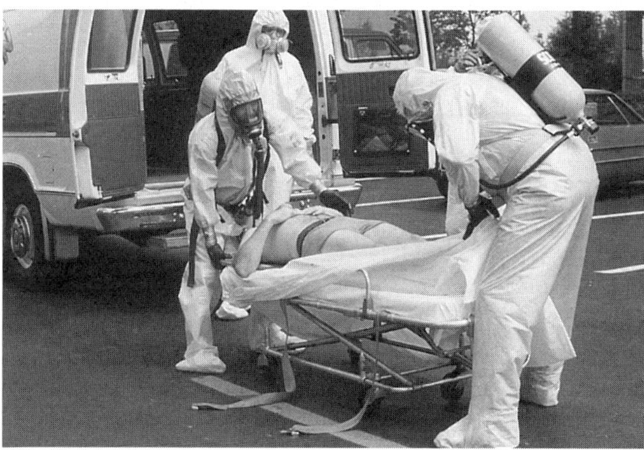

FIG. 18-3 Patient and reverse isolation procedures.

Protective Equipment

EMS personnel may wish to wear respiratory-protective and chemical-protective clothing (CPC) when transporting patients who may have been contaminated. Protective equipment should never be used as a reason or excuse not to decontaminate the patient before transport. Lightweight, disposable CPC or body substance isolation equipment can easily be used to reduce the chance of skin exposure and protect the responders' uniform and shoes. Two pairs of gloves (examination and chemical) can provide hand exposure protection. Respiratory protection is not nearly so easy. Many EMS responders have not been trained and fit-tested to wear air-purifying respirators (APRs) other than disposable high efficiency particulate air (HEPA) respirators commonly used for protection against tuberculosis. HEPA respirators will provide protection against particulates but not chemical vapors or gases. APR filters and cartridges must be specific for the chemical threat. It is difficult and expensive to try to stock a complete selection of respirator cartridges on the ambulance. Remember that some chemicals cannot be filtered or rendered harmless by APRs. Respiratory protection with APRs cannot be ensured unless the responder has been fit-tested into that specific respirator brand, model, and size respirator. Air-supplied units (self-contained breathing apparatuses [SCBAs] or air lines) are almost impossible to use during transport unless your ambulance has been specially designed with an air-line system, which is expensive. In addition to the logistical concerns, the use of chemical-protective equipment, such as respirators and heavy chemical gloves, will complicate patient care procedures. If protective equipment is to be used, responders should practice with the equipment before actual use. In all cases, responders should never attempt to wear respirators or protective clothing unless they have received specific training and fit testing, as necessary, on that piece of equipment. Consider coordinating with the local hazardous materials (HAZMAT) team for training and provision of the proper types of protective equipment.

Even patients with toxic ingestions and no other exposure may present a secondary contamination hazard.

The patient may vomit during transport. The vomitus may contain volatile compounds, leading to an inhalation hazard. Any vomitus should be isolated immediately in a sealed plastic bag.

Air Transportation

Transporting patients from hazardous materials incidents by air involves risk. The helicopter may travel through an unsafe area, or the rotor wash from the helicopter may affect vapors or fumes at the scene. If decontamination is not complete, the flight crew could experience symptoms of exposure. Because of this, air transportation of patients from a hazardous materials emergency usually is considered to be contraindicated unless rapid transport is absolutely necessary and the patient is *completely* decontaminated or was exposed to a chemical with no risk of secondary contamination. Many flight services are apprehensive about transporting patients from any hazardous materials scene. If helicopter transport is necessary in your area, preincident planning should be carried out with the flight service. Decontamination procedures and safe scene practices should be explained and demonstrated. This preplanning and training may help in reducing potential problems.

Flight services should not be ignored in hazardous materials response planning. They may be the only reasonable way to transport severely injured patients from rural areas or to distant special care centers. Air medical crews may be called to an unrecognized hazardous materials incident and be on scene very quickly. Just like all field responders, air medical crews should receive adequate training in hazardous materials recognition and safe response practices. As in ground transport, vomitus may still pose a threat, and measures should be in place for immediate isolation of emesis. The helicopter landing area should be a safe distance from the hot zone to avoid spreading the contamination with the rotor wash. Because many hazardous materials are invisible to the eye, pilots must be advised of scene conditions to ensure a safe approach. With proper preplanning, training, and complete patient decontamination, air transport can be a safe alternative when rapid transportation is essential.

Summary

Hospitals must receive early warning when a hazardous materials event has occurred. Many patients may make their own way to a medical center, and the facility may easily be overwhelmed. Time is needed to gather information, resources, and staff. The regional poison center may be a valuable resource and can assist with information and coordination needs. Because it is difficult to ensure that full decontamination has been achieved in the field, certain procedures will help reduce the chance of responder and equipment exposure during transport. Ambulance preparation, adequate ventilation, responder protection, and reverse isolation techniques all will reduce the chance of secondary exposure. In areas where air transport may be needed, preplanning should address how to minimize the complications that may arise when aircraft are used to transport patients from hazardous materials scenes.

CHAPTER REVIEW QUESTIONS

1. Why is early hospital notification necessary when dealing with hazardous materials incidents?
2. List at least eight items that should be included in the report to the hospital.
3. How can the regional poison center be utilized during a hazardous materials emergency?
4. What are the types of exposure for which patients may need to be isolated and transported before decontamination?
5. List at least three conditions that may result in less than adequate patient decontamination.
6. Why won't opening of the windows in the patient care compartment of an ambulance ensure adequate respiratory protection?
7. Why can covering the walls in the patient compartment of the ambulance with plastic increase the chance of secondary exposure?
8. How can reverse isolation procedures increase patient exposure?
9. What are the advantages and disadvantages of the use of protective equipment during transport?
10. What are the disadvantages of using air transport for patients at a hazardous materials emergency?

BIBLIOGRAPHY

Agency for Toxic Substances and Disease Registry: *Managing hazardous materials incidents, emergency medical services: a planning guide for the management of contaminated patients,* Atlanta, Ga, 1992, US-DHHS.

Bronstein AC, et al: Measurements of ambulance ventilation rates: impact on chemical exposure. Annual meeting of the AACT/AAPCC/ABMT/CAPCC, Toronto, Ontario, Canada, Oct 1-4, 1991.

Bronstein AC, Currance PL: *Emergency care for hazardous materials exposure,* ed 2, St Louis, 1994, Mosby.

Bronstein AC, Currance PL: Module 4: emergency medical operations. In Ayers S, Christopher J, editors: *Medical response to chemical emergencies,* Washington, DC, 1994, Chemical Manufacturers Association.

California EMS Authority. *Hazardous materials medical management protocols.* 1991.

Currance PL: *Hazmat for EMS,* St Louis, 1995, Mosby (videotape and guidebook).

Guidelines for public sector hazardous materials training. 1998 ed, HMEP Curriculum Guidelines, Emmitsburg, Md, 1998, National Emergency Training Center.

National Fire Protection Association: *NFPA 473, Standard for professional competence of EMS responders to hazardous materials incidents,* Quincy, Mass, 1992, The Association.

Ricks RC, Leonard RB: *Hospital emergency department of radiation accidents,* Washington, DC, 1984, Emergency Management Institute, National Emergency Training Center.

SECTION FOUR

Incident Termination

19

Postincident Concerns

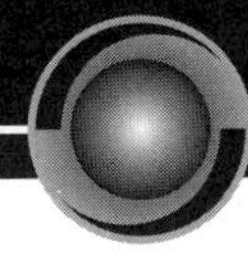

Phil Currance

CHAPTER OBJECTIVES

At the conclusion of this chapter the student will be able to:

- Identify items that may present a secondary contamination risk.
- Identify tests that can be carried out to ensure that equipment decontamination is complete.
- Discuss the proper way to handle contaminated uniforms and personal protective equipment (PPE).
- Discuss federal regulations regarding hazardous waste and what effect they may have on emergency medical services (EMS) agencies.
- Identify agencies that can provide advice and assistance regarding handling contaminated articles.
- Explain the importance of medical follow-up for EMS responders.
- Discuss the purpose of an incident debriefing following every hazardous materials incident.
- Identify common questions to be addressed in the postincident review.
- Explain why stress factors may be higher at a hazardous materials incident.

CASE STUDY

Patients have been transported from the scene of an accident involving a tanker truck and an automobile. It is wintertime. Patients were contaminated with xylene at the accident site, but they were decontaminated before transport. Because of weather conditions, decontamination may not have been 100% complete. EMS responders used protective suits during transport. The patients have been delivered to the hospital emergency department, where they have undergone a secondary decontamination.

- ◆ What should be done with contaminated PPE and patient care equipment?
- ◆ Who can be contacted for decontamination and hazardous waste disposal advice?
- ◆ What topics should be covered in a postincident debriefing?

After a hazardous materials incident has ended, numerous things must still be addressed. Procedures must be in place to prevent secondary contamination after the incident is concluded. Residual contamination may still exist on the ambulance and patient care equipment, and present a significant hazard. An incident debriefing and postincident analysis and review should follow every hazardous materials response. The cause of the incident and response procedures should be assessed. Procedures also should be in place to deal with any emotional stress created by the incident.

Secondary and Residual Contamination

All articles that possibly are contaminated must be isolated for further decontamination, testing, and/or proper disposal according to federal, state, and local regulations.

These items may include patient clothes and personal possessions, any contaminated patient care equipment, and the responder's contaminated uniforms or PPE. Patient clothes and personal possessions must be completely decontaminated before being returned to the owner or disposed of properly. Any contaminated patient care equipment must be decontaminated before it can be reused. Contaminated uniforms or PPE must be handled properly. Contaminated clothing should never be taken home and laundered or disposed of. It should be disposed of as hazardous waste or isolated for cleaning at a designated facility. Many cities have private laundry companies that are able to launder clothing contaminated with hazardous materials. These locations should be identified as a part of preplanning.

Patient care equipment is another concern. If equipment is to be reused, decontamination must be complete. The local or state health department, CHEMTREC, or the Agency of Toxic Substances and Disease Registry (ATSDR [see Chapter 6]) may be able to provide advice on complete decontamination procedures. Wipe samples from decontaminated surfaces can be sent for laboratory analysis to ensure that decontamination is complete. Most laboratories will provide sample wipes, containers, and instructions on how to obtain and preserve the sample.

Hazardous Waste Disposal

Any contaminated items that cannot be decontaminated must be disposed of as hazardous waste. Environmental Protection Agency (EPA) law regulates the handling of hazardous waste. The Resource Conservation and Recovery Act (RCRA), passed in 1976, strictly controls the generation, transportation, and disposal of hazardous waste. RCRA mandates that whoever generates the waste is ultimately responsible for its proper disposal. Under other EPA regulations, the cleanup of hazardous materials spills, including the disposal of any waste created during the response, is the responsibility of whomever caused the spill. The Comprehensive Environmental Response, Compensation and Liability Act (CERCLA but better known as *Superfund*) and its amendment, the Superfund Amendment and Reauthorization Act (SARA), impose strict liability for the cleanup of a hazardous materials spill. Individual states also may enact laws that are at least as stringent or more stringent than federal laws. EMS agencies must ensure that items used during the response that must be disposed of as hazardous waste become the responsibility of whomever caused the emergency in the first place. The best way to ensure that this happens is to isolate contaminated items and leave them at the scene for proper cleanup and disposal. Items that must be removed from the scene, such as responder uniforms and patient care equipment used during transport, should be isolated and the responsible party contacted for pickup and disposal. If this is not done, under RCRA, the liability and cost of disposal may end up being the responsibility of the emergency response agency. Your state health department, hazardous waste division, can offer valuable assistance and advice on handling hazardous waste properly.

Equipment and Responder Decontamination

The ambulance also may be contaminated. Returning the unit to service prematurely will prolong the exposure to EMS personnel and create a hazard for other patients. The unit should be isolated until it can be decontaminated, including a thorough decontamination of the patient compartment, as well as mechanical and exterior decontamination. Tests, such as wipe sampling, can be carried out to ensure proper decontamination. In most cases, soap and water are adequate for vehicle decontamination. CHEMTREC, ATSDR, and the local health department can assist with decision making. This is another reason to ensure safe scene practices and adequate decontamination before transport. If the patient is clean and the ambulance remained a safe distance from the release, then the ambulance and equipment also will be clean.

EMS responders also must undergo decontamination as necessary. The best protection for responders is to avoid contact with the hazardous material because then responder decontamination is unnecessary. If the responders were contaminated or their protection from contamination was uncertain, they should follow a procedure that will ensure proper decontamination. Detailed decontamination procedures can be found in Chapter 13. Contaminated articles (clothing, personal possessions, equipment) should be isolated in polyethylene bags or steel drums until they can be properly decontaminated or disposed of as necessary. All scene responders should shower and change into clean clothes as soon as possible after incident response is terminated.

Medical Follow-up

Medical follow-up for EMS personnel should be carried out as needed. The Occupational Safety and Health Administration (OSHA) Hazardous Waste Operations and Emergency Response (HAZWOPER) regulation requires exposure-specific examinations for any personnel who were exposed and injured during a hazardous materials response. A detailed discussion of medical surveillance requirements can be found in Chapter 7. Every EMS responder should complete a personnel exposure record. This record should include the type of chemical involved in the incident. Any possibility of exposure and the type of PPE used should be recorded. Any signs and symptoms that are experienced and the type of immediate medical care received also should be recorded.

Fortunately, we do not have many hazardous materials incidents. However, this limited number of responses does present problems. We do not have enough responses to adequately test procedures and maintain proficiency of special skills. Therefore, every hazardous materials incident should be followed up with specific termination procedures. All responders should be debriefed immediately following the incident so that they know to what they have been exposed and so that any necessary precautions can be taken. Any equipment that was damaged or needs specialized decontamination also should be addressed. Responsibilities for information gathering for a postincident analysis and review can be assigned. The need for a critical incident stress management meeting should be assessed.

BOX 19-1

REVIEW KEY QUESTIONS

What caused the incident?
Was proper notification made?
Were adequate personnel available?
Was adequate equipment available?
Were communication systems adequate?
What areas need improvement?

Postincident Analysis

The second step is to conduct a postincident analysis (PIA). The PIA is an in-depth look at the response from start to finish. It usually is conducted by one or two people who reconstruct the incident to establish a clear picture of the events. The purpose of the PIA is to ensure that the incident has been properly documented and reported and determine the level of financial responsibility. It establishes a clear picture of the response practices and procedures for further study. It also provides a foundation for the development of formal investigations and establishes information that can be used to guide the incident review.

Incident Review

The final step is to hold an incident review. Because multiple agencies are involved at these incidents, all responders should participate. Questions asked during the review should include what caused the incident, other locations that may have the same problem, and how to keep the situation from recurring. Communications during the incident should be examined. A major problem at many incidents is a lack of essential personnel, equipment, and supplies. Reviews can give administrators a realistic list of equipment and other resources that were actually needed at the incident. An incident review can identify what areas of an emergency response plan need changing. Emergency response plans should constantly be rehearsed or examined after an incident, changed as necessary, and rehearsed again. One very important note: the review must be well managed, and it should never be used to assign blame. The review should promote teamwork and be a valuable learning experience (Box 19-1).

Incident Stress Factors

Another factor to consider is the effect of stress on EMS personnel. Stress factors may be higher at hazardous materials incidents because of the nature of the incident and its many complicating factors. The inability to intervene at the scene because of inadequate equipment or training is a major factor. Medical training has always emphasized the need for quick intervention and transport. In hazardous materials incidents, EMS personnel may find themselves waiting for an extended period for patients to be rescued and decontaminated. Multiple victims may necessitate making triage decisions, leading to increased stress. Concerns for response team member safety may have been a factor at the scene. There may also be questions and concerns regarding possible exposure and delayed health effects. Stress level should not be judged by the magnitude of the incident alone. All possible stress factors must be evaluated, and the services of a qualified critical incident stress management team should be obtained as needed.

Summary

The conclusion of field operations at a hazardous materials incident does not mean that all response activities are over. Many concerns will remain to be addressed. All articles that may have been contaminated must be decontaminated or isolated for proper disposal. In addition, several administrative items must be addressed. A debriefing to address immediate concerns should be conducted before responders leave the scene. Then a postincident analysis should be conducted to look at every part of the response. Finally, an incident review should be held and should include the participation of all involved responders. Termination activities will help ensure the safety of responders at the present incident as well as improve response activities in future incidents.

CHAPTER REVIEW QUESTIONS

1. What should be done with possibly contaminated items such as patient care equipment and PPE?
2. Can contaminated uniforms be taken home for cleaning or disposal?
3. Who can be contacted for advice on decontamination and hazardous waste disposal?
4. How can responders tell if equipment decontamination procedures were effective?
5. Who is responsible for disposing of the hazardous waste created during a hazardous materials emergency response?
6. How does the HAZWOPER law requirement for medical surveillance pertain to EMS responders?

7. Why should a debriefing be held after each hazardous materials incident?
8. List at least four things that should be included in a postincident analysis.
9. How can the postincident review be used to improve the agency's emergency response plan?
10. List at least three things that will increase stress factors at a hazardous materials incident.

BIBLIOGRAPHY

Agency for Toxic Substances and Disease Registry: *Managing hazardous materials incidents, emergency medical services: a planning guide for the management of contaminated patients,* Atlanta, Ga, 1992, USDHHS.

Andrews LP, editor: *Emergency responder training manual for the hazardous materials technician,* New York, 1992, Van Nostrand Reinhold.

Bronstein AC, Currance PL: *Emergency care for hazardous materials exposure,* ed 2, St Louis, 1994, Mosby.

Currance PL: *Hazmat for EMS,* St Louis, 1995, Mosby (videotape and guidebook).

Guidelines for public sector hazardous materials training. 1998 ed, HMEP Curriculum Guidelines, Emmitsburg, Md, 1998, National Emergency Training Center.

National Fire Protection Association: *NFPA 471, Recommended practice for responding to hazardous materials incidents,* Quincy, Mass, 1992, The Association.

National Fire Protection Association: *NFPA 473, Standard for professional competence of EMS responders to hazardous materials incidents,* Quincy, Mass, 1992, The Association.

Noll GG, Hildebrand MS, Yvorra JG: *Hazardous materials: managing the incident,* ed 2, Stillwater, Okla, 1995, Fire Protection Publications.

SECTION FIVE

Hazardous Materials Response Situations

20

Examples of Locations/Situations and Chemicals Involved

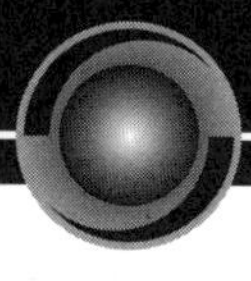

Phil Currance

CHAPTER OBJECTIVES

At the end of this chapter the student will be able to:

- Identify possible locations at which hazardous materials may be encountered.
- Identify the major types of hazardous materials that can be found in each described location.

CASE STUDY

Emergency Medical Services (EMS) units have been dispatched to a local power-generating station for a report of several persons with respiratory distress. A possible chemical release may have occurred at the scene.

- ◆ What types of chemicals are commonly found at power-generating stations?
- ◆ Are there chemicals at that location that, if released, could possibly affect the surrounding population?
- ◆ How can this information be obtained?

Incidents involving hazardous materials may occur in transportation or in fixed facilities. Hazardous materials may be found in industrial locations, retail establishments, swimming pools, hospitals, agricultural areas, and homes. Illegal drug laboratories present a serious hazard to EMS responders. Every year rescue personnel are injured or killed during rescues from confined spaces. Hazardous materials also are moved by every mode of transportation. Transport trucks often carry hazardous materials and commonly are involved in accidents. When emergency personnel respond to a hazardous materials incident, they must be able to assess the nature of the incident quickly and make sound decisions.

Hazardous materials incidents can occur with any type of transportation mode. Truck accidents involving gasoline account for many hazardous materials responses. However, a large percentage of spills other than fuel products occurs in fixed facilities. Past Environmental Protection Agency (EPA) studies designed to look at hazardous chemicals and their sources of release have shown that 75% of nonfuel spills occur at fixed facilities. Frequently released hazardous materials (other than fuel products) include:

- ◆ Sulfuric acid
- ◆ Anhydrous ammonia
- ◆ Chlorine

BERRY 92 ©
FOR GAWD'S SAKES, OWEN... WHERE'S YOUR SPIRIT OF ADVENTURE?

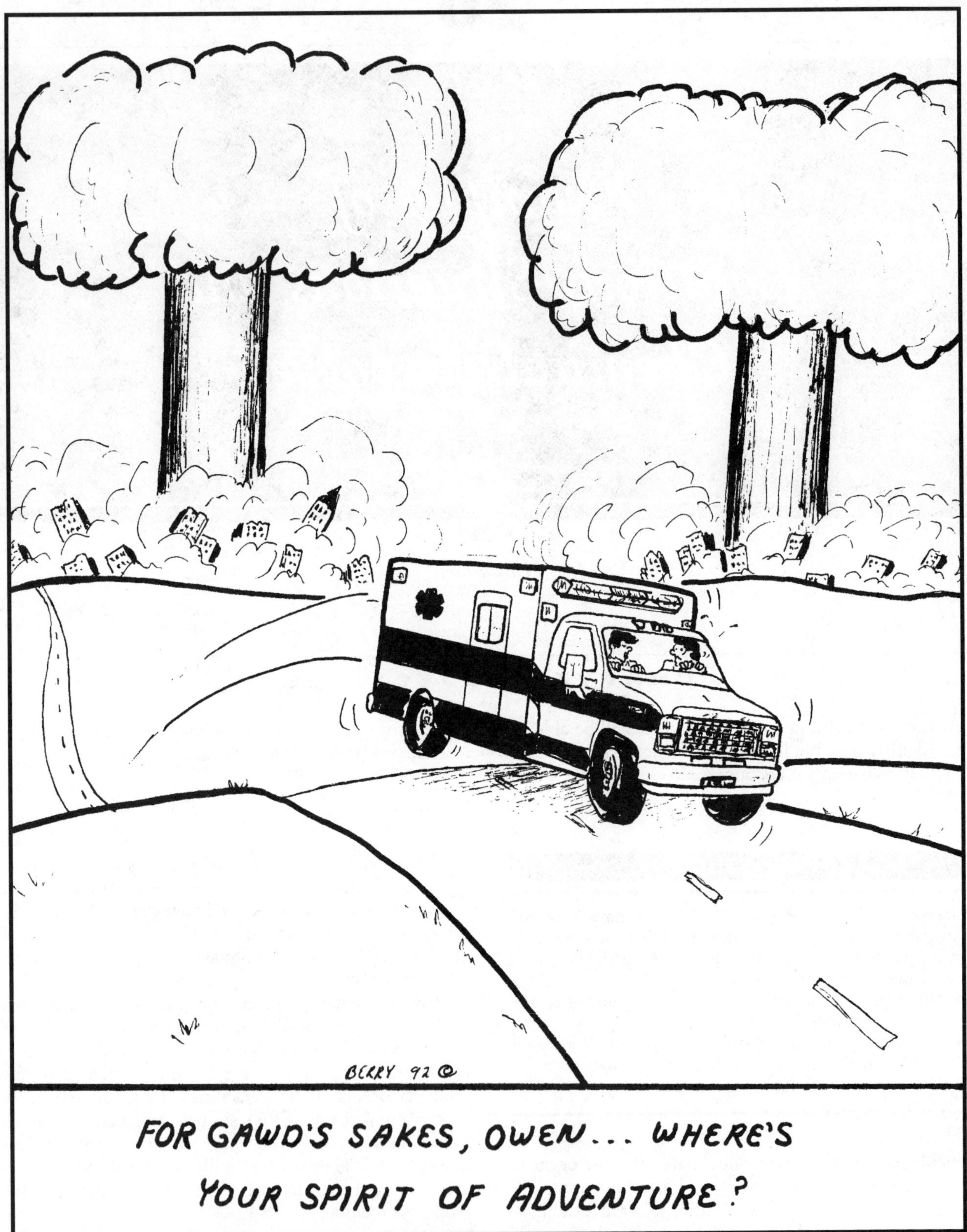

Reprinted with permission from Steve Berry's *I'm Not an Ambulance Driver* cartoon book series.

- Hydrochloric acid
- Sodium hydroxide
- Methanol/methyl alcohol
- Nitric acid
- Toluene
- Methyl chloride

A knowledge of common locations where hazardous materials are used or stored and the types of hazardous materials that can be found in those locations is essential to a safe and effective response. All too often responders must settle for obtaining this information on arrival at the scene. A better approach is to assemble this information during preplanning. Superfund Amendment and Reauthorization Act (SARA) Title III reporting and meetings of the Local Emergency Planning Committee (LEPC) are valuable sources of information on what are determined to be extremely hazardous substances (EHS) in the community. Inspections of local industries and discussions with their health and safety staff or emergency response personnel will provide a wealth of information. Although it is not feasible, or even possible, to discuss every location at which hazardous materials may be found, this chapter will discuss some of the occupations or situations that could potentially be involved in a hazardous materials incident. EMS responders should remember that the use of hazardous materials is so common that they probably are found in almost every location at which emergencies may occur.

Agricultural Areas

Agricultural work is one of the most dangerous occupations in the United States. Workers are at risk from trauma, respiratory illness, skin disorders, muscle and joint problems, and toxic exposures. Workers in agricultural settings may be exposed to various chemicals. We cannot possibly list all of them here but will discuss some of the more commonly encountered substances.

The bulk of agricultural chemicals are fertilizers, insecticides, fumigants, rodenticides, herbicides, and fungicides. Fertilizers can include anhydrous ammonia, iron and zinc compounds, nitrates and nitrites, and phosphate compounds (Fig. 20-1). Although the iron, zinc, and phosphate compounds are relatively safe, exposure to anhydrous ammonia can result in serious soft-tissue, eye, and respiratory tract damage. Exposure to many nitrate and nitrite compounds can result in hypotension, chemical asphyxiation, and respiratory tract damage.

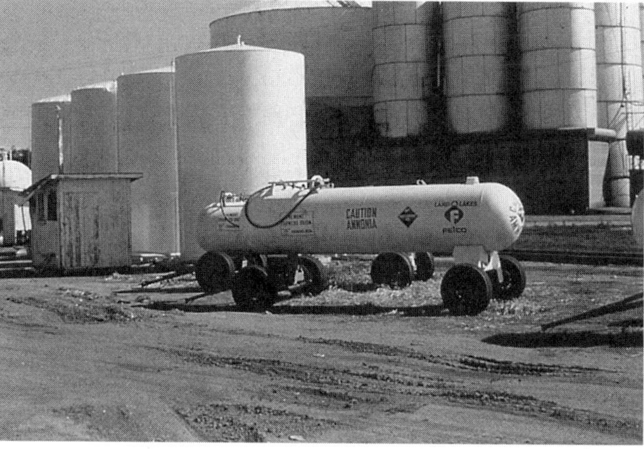

FIG. 20-1 Fertilizers can contain anhydrous ammonia, iron and zinc compounds, nitrates, nitrites, and phosphate compounds.

Many types of insecticide compounds are available. The most commonly used are of the organophosphate family, including malathion, parathion, TEPP, Disulfoton, diazinon, and Naled. Carbamates are related to the organophosphate family and also are widely used. This family includes Aldicarb, Carbyl, and Mexacarbate. Chemicals from the organophosphates and carbamates can cause overstimulation of the parasympathetic nervous system and the classic SLUDGE (*s*alivation, *l*acrimation, *u*rination, *d*efecation, *g*astrointestinal pain/spasm, and *e*mesis) syndrome. Another common family of insecticides is the chlorinated hydrocarbon insecticides. These include chemicals such as DDT, chlordane, heptachlor, aldrin, dieldrin, and toxaphene. DDT and chlordane use has been restricted in the United States because of their persistence in the environment. Others in this family are allowed on a limited basis. Overexposure to these chemicals can result in seizures and respiratory failure. Pyrethrins, pyrethroids, and plant-derived pesticides compose another family of insecticides. This family includes chemicals such as pyrethrin, decamethrin, permethrin, and rotenone. Most of the chemicals in this family present a low level of human toxicity. They usually are mixed in a hydrocarbon solution, and the hydrocarbon may present the biggest hazard. Other members of the plant-derived insecticide family, such as nicotine, can pose a significant human health hazard. Nicotine exposures can result in respiratory arrest and cardiac standstill.

Many types of chemicals are used as fumigants. Some of these, including cyanide, acrylonitrile, phosphine, boron trifluoride, and methyl bromide, present an extreme human health hazard. Exposure to cyanide and acrylonitrile will block the body's use of oxygen at the cellular level. Exposure to phosphine, boron trifluoride, and methyl bromide may result in pulmonary edema. In addition, methyl bromide is a neurotoxin that may cause coma and convulsions. Rodenticides can include chemicals such as strychnine, sodium fluoroacetate, and warfarin. Exposure effects will be different with each of these. For example, strychnine exposure may result in convulsions leading to acidosis and respiratory arrest. Exposure to sodium fluoroacetate may lead to respiratory failure, pulmonary edema, and cerebral edema. Warfarin exposure can impair the clotting ability of the blood and result in internal hemorrhage.

Many different herbicides are used in agriculture. These include but are not limited to 2,4-Ddichlorophenoxyacetic acid (2,4-D), Dicamba, Silvex, pentachlorophenol, paraquat, and diquat. Exposure to 2,4-D and Dicamba can lead to hypo or hyperexcitation of the nervous system and respiratory failure. Pentachlorophenol exposure can result in respiratory and circulatory collapse and a severe increase in body temperature. Paraquat and diquat exposure can lead to multiple organ system damage, including the lungs, heart, and brain.

Fungicides used in agriculture include chemicals such as Thiram, Maneb, Zineb, thiabendazole, Dicloran, and organotin fungicides. Thiram, Maneb, and Zineb are dithiocarbamates and may cause hypotension and respiratory failure. Exposure to thiabendazole can result in cardiovascular collapse and respiratory tract irritation. Organotin fungicide exposure can result in respiratory failure, pulmonary edema, and cerebral edema. Other chemical groups found in these settings can include cleaning compounds, solvents, and fuels. Although we have discussed numerous chemicals in this section, many more can be found in agricultural settings. Local and regional agriculture commissioners or similar authorities can be an excellent resource for agricultural chemicals. Always consult references and medical control for the exact effects and treatment of each chemical threat.

Clandestine Drug Laboratories

The number of clandestine drug laboratories producing methamphetamine has been steadily rising for the past 10 years. EMS personnel may find themselves at a clandestine laboratory in support of a law enforcement operation or may be called because of illness or injuries involving the people operating the laboratory. Common injuries can include exposure to acids and bases, thermal burns from fire or explosion, or drug exposure. Many drug laboratories are located in rural areas. In other cases, mobile homes and self-storage units have been used. Drug laboratories often are discovered after a fire or explosion has occurred. Maintain a high index of suspicion when responding to these types of calls. Another common cue is the presence of a strong odor resembling cat urine. EMS personnel discovering the presence of one of these laboratories should immediately withdraw from the area and notify law enforcement authorities. If you have already entered the scene, use extreme caution when exiting. Many of the chemicals used in these processes are shock sensitive. Do not touch or knock over anything as you leave. Also, some operators have been known to protect their laboratories with booby traps. EMS personnel who have inadvertently entered a laboratory should consider personal decontamination as soon as possible. Refrain from eating, drinking, or smoking until decontamination is complete. Chemicals used during the manufacture of methamphetamine include corrosive, flammable, and reactive agents (Box 20-1). Common acids, such as hydrochloric, sulfuric, and nitric, may be present. Bases, such as sodium hydroxide, potassium hydroxide, and ammonium hydroxide, are common. Exposure to these chemicals may result in skin and soft-tissue burns. Many of these corrosive chemicals will evaporate into a corrosive vapor, which may cause respiratory burns and pulmonary edema when inhaled. Many flammable solvents also are used during drug manufacturing. These can include acetone, isopropyl alcohol, naphtha, benzene, chloroform, and diethylether. These solvents all are extremely flammable, and exposure in large amounts can lead to myocardial irritability and depression of the central nervous system (CNS). Diethylether presents an additional explosion hazard when it drys out. Dried diethylether forms peroxide salts, which may explode when subjected to heat, shock, or friction. Containers holding this product have been known to explode when opened, knocked over, or even picked up. Common reactive chemicals include lithium aluminum hydride, potassium permanganate, and sodium metals such as sodium dicromate. These chemicals are water reactive and release extreme heat when mixed with water. Care must be exercised in decontamination procedures. Any visible powder on patients or responders must be thoroughly brushed off before any water is applied. After physical removal of any powder, flooding quantities of water

BOX 20-1

Common Chemicals Found at Clandestine Drug Laboratories

Acetic acid
Acetone
Ammonium hydroxide
Benzene
Calcium hydroxide
Chloroform
Cyanide
Diethylether
Ethanol
Ethyl amine
Formaldehyde
Hydrochloric acid
Hydrogen gas
Isopropyl alcohol
Lithium aluminum hydride
Magnesium shavings
Methyl amine
Methylene chloride
Naphtha
Nitric acid
Phosphorous pentachloride
Potassium hydroxide
Potassium permanganate
Propane
Pyridine
Sodium dichromate
Sodium hydroxide
Toluene

should be used to remove quickly any residual product and overcome reactions.

We have discussed only a handful of the many chemicals that can be encountered at an illegal drug laboratory. Responding to an emergency at one of these locations is one of the most dangerous things that EMS responders will ever do. The illegal nature of the operation itself implies extreme danger, not to mention the possibility of booby traps and the threat from exposure to multiple chemicals. Extreme caution must be used in any response to these locations.

Confined Spaces

Every year workers are killed or injured in accidents that occur in confined spaces (Fig. 20-2). The National Institute of Occupational Safety and Health (NIOSH) reports that an average of 60 people a year die in confined spaces. Other estimates run much higher. Rescuers routinely rush into the confined spaces on unplanned and unprepared rescues. Statistics have shown that would-be rescuers (co-workers and professional rescue personnel) account for 60% of the deaths in confined spaces (Box 20-2).

BOX 20-2

HAZARDS FOUND IN CONFINED SPACES

- Atmospheric hazards
  - Abnormal oxygen levels
  - Flammable atmospheres
  - Toxic atmospheres
- Engulfment hazards
- Entrapment hazards
- Work-induced hazards
- Electrical, machinery, or other physical hazards

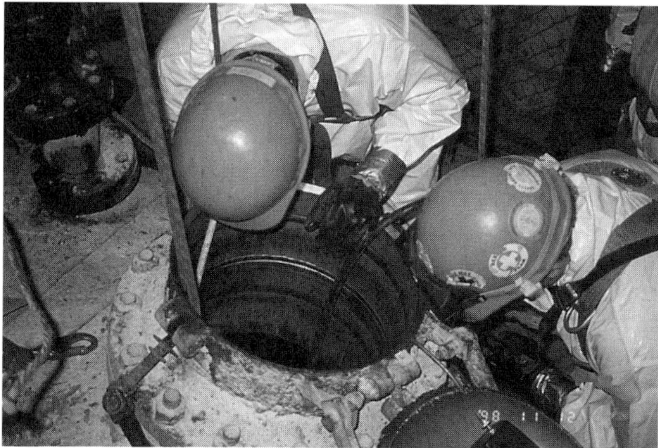

FIG. 20-2 Each year an average of 60 people die in confined spaces.

An estimated 80% to 85% of deaths occurring in confined spaces result from atmospheric hazards. In the vast majority of cases, oxygen deficiency is the main problem. Methane or another simple asphyxiant has displaced the air, resulting in a decrease in oxygen. The Occupational Safety and Health Administration (OSHA) has established 19.5% as the minimal concentration needed for workers without specific respiratory protection. Oxygen-enriched atmospheres (>23.5%) also can create a hazard by causing a severe fire hazard.

Flammable atmospheres also are a problem. Methane is an extremely flammable gas created by the decay of organic matter. Although it often creates an oxygen-deficient atmosphere, in lower concentrations, methane presents a major fire hazard. Confined spaces, such as tanks, often are used to store many other flammable liquids and gases. Toxic gases and vapors also create a hazard in confined spaces. The two toxic gases most often encountered are carbon monoxide and hydrogen sulfide. Both of these gases are chemical asphyxiants that interfere with the body's use of oxygen. Carbon monoxide prevents the bonding of oxygen with hemoglobin, and hydrogen sulfide interferes with the use of oxygen at the cellular level. Responders should identify any chemicals that were stored in the space and all chemicals that are used or stored around the space. Patient treatment will depend on the chemicals that are involved. Amyl nitrite and sodium nitrite, found in cyanide antidote kits, can be used to treat hydrogen sulfide toxicity.

In many cases, the work that was being performed in the space created the hazard. Solvents, paints, and cleaning compounds are all possible problems. Welding or cutting operations may release a flammable gas or deplete available oxygen. In addition to atmospheric hazards, OSHA has identified certain physical hazards as being extremely dangerous. Engulfment in loose materials and entrapment by sloping floor tanks are frequent hazards. In addition to these, any other serious safety hazards, such as electricity and operating machinery, must be identified. EMS responders should never enter a confined space unless they have received proper training, have the proper safety equipment, and have an attendant available. Because the majority of deaths in confined spaces are due to atmospheric hazards, defensive actions, such as ventilation, can provide the time needed for trained rescue crews to set up and enter the space.

Oil Refineries

Many refinery operations involve the use of hazardous chemicals (Fig. 20-3). These include corrosive and toxic chemicals as well as the expected flammable liquids. Inventories can include several hundred chemicals. We will discuss some of the most common chemicals that when released, may cause injuries that will require EMS involvement (Box 20-3). Some of these chemicals occur as liquids, whereas others are found in the gaseous state.

Anhydrous ammonia, chlorine, and sulfur dioxide are

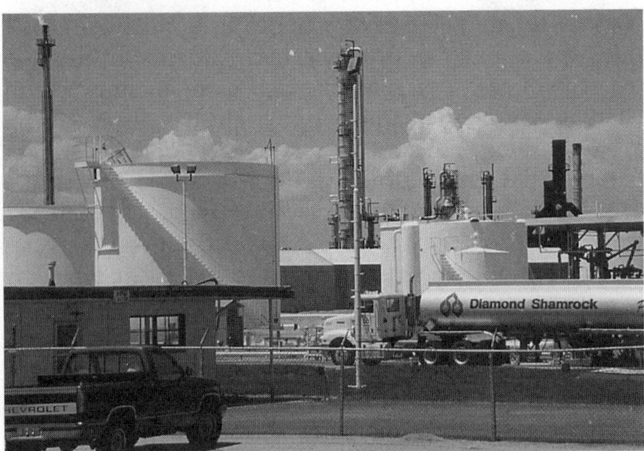

FIG. 20-3 Oil refinery.

BOX 20-3

Examples of Common Refinery Chemicals

Anhydrous ammonia
Carbon monoxide
Caustic soda
Chlorine
Hydrogen sulfide
Hydrofluoric acid
Nitrogen
Sulfur dioxide
Sulfuric acid
Tetra-ethyl lead

corrosive gases that are widely used at oil refineries. Exposure to these gases will result in skin, mucous membrane, and pulmonary tissue irritation and burns. Anhydrous ammonia is used in almost all operating areas in refineries. It is stored and handled as a liquid but will rapidly change into a gas when released from its container. Its massive expansion ratio will result in widespread exposure when it is released. Chlorine can be found in cylinders of various sizes at the refinery. One hundred-pound cylinders, 1-ton containers, and occasional 90-ton railcars all can be encountered. Like anhydrous ammonia, chlorine also has a large expansion ratio. A large vapor cloud will result even if a small amount of liquid is released. Sulfur dioxide is another corrosive chemical that commonly is used in water treatment operations. It is found as a liquid in 1-ton cylinders and when released, will rapidly turn into sulfuric acid on moist tissue. EMS response to injuries caused by these chemicals should include self-protection, decontamination as necessary, and supportive management.

Carbon monoxide and hydrogen sulfide are chemical asphyxiants that are common at oil refineries. Carbon monoxide is a chemical asphyxiant that binds hemoglobin. It is found in the exhaust of internal-combustion engines and the flue gases of furnaces and heaters. Because it is colorless, odorless, and tasteless, it has no warning properties. Because carbon monoxide is so prevalent at refineries, its involvement should be considered when workers are stricken in process areas or when multiple patients have similar complaints such as headaches, nausea, and ringing in the ears. Hydrogen sulfide is a colorless gas with a strong odor of rotten eggs. In higher concentrations it may cause olfactory fatigue, resulting in a decrease in the ability of exposed patients to detect its odor. At refineries it may be encountered in storage vessels, tanks, flare lines, and sewers. It also acts as a chemical asphyxiant by interfering with the cellular use of oxygen. Caustic soda (sodium hydroxide) and sulfuric acid are supplied to many refinery units. Hydrofluoric acid is used in many refineries for high-octane gasoline blending. They all are strong corrosives that can cause soft-tissue injuries and respiratory burns. Caustic soda is used extensively throughout refineries and can be found in lines, storage vessels, and other equipment. When supplied to operating units, caustic soda commonly is known as *fresh caustic,* and after it is contaminated or diluted it is known as *spent caustic.* Sulfuric acid is a heavy, oily, corrosive liquid that may be encountered throughout the refinery. When contaminated it is referred to as *spent acid.* Hydrofluoric acid has the added hazard of resulting in systemic fluoride toxicity when absorbed into the body.

Nitrogen is used at refineries for gas blanketing, and purging lines and instruments. Because it is a major component of the air, its hazards often are overlooked. Nitrogen is an extremely effective simple asphyxiant and possesses an additional cryogenic hazard. Tetra-ethyl lead and tetra-ethyl lead compounds are used at refineries in connection with the blending of finished motor gasoline. These heavy, oily liquids are poisonous by inhalation, absorption, or ingestion.

Plastics Manufacturing

The plastics industry has greatly affected our lives. Plastics are used to manufacture many items that we use every day. Automobiles, toys, furniture, clothing, and food and beverage containers all are made of plastic. Plastics are made from small molecular units (monomers) that are linked together to become larger molecules (polymers). This process is called *polymerization.* The manufacture of plastics involves many chemicals (Fig. 20-4). Vinyl chloride monomer is used to produce polyvinyl chloride (PVC). Exposure to vinyl chloride monomer can result in CNS depression, respiratory arrest, and circulatory collapse. Styrene and acrylonitrile are used to manufacture polystyrene and synthetic rubber. Overexposure to styrene can result in respiratory and mucous membrane irritation. CNS depression also may be seen. Acrylonitrile also causes skin irritation but more importantly is metabolized to cyanide in the body. Acrylic acid and methyl acrylate are used to produce acrylics. Exposure to these chemicals can result in skin and mucous membrane irri-

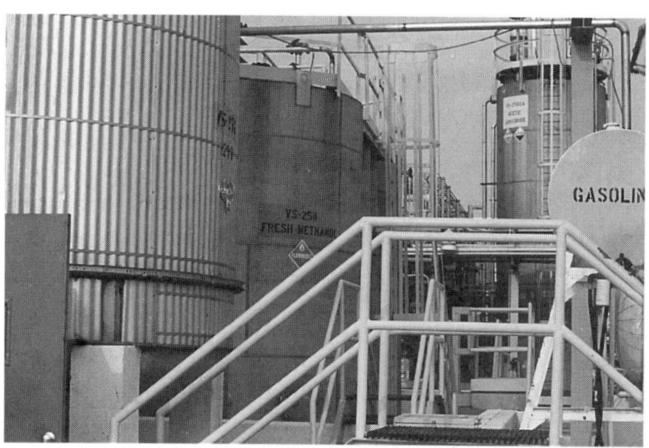

FIG. 20-4 Chemical storage area at plastics manufacturer.

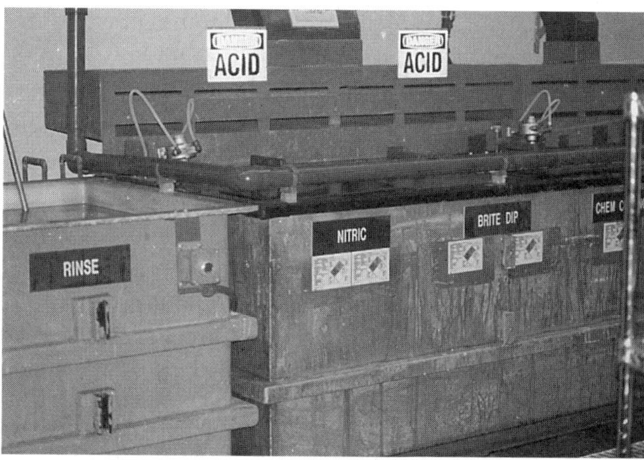

FIG. 20-5 Plating line operations.

tation. Exposure to methyl acrylate also can cause headache, fatigue, and skin sensitization.

Fluoropolymers are used to produce nonstick cookware and wire coatings. Various hydrocarbons, hydrogen fluoride, and hydrofluoric acid are used to produce fluoropolymers. Hydrogen fluoride and hydrofluoric acid exposure can lead to serious, deep skin burns and lung and mucous membrane irritation. Systemic fluoride toxicity also can result. Phenol and formaldehyde are common chemicals used to produce phenolic resins. Phenolic resins are used to produce plywood, adhesives, and coating of fabrics. Phenol and formaldehyde can cause skin irritation and burns, and are skin absorbable. In addition, phenol can cause CNS depression, cardiac arrhythmias, and pulmonary edema. Formaldehyde exposure can result in seizures, respiratory failure, and pulmonary edema. Isocyanates, such as toluene diisocyanate, hexamethylene diisocyanate, and isophorone diisocyanate, are used to produce polyurethane and urethane, which, in turn, are widely used to make furnishings and coatings. Exposure to most isocyanates can result in mucous membrane irritation, pulmonary edema, CNS depression, and paralysis of the respiratory center.

The foregoing is only an overview of chemicals commonly used in the manufacture of plastics. The different processes involve many other chemicals and can produce many by-products and hazardous wastes. In addition to the primary hazards associated with these chemicals, plastics present a major hazard when they are thermally decomposed in heat or fire. Some decomposition products, such as hydrochloric acid and aldehydes, can cause respiratory irritation. Others, such as nitrogen oxides and phosgene, can cause severe pulmonary damage. Carbon monoxide and cyanide also are released by burning plastics. Be sure to identify and assess each and every chemical that is involved in each emergency.

Plating Operations

Metal-plating operations are common in industry. Plating operations commonly are found in the semiconductor industry, at automobile and aircraft manufacturers, and anywhere that small metal parts are manufactured. In plating operations, chemical vats are prepared along a "plating line" (Fig. 20-5). Parts are then prepared and coated by dipping them into the appropriate vats along the line.

Common plating operations include chemicals such as acids, bases, solvents, and poisons (Box 20-4). Acids can include nitric, hydrofluoric, sulfuric, and hydrochloric. Common bases used are sodium hydroxide, potassium hydroxide, and ammonium hydroxide. Exposure to any of these corrosives can result in skin, soft-tissue, and respiratory tract burns. Isopropyl alcohol, acetone, methanol, and methyl chloride are common flammable solvents. In addition to the fire hazard, they can cause myocardial irritability and CNS depression.

Cyanide is one of the most toxic chemicals used in

BOX 20-4

Common Chemicals Used in Plating Operations

Acetone
Anhydrous ammonia
Caustic soda
Chlorine
Hydrochloric acid
Hydrofluoric acid
Hydrogen peroxide
Nitric acid
Phosphoric acid
Potassium cyanide
Potassium hydroxide
Sodium cyanide
Sulfuric acid
Trichloroethylene
Zinc cyanide

these operations. It is toxic through all routes of exposure. A major hazard exists if workers add cyanide to acid or acid to cyanide when preparing the vats. Cyanide and acid together will create hydrogen cyanide gas. Plating operations also will involve chemicals, such as sulfuric acid, sodium hydroxide, and chlorine, in large quantities to treat water.

Power-Generating Stations

Coal-fired, power-generating stations are associated with a wide variety of hazardous chemicals, many of which are used for the stations' water treatment needs. The greatest hazard found at these sites is the large quantities of chlorine (Fig. 20-6). Many facilities may have up to six 1-ton cylinders of liquified chlorine. Because chlorine has an expansion ratio of approximately 1 cubic foot of liquid to 450 cubic feet of pure vapor, even a small leak in one of these cylinders can create a major problem. In addition to the chlorine, most facilities have large quantities of sulfuric acid and sodium hydroxide. As in most maintenance shops, many solvents, cleaners, degreasers, and flammable liquids can be found at power-generating stations. Flammable gases found at these facilities include acetylene, which is used for repair operations, and hydrogen, which is used in coal combustion.

Semiconductor Industry

Electronics is the world's fourth largest industry. Many of the chemicals used in the semiconductor industry are the most dangerous to which EMS personnel may have to respond. Fortunately, most semiconductor businesses have established extensive safety procedures. Large semiconductor facilities may use several hundred or even thousands of chemicals (Fig. 20-7). Although it is not feasible to review every one of the possible chemical threats, we will discuss some of the more common dangers found industrywide.

If an accidental release does occur, workers may be exposed to flammable solvents and gases, corrosive liquids, poisonous liquids, and poisonous gases. Flammable liquids, such as acetone and isopropyl alcohol, are used in wave solder machines and as solvents. Other flammable solvents can include trichloroethylene, perchloroethylene, methanol, xylene, and N-methyl pyrrolidone. Hydrogen and silane are widely used flammable gases. Silane is a pyrophoric gas used in the electronics industry. When it is released from its container, it usually will ignite immediately. In rare cases, it may form into a pocket of expanding gas before it can ignite. In these cases, the silane can detonate. The corrosive liquids used in the industry include both acids and bases. Sulfuric, nitric, hydrochloric, hydrofluoric, and chromic acid all are common. All acids can cause soft-tissue injury on contact and lung injury when inhaled. Hydrofluoric acid also can act as a skin-absorbable systemic poison, resulting in fluoride toxicity. Common bases include sodium hydroxide, potassium hydroxide, and ammonium hydroxide. Poisonous liquids and gases may be found. Acutely toxic liquids in-

TABLE 20-1
COMMON TOXIC GASES USED IN THE SEMICONDUCTOR INDUSTRY

GAS	PEL	IDLH
Arsine	0.05 ppm	3 ppm
Bromine	0.1 ppm	3 ppm
Chlorine	0.5 ppm	10 ppm
Diborane	0.1 ppm	15 ppm
Phosphine	0.3 ppm	50 ppm
Trifluoroboron	1 ppm (ceiling)	25 ppm
Tetrachlorocarbon	10 ppm	200 ppm
Hydrogen chloride	5 ppm (ceiling)	500 ppm

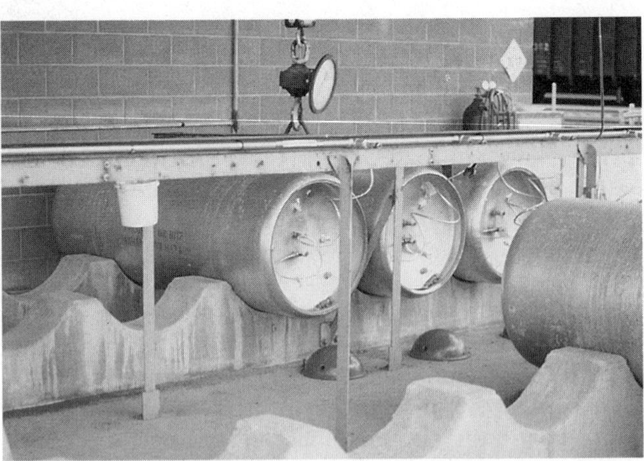

FIG. 20-6 Chlorine cylinders at power-generating facilities pose the greatest hazard.

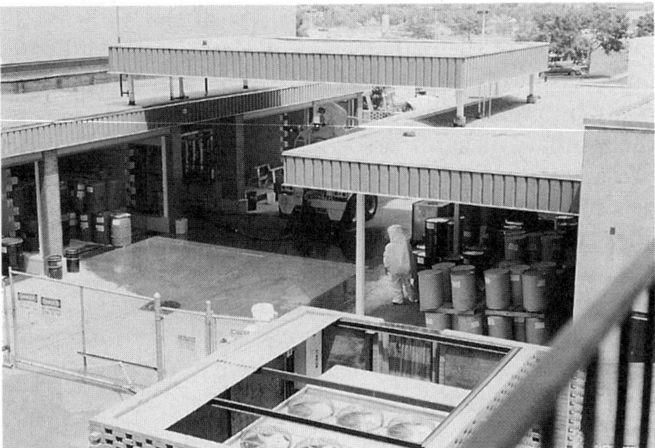

FIG. 20-7 Large facilities may use thousands of chemicals.

clude cyanide, which is used in gold etching operations, and arsenic compounds. Others, such as glycol ethers and photoresist compounds, present a chronic exposure hazard and reproductive or possible carcinogenic threats. Some of the gases used in this industry are the most poisonous that workers use (Table 20-1). Arsine gas is a perfect example. Exposure to arsine gas can result in red blood cell destruction and renal failure. It currently has a permissible exposure limit (PEL) of 0.05 ppm and an immediately dangerous to life and health limit (IDLH) of 3 ppm. Other gases, such as nitrogen and argon, are not considered to be poisons but are extremely effective simple asphyxiants. Because of the nature of chemicals in this industry, EMS responders should exercise extreme caution when responding to emergencies at these facilities.

Terrorist Activities (Purposeful Release of Biological or Chemical Agents)

The use of biological warfare dates back to 1346. During a war in Kaffa (now Feodossia), Tartar soldiers who had died from the plague were thrown over the walls of the besieged city. Some medical historians believe that this action led to the plague epidemic, which spread over all of Europe from Genoa, via the Mediterranean ports. Biological and chemical warfare has come a long way since then. Except for nuclear weapons, chemical and biological weapons (or *weapons of mass destruction,* which is the current politically correct term) are the most destructive weapons in most warfare inventories. These agents have not been widely used in war, having seen limited application during World War I and only sporadic use since then. Unfortunately, the threat of terrorist use of these weapons is growing. The March 1995 incident in which Japanese subway passengers were exposed to the highly toxic nerve agent sarin in a terrorist attack is a perfect example of how relatively easy it is to place a weapon of mass destruction in a public area. The size and portability of biological and most chemical agents make them the perfect terrorist weapon. Although most chemical agents are difficult to acquire, some agents, such as sarin, can be easily made in laboratories by experienced chemists. The recipe and instructions are available on the Internet.

Biological weapons are even easier to obtain. They sometimes are obtained under the false pretense of research studies; also, some can be manufactured easily. Many biological agents, including anthrax, plague, ricin, and smallpox, are well recognized for their potential as biological weapons (Box 20-5). Almost all of these agents will present with an incubation period of anywhere from 1 to 30 days, depending on the specific agent. Signs and symptoms will vary, depending on the agent. This overview does not allow for discussion of each agent; however, a wealth of information is available in the literature.

Because delayed symptoms are the norm with these agents, the fact that an exposure has occurred will not be known for several days and possibly weeks.

Numerous chemical agents can be used as weapons also. These include nerve agents; blister agents, or vesicants; riot control agents; choking agents; and blood agents or chemical asphyxiants. Nerve agents are probably the best known chemical weapons. They are related to the organophosphate class of pesticides and function as cholinesterase inhibitors. Cholinesterase deactivates acetylcholine (ACh), the primary neurotransmitter in the parasympathetic nervous system. Cholinesterase breaks down and stops the action of ACh. When cholinesterase is inhibited, it is unable to perform its function; consequently, ACh continues to overstimulate the parasympathetic nervous system. The classic SLUDGE syndrome of organophosphate poisoning commonly is seen. This group of agents includes sarin (GB), tabun (GA), soman (GD), and VX. Sarin, tabun, and soman are absorbable through inhalation and the skin. They usually are dispersed as a vapor or mist. VX is formulated to be more persistent in the environment. It is dissolved in an oily base so that it does not evaporate as easily as the other nerve agents. It most commonly is absorbed through the skin. Antidotes for this group of chemicals includes a combination of atropine, pralidoxime chloride (2PAM), and Valium.

Riot control agents, also known as *irritants, lacrimators,* and *tear gas,* produce transient discomfort and irritation of the skin, eyes, and mucous membranes. Law enforcement agencies use these agents for crowd control. The most common of these agents are CS gas, CN gas, and pepper spray. Their major effect is to cause pain, burning, or discomfort to exposed mucous membranes and skin. These effects typically occur within seconds of

BOX 20-5

Possible Biological Warfare Agents

Anthrax toxin
Botulinum toxin
Brucellosis
Cholera toxin
Clostridium perfringens toxins
Crimean-Congo hemorrhagic fever
Melioidosis
Plague
Q fever
Ricin
Rift Valley fever
Saxitoxin
Smallpox
Staphylococcal enterotoxin B
Trichothecium mycotoxins
Tularemia
Venezuelan equine encephalitis

exposure and have a limited duration of action. Exposures to high concentrations can cause severe respiratory tract irritation. These agents (especially pepper spray) commonly are used by pranksters in public areas such as schools, shopping malls, or public restrooms.

Blister agents, or vesicants, are another type of chemical warfare agent. This group includes sulfur mustard (H, HD, HS, HL, HT), nitrogen mustard (HN1, HN2, HN3), lewisite (L), and phosgene oxime (CX). The mustard agents pose a threat in liquid and vapor forms. They usually present with an asymptomatic period of hours and later cause burns and blisters on exposed skin and eyes. Respiratory effects can occur immediately and can range from mild irritation to extreme airway damage. Systemically absorbed mustard may produce effects in the bone marrow, the gastrointestinal (GI) tract, and the central nervous system (CNS). There is no antidote for the mustard agents. Lewisite is a blister agent that damages the eyes, skin, and airways by direct contact. It can be dispersed as a liquid or mist. After it is absorbed, it can cause an increase in capillary permeability, resulting in hypovolemia. Exposure causes immediate irritation and pain, although skin lesions may take hours to reach full damage potential. British-Anti-Lewisite (BAL) is an antidote for lewisite that will alleviate some of the effects. CX is a warfare agent that causes a corrosive-type burn. It does not cause blisters like the other agents. Below 95° F it is a solid, but the vapor pressure of the solid is high enough to produce symptoms. It causes immediate burning and irritation of the skin, eyes, and respiratory tract. There is no antidote for CX exposure. Immediate decontamination for patients exposed to any of these agents is essential.

Choking agents cause respiratory irritation and varying degrees of pulmonary edema. Included in this class are phosgene (CG), diphosgene (DP), chlorine (CL), and chloropicrin (PS). These agents are a gas at room temperature but may be stored as a liquid under pressure. They typically have a high expansion ratio and when released, convert into a large amount of gas. Exposed patients will present with eye and airway irritation, dyspnea, and a delayed onset of pulmonary edema. These agents can damage the alveolar-capillary membrane, resulting in fluid passing into the alveolar spaces of the lungs. The gas also will become a solution on moist areas of the body, resulting in soft-tissue injury. Triage protocols should be modified to account for the delayed onset of pulmonary edema.

Blood agents, or chemical asphyxiants, interfere with the body's use of oxygen. Blood agents that could be used for chemical warfare include hydrogen cyanide (AC) and cyanogen chloride (CK). These agents commonly are liquids at room temperature but will vaporize rapidly into gas. The cyanide ion has a high affinity for iron (Fe^3) in the cytochrome oxidase complex, which is vital for the cellular use of oxygen. When the cyanide binds with the iron in this complex, it effectively prevents the cellular use of oxygen. At higher concentrations these agents have an extremely rapid onset of symptoms. After approximately 15 seconds' exposure to a high concentration, there is a transient increase in respirations (hyperpnea) followed in 15 to 30 seconds by convulsions. Respiratory activity stops 2 to 3 minutes later, and cardiac activity ceases several minutes after that. The onset and progression of signs and symptoms after ingestion of cyanide or after inhalation of a lower concentration of vapor are slower. The first effects may not occur until several minutes after exposure, and the progression of effects depends on the amount and rate of absorption. The initial transient hyperpnea may be followed by a feeling of anxiety or apprehension, agitation, vertigo, nausea, vomiting, and muscle tremors. Later, consciousness is lost, respirations decrease in rate and depth, and convulsions and cardiac dysrhythmias follow. Because the progression of events is delayed, diagnosis and successful treatment are feasible. A possible clue of cyanide involvement is the odor of bitter almonds. However, an estimated 50% of the population is genetically unable to detect the odor of cyanide. Once patients are removed from a gas exposure to a blood agent, decontamination usually is not needed. If patients are wet or their clothes are wet, decontamination is needed. Delayed signs and symptoms are not a typical problem with these agents. Treatment of patients exposed to these agents may include administration of the cyanide antidote kit.

Wastewater Treatment Facilities

Surveys reveal that approximately 100 different chemicals are commonly used at sewage treatment plants. These can include disinfectants, cleaning products, laboratory chemicals, water treatment chemicals, solvents, lubricants, and pesticides (Fig. 20-8). Most accidents will involve disinfectants and water treatment chemicals. Disinfectants and cleaning products include ammonia, alcohols, and liquid chlorine cleaners. Chlorine, aluminum sulfate, and ferric chloride are common water treatment

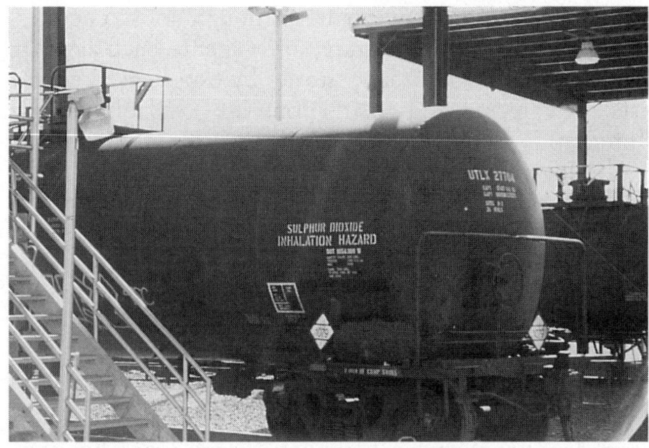

FIG. 20-8 Chlorine and sulfur dioxide railcars at a wastewater treatment facility.

chemicals. Among the latter, chlorine presents the greatest hazard. It usually is stored in 1-ton cylinders or 90-ton railcars. Aluminum sulfate can produce sulfuric acid when mixed with water. Ferric chloride decomposes to hydrochloric acid when mixed with water. Perhaps the greatest hazard at these facilities are the gases that are produced during the wastewater treatment process. Hydrogen sulfide is a gas commonly found in these locations. It is an extremely toxic chemical asphyxiant and also is a flammable gas. Carbon monoxide, produced by malfunctioning equipment, occasionally is encountered when maintenance crews are working on sewage digesters. Ammonia and methane are produced by the natural breakdown of sewage. Ammonia can be extremely irritating and becomes ammonium hydroxide when it contacts moist tissue or mucous membranes. Methane is an extremely flammable gas and a simple asphyxiant. Other simple asphyxiants commonly found at these facilities include nitrogen and carbon dioxide. Workers at wastewater treatment facilities often perform work in confined spaces. EMS responders must exercise extreme caution when responding to these types of emergencies. Rescues should be performed only by trained personnel using proper personal protective equipment.

Summary

This chapter has provided an overview of some of the many locations or situations that may involve hazardous materials. Almost every industry, as well as most homes, use some hazardous materials. EMS responders should be proactive in obtaining information regarding hazards in their response area. Information on the types of chemical and physical hazards to be expected is vital for a safe and effective response. The time to prepare for a hazardous materials response is before it happens. When the call comes in, your time may have just run out.

CHAPTER REVIEW QUESTIONS

1. Where can information regarding the types of chemicals that may be present in your response area be found?
2. What types of chemical hazards may be found at agricultural areas?
3. What types of hazards may be encountered when responding to emergencies in confined spaces?
4. What types of chemicals may be found at clandestine drug laboratories?
5. What types of chemicals may be found at oil refineries?
6. What types of chemicals may be found at plastics manufacturing facilities?
7. What types of chemicals may be found at facilities that conduct plating operations?
8. What types of chemicals may be found at power-generating facilities?
9. What types of chemicals may be found in the semiconductor industry?
10. What types of chemical and biological agents may be released in terrorist activities?
11. What types of chemicals may be found at wastewater treatment plants?

BIBLIOGRAPHY

Agency for Toxic Substances and Disease Registry: *Managing hazardous materials incidents, emergency medical services: a planning guide for the management of contaminated patients,* Atlanta, Ga, 1992, USDHHS.

Brackett D: *Holy terror: Armageddon in Tokyo,* New York, 1996, Weatherhill Inc.

Chemical Casualty Care Office: *Medical management of chemical casualties handbook,* Aberdeen, Md, 1995, MRICD, Aberdeen Proving Ground.

Currance PL: *Hazmat for EMS,* St Louis, 1995, Mosby (videotape and guidebook).

Franz D: *Defensive against toxic weapons,* Fredrick, Md, 1996, US Army Medical Research Institute of Infectious Diseases.

Haddad LM, Shannon MW, Winchester JF: *Clinical management of poisoning and drug overdose,* ed 3, Philadelphia, 1998, WB Saunders.

Medical management of biological casualties handbook, Fredrick Md, 1993, US Army Medical Research Institute of Infectious Diseases.

Noll GG, Hildebrand MS, Yvorra JG: *Hazardous materials managing the incident,* ed 2, Stillwater, Okla, 1995, Fire Protection Publications.

Somani S, editor: *Chemical warfare agents,* San Diego, 1992, Academic Press.

Sullivan JB, Kreiger GR, editors: *Hazardous material toxicology: clinical principles of environmental health,* Baltimore, 1992, Williams & Wilkins.

10-90 Gold NBC Response Plan: *Procedures and support activities developed by the defense protective service to a nuclear, biological, or chemical incident within DPS jurisdiction,* Washington, DC, 1996, Defense Protective Service.

Glossary

A

absorbents Materials designed to pick up and hold liquid hazardous materials.

ACGIH The American Conference of Governmental and Industrial Hygienists (ACGIH). A private consortium of governmental, university, and industrial members has developed a system called *threshold limit values (TLVs).*

adsorbents Materials designed to adhere liquid and vaporous hazardous materials on their surface area.

aerosols Suspension of solids or liquids in air.

alpha particle A positively charged particle emitted by certain radioactive materials.

APR Air-purifying respirator.

asphyxiant A substance that can cause death by depriving the body of oxygen. Asphyxiants may be classified as either simple or chemical (see following two entries).

asphyxiant, chemical Chemicals that have systemic actions impairing the body's ability to either supply oxygen to the tissues or prevent oxygen from being used during metabolism. Examples include cyanide and carbon monoxide.

asphyxiant, simple Chemicals that deprive the body of oxygen by displacing oxygen in ambient air. The simple asphyxiant has no chemical action other than functioning as an oxygen displacer. Examples include argon, neon, and helium.

asphyxiation Oxygen deprivation within the body. Simple asphyxiants displace oxygen, and chemical asphyxiants interfere with oxygen transportation or use inside the body.

atmospheric storage tanks Fixed-facility storage tanks that hold liquid at atmospheric pressure.

awareness level Training level established by OSHA 29 CFR 1910.120. Responders who may be the first on the scene of a hazardous materials emergency. Awareness-level responders are trained to recognize the presence of hazardous materials, protect themselves, call for help, and secure the area.

B

beta particle A negatively charged particle emitted by certain radioactive materials.

buddy system Personnel organization system in which each responder is working with and observed by at least one other employee in the response group.

bulk containers Cargo containers that may be transported by truck, rail, or ocean-going vessel designed to transport large quantities of a single product.

C

CGI Combustible gas indicator.

cold zone The cold zone (support) is a safe area that is isolated from the area of contamination. This zone has safe and easy access. It contains the command post, staging areas for personnel, vehicles, and equipment. EMS personnel are stationed in the cold zone.

combustible liquids Any liquid having a flash point above 141° F (60.5° C) and below 200° F (93° C). Examples include brake fluid, glycol ethers, and camphor oil.

corrosive substance Any liquid or solid that can destroy human flesh on contact or has a severe corrosion rate on steel.

CPC Chemical-protective clothing.

cryogenics Gases that have been liquified with a boiling point of less than −130° F (−90° C). Cryogenic liquids have a great expansion ratio and will vaporize rapidly when heated.

D

decon Abbreviation for decontamination.

decontamination The physical and chemical process of reducing and preventing the spread of contamination from persons and equipment used at a hazardous materials incident. Also referred to as *contamination reduction.*

defensive actions Actions carried out at a hazardous materials incident that do not involve direct intentional contact with the material. Actions carried out from a safe distance that are focused at slowing down the progression of the incident.

degradation The physical breakdown of chemical-resistant clothing because of exposure to chemicals, use, or improper storage conditions.

DOT Department of Transportation.

dusts Solid particles of various sizes.

E

EHS Extremely hazardous substances.

EMS Emergency Medical Services.

Emergency Medical Services (EMS) Functions as required to provide emergency medical care for ill and/or injured persons by trained providers.

EPA Environmental Protection Agency.

etiology The causes or origin of a disease or disorder.

evaporation The process of a solid or liquid turning into a gas.

explosive substance Any chemical compound, mixture, or device, the primary or common purpose of which is to function by detonation or rapid combustion (i.e., with substantial instantaneous release of gas and heat). Found in liquid or solid forms. Includes dynamite, TNT, black powder, fireworks, and ammunition.

extremely hazardous substances (EHS) Chemicals determined by the Environmental Protection Agency, in the Superfund Amendment and Reauthorization Act, to be extremely hazardous to a community during an emergency spill or release as a result of their toxicities and physical and chemical properties.

F

FID Flame ionization device.
flammable The capacity of a substance to ignite.
flammable gases Any compressed gas that meets requirements for lower flammability limit, flammability limit range, flame projection, or flame propagation as specified in CFR Title 49, Sec. 173.300(b). Examples include acetylene, butane, hydrogen, and propane.
flammable liquids Any liquid having a flash point below 141° F (60.5° C). Examples include benzene, gasoline, and acetone.
flammable solids A solid material other than an explosive that is liable to cause fires through friction, retained heat from manufacturing or processing, or that can be ignited readily. When these substances are ignited, they burn so vigorously and persistently that they create a serious transportation hazard. Examples include phosphorus, lithium, magnesium, titanium, and calcium resinate.

G

gamma A type of electromagnetic radiation.

H

hazardous material A substance (solid, liquid, or gas) capable of posing an unreasonable risk to health, safety, environment, or property.
Hazardous Materials Communication Standard OSHA regulation (29 CFR 1910.120), which requires chemical manufacturers to develop material safety data sheets (MSDS) on specific types of hazardous chemicals and requires employers to provide chemical health information to employees.
Hazardous Materials Identification Guide (HMIG) A marking system used to provide hazard information to users. Provides information on health, fire, and reactivity hazards, and protective equipment needs.
Hazardous Materials Identification System (HMIS) A marking system used to provide hazard information to users. Provides information on health, fire, and reactivity hazards, and protective equipment needs.
heat cramps Cramps in the extremities or abdomen caused by excessive sweating and depletion of body fluids and electrolytes.
heat exhaustion A form of shock caused by excessive sweating and fluid loss. May lead to heat stroke.
heat fatigue Most mild form of heat illness. Characterized by extreme fatigue and occasionally, heat rash.
heat stroke Severe and sometimes fatal condition caused by prolonged exposure to heat and excessive sweating, leading to a failure of the body's cooling system. Core body temperature is greater than 105° F (40.5° C). Rapid intervention and transport to a medical facility is required.
HMIG Hazardous Materials Identification Guide.
HMIS Hazardous Materials Identification System.
hot zone The hot (exclusion) zone is the area where contamination exists. Patients are removed from this area to the warm zone for decontamination. Entrance to the hot zone requires proper personal protective equipment.
hypothermia A breakdown in temperature regulation of the body. Core body temperature is below 95° F (35° C). First sign is uncontrollable shivering. Rapid rewarming of the patient is necessary.
hypoxia Lack of an adequate amount of oxygen in inspired air; reduced oxygen concentration or tension.

I

IDLH Immediately dangerous to life or health. The maximum air concentration of a chemical from which one could escape within 30 minutes without impairing symptoms or irreversible health effects. Used to determine respirator selection. (Possible carcinogenic effects were not considered in setting these values.)
IMS Incident management system.
incident command level Responders who will assume control of an incident scene beyond the level of the first responder operations.
infectious substance A viable microorganism, or its toxin, that causes, or may cause, human disease. Examples include anthrax, rabies, tetanus, botulism, polio, and specimens obtained from patients with acquired immunodeficiency syndrome (AIDS).
inorganic compound Chemical compounds that do not contain carbon.
intrinsically safe Equipment that is incapable of releasing sufficient electrical energy to cause the ignition of a flammable mixture.
IP Ionization potential.
irritating material A liquid or solid substance that on contact with fire or when exposed to air gives off dangerous or intensely irritating fumes, but not including any poisonous material. Examples include tear gas, xylyl bromide, phenacyl chloride, CN gas, and chemical mace.

L

labels Written or printed matter accompanying an article or substance to furnish identification.
LC_{50} Lethal concentration 50% (LC_{50}). The inhaled dose of a substance that causes death in 50% of the test animal population.
LD_{50} Lethal dose 50% (LD_{50}) The absorbed dose (oral or dermal) of a substance that causes death in 50% of the test animal population.
LEL Lower explosive limit.
LEPC Local Emergency Planning Committee.
lethal concentration 50% (LC_{50}) The inhaled dose of a substance that causes death in 50% of the test animal population.
lethal dose 50% (LD_{50}) The absorbed dose (oral or dermal) of a substance that causes death in 50% of the test animal population.
level A Fully encapsulated, vapor-tight suit with SCBA or positive-pressure air line and chemically resistant boots and gloves. Provides protection against vapors and skin-toxic chemicals.
level B Chemical splash suit with SCBA or positive-pressure air line and chemically resistant boots and gloves. Provides protection against inadvertent chemical splash and particulates.
level C Chemical splash suit, with APR and chemically resistant boots and gloves. Provides protection against known chemical concentrations below IDLH concentrations.

level D Work uniform. Provides no protection against chemical exposure.

limited-use garments Chemical-protective clothing that is used and then discarded as hazardous waste. Although limited-use garments can be worn several times based on use and exposure patterns, they commonly are discarded after one wearing.

liquified gases Gases that are liquified at normal temperature by applying pressure.

LOC Level of concern.

local emergency planning committee (LEPC) A committee appointed by a state emergency response commission (SERC), as required by SARA Title III, to formulate a comprehensive emergency plan for its region.

M

manifests A shipping document that lists the commodities being transported. Hazardous waste manifests are required by the EPA.

MC 306 Motor carrier 306 atmospheric pressure storage tank truck. Oval cross section, usually single-shell aluminum construction. Generally 9000 gallons maximum capacity.

MC 307 Motor carrier 307 low-pressure chemical cargo tank truck. Circular cross section with pressures up to 25 psi. Double-shell construction with insulation most common. Insulated tanks may not appear circular in cross section. One or two compartments. Generally 6000 to 7000 gallons maximum capacity.

MC 312 Motor carrier 312 corrosive cargo tank truck. Circular cross section, smaller diameter with external reinforcing ribs often visible. May also be found in double-shell configuration. Insulated tanks may not appear circular in cross section. Generally 5000 to 6000 gallons maximum capacity.

MC 331 Motor carrier 331 high-pressure gas cargo tank truck. Circular cross section with rounded ends or heads. Single shell, noninsulated tank. Usually painted white or highly reflective color. Capacity ranges from 2500-gallon "bobtail" delivery truck to 11,500-gallon cargo tank truck.

migration Movement of a hazardous material.

mists Condensation of liquid droplets on particles.

MSDS Material safety data sheet. A document that contains information about the specific identity of a hazardous chemical. Information includes exact name and synonyms, health effects, first aid, chemical and physical properties, and emergency telephone numbers.

N

National Fire Protection Association (NFPA) International voluntary membership organization to promote improved fire protection and prevention, and establish safeguards against loss of life and property by fire. Writes and publishes national voluntary consensus standards.

National Response Center (NRC) Communications center operated by the United States Coast Guard in Washington, DC. It is the federal spill notification point.

NFPA National Fire Protection Association.

NIOSH National Institute for Occupational Safety and Health. The agency of the Public Health Service, Department of Health and Human Services that tests and certifies respirators and air sampling devices. It recommends exposure limits to OSHA for substances, investigates incidents, and researches occupational safety.

nonflammable gas Any compressed gas other than a flammable gas. Examples include ammonia, nitrogen, and carbon dioxide.

O

offensive actions Actions taken at a hazardous materials incident that involve direct, intentional contact with the hazardous material. Actions are focused on mitigation of the problem.

operations level Training level established by OSHA 29 CFR 1910.120. Personnel who respond to a hazardous materials incident to protect nearby persons, property, or the environment from the effects of the release. They respond in a defensive fashion to control the release from a safe distance and keep it from spreading.

organic compounds Chemical compounds that contain carbon.

OSHA Occupational Safety and Health Administration. A unit of the U.S. Department of Labor. OSHA establishes protective standards, enforces those standards, and reaches out to employers and employees through technical assistance and consultation programs.

overpack Use of a specially designed container to isolate and control a leaking container, usually a drum.

oxidizing substances Substances that yield oxygen readily to stimulate the combustion of matter. Examples include lithium peroxide and calcium chlorite.

P

packing group Classification of hazardous materials based on the degree of danger represented by the material. Packing Group I indicates great danger, Packing Group II indicates medium danger, and Packing Group III indicates minor danger.

PEL Permissible exposure limit. Occupational exposure limits established by OSHA. These may be expressed as time–weighted average (TWA) limit, ceiling (C) limit, or short term exposure limit (STEL). OSHA PELs are legally enforceable. These exposure limits may be different from ACGIH TLVs or NIOSH RELs.

penetration The flow of a chemical substance through openings in CPC such as zippers, seams, stitches, holes, or tears in the material.

permeation The process by which a chemical moves through a chemical-resistant fabric on a molecular level, or diffusion.

PID Photo ionization device.

placards Diamond-shaped, 10¾-square inch markers required on a bulk container or transport vehicle such as a truck, tank car, or freight container.

poisonous substances Poisonous gases, liquids, or other substances of such nature that exposure to a very small amount of the substance is dangerous to life or is a hazard to health. Examples include cyanide, arsenic, phosgene, aniline, methyl bromide, insecticides, and pesticides.

PPE Personal protective equipment.

ppm Parts per million.

Process Safety Management Standard OSHA regulation 29 CFR 1910.119 that applies management principles, methods, and practices to prevent and control releases of hazardous chemicals or energy.

psi Pounds per square inch.
pyrophoric liquid Any liquid that ignites spontaneously in dry or moist air at or below 130° F (54.4° C).

R

radioactive The ability to emit ionizing radioactive energy.
radioactive substances Any material or combination of materials that spontaneously emit ionizing radiation, and have a specific activity greater than 0.002 μCi/g. Examples include plutonium, cobalt, uranium 235, and radioactive waste.
reactive The ability to undergo a chemical reaction with the release of energy when exposed to air, water, or other chemicals. Also the ability to explode when subjected to heat, shock, or friction.
REL Recommended exposure limit. Developed by NIOSH, the highest allowable airborne concentration of a chemical that is not expected to injure a worker. RELs may be expressed as a ceiling limit or as a time–weighted average (TWA), usually for 10-hour work shifts.
reportable quantity (RQ) The designated amount of a hazardous substance that if spilled or released requires immediate notification to the National Response Center.
RQ Reportable quantity.

S

SAR Supplied-air respirator, or air line.
SARA Superfund Amendment and Reauthorization Act.
SCBA Self-contained breathing apparatus.
secondary contamination The risk of another person or health care provider becoming contaminated with a hazardous material by contact with a contaminated victim.
shipping papers Documents that must accompany all shipments of goods for transportation. Under new DOT regulations, hazardous materials shipping papers must include a 24-hour emergency number.
specialist level Training level established by OSHA 29 CFR 1910.120. Personnel who respond with and provide support to hazardous materials technicians. Their actions usually parallel those of technicians; however, they have specialized knowledge of chemicals, transportation modes, or processes that may be involved. They also act as liaisons with federal, state, and local governmental agencies.
Superfund Amendment and Reauthorization Act EPA regulation that reauthorized the Superfund (Comprehensive Environmental Response, Compensation and Liability Act, or CERCLA) program. Also established federal status for community right-to-know standards and emergency response to hazardous materials accidents.

T

technician level Training level established by OSHA 29 CFR 1910.120. Personnel who respond to releases of hazardous materials to control the release. They use specialized chemical-protective clothing and specialized control equipment. Technician-level responders take offensive actions.
TLV Threshold limit values refer to airborne concentrations of substances and represent conditions under which it is believed that nearly all workers may be repeatedly exposed day after day without adverse health effects. Because of wide variation in individual susceptibility, a small percentage of workers may experience ill effects at concentrations below the TLV. There are three categories of TLVs: TLV–TWA, TLV–STEL, and TLV–C (see individual definitions).
TLV–C Threshold limit value–ceiling. The airborne concentration that should not be exceeded during any part of the working exposure.
TLV–STEL Threshold limit value–short term exposure limit. The concentration to which workers can be exposed continuously for a short period without suffering (1) irritation, (2) chronic or irreversible tissue damage, or (3) narcosis of sufficient degree to increase the likelihood of accidental injury, impair self-rescue, or materially reduce work efficiency, and provided that the daily TLV–TWA is not exceeded. A STEL is defined as a 15-minute TWA exposure that should not be exceeded at any time during a workday even if the 8-hour TWA is within the TLV–TWA. Exposures above the TLV–TWA up to the STEL should be for no longer than 15 minutes and should not occur more than four times a day. There should be at least 60 minutes between successive exposures in this range.
TLV–TWA Threshold limit value–time weighted average. The time-weighted average concentration for a normal 8-hour workday and a 40-hour workweek, to which nearly all workers may be repeatedly exposed, day after day, without adverse health effects.
toxin A product that can cause injury to biological tissue.
toxicology Division of science and biology that studies poisonous substances, how to detect them, their chemistry and pharmacological actions, and antidotes and treatment methods. Medical toxicologists apply this knowledge to human poisoning victims.

V

vapor pressure (VP) The ability of a material to evaporate in air. Vapor pressure is proportional to temperature. The vapor pressure increases with increasing temperature.

W

warm zone The warm (contamination reduction) zone is the area surrounding the hot zone. It functions as a safety buffer area, decontamination area, and as an access and egress point to and from the hot zone.
warning property An odor, taste, or mucous membrane irritation from chemical exposure that is detectable below the PEL and persists to above the IDLH air concentration. A chemical that meets this definition is said to have adequate warning properties.

Appendix 1

ACLS Algorithms

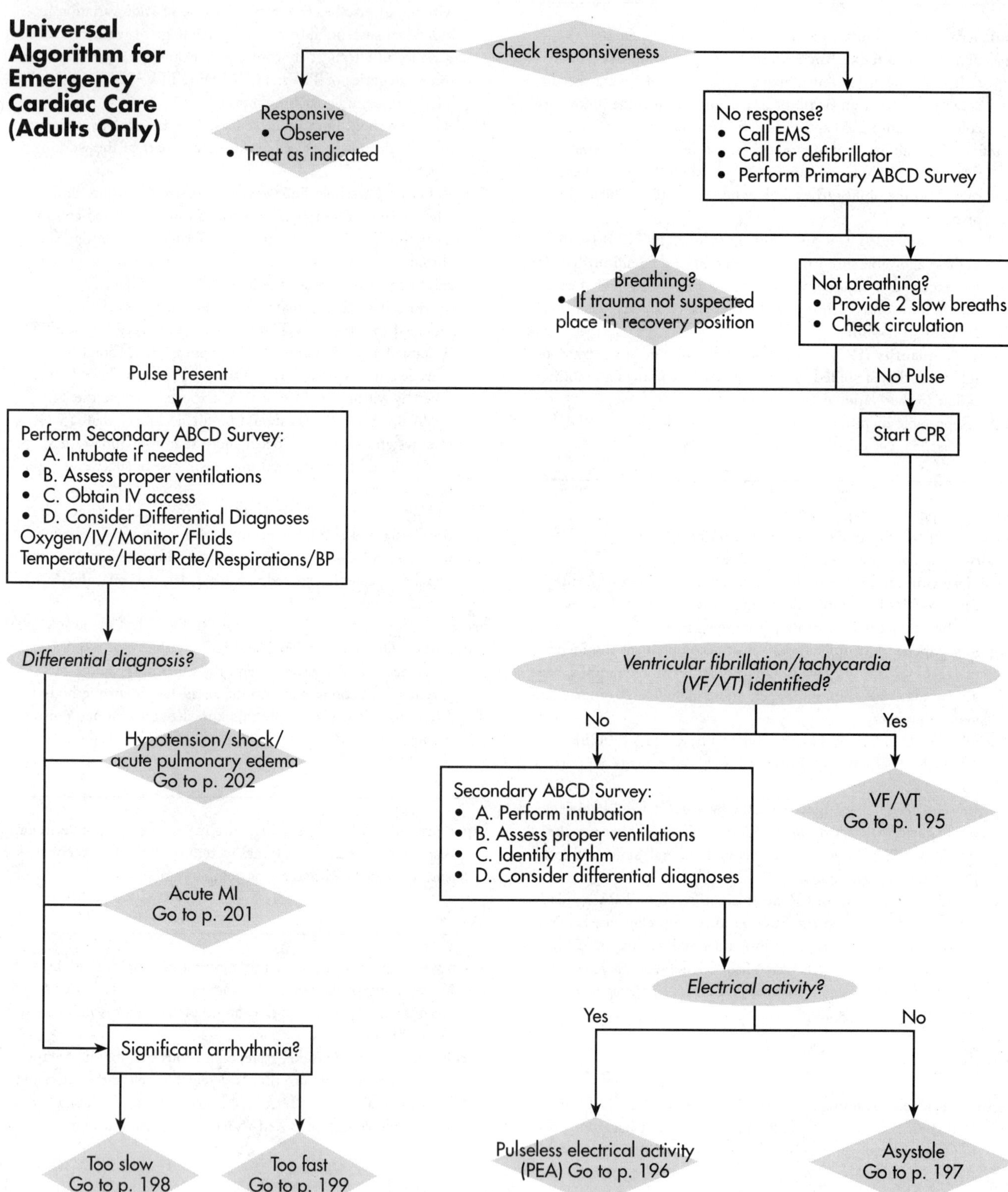

Modified from Guidelines for Cardiopulmonary Resuscitation and Emergency Cardiac Care, *JAMA* 268:2216, 1992.

Ventricular Fibrillation and Pulseless Ventricular Tachycardia Algorithm

Primary ABCD Survey:
- Basic CPR
- Attach Defibrillator[a]
- Check Rhythm

↓

- Ventricular fibrillation or pulseless Ventricular tachycardia (VF/VT) is present

↓

Defibrillate
Rapid shocks (up to three) if VF/VT persists
(200 J, 200 to 300 J, 360 J)

↓

Check rhythm following initial shocks[b]

↓

VF/VT continues

- Continue CPR
- Intubate as soon as possible
- Start IV

↓

- *Epinephrine* 1 mg IV push[c,d] repeat every 3 to 5 min

↓

- Defibrillate 360 J within 30 to 60 sec[e]

↓

- Add antiarrhythmics of probable benefit (Class IIa) if VF/VT continues or recurs[f,g]

↓

- Defibrillate 360 J, 30 to 60 sec after each medication[f]
- Sequence should be drug-shock, drug-shock

Return of spontaneous circulation

- Check vital signs
- Maintain airway
- Provide ventilations
- Give medications as indicated for blood pressure, heart rate, and rhythm

PEA
Go to p. 196

Asystole
Go to p. 197

Class I: Definitely helpful
Class IIa: Acceptable, probably helpful
Class IIb: Acceptable, possibly helpful
Class III: Not indicated, may be harmful

(a) Precordial thump is a Class IIb action in witnessed arrest, no pulse, and no defibrillator immediately available.

(b) Hypothermic cardiac arrest is treated differently after this point. *See Fig. 14.1*

(c) The recommended dose of **epinephrine** is 1 mg IV push every 3-5 min. If spontaneous circulation does not return, consider several Class IIb dosing regimens:
- Intermediate: **Epinephrine** 2-5 mg IV push, every 3-5 min.
- Escalating: **Epinephrine** 1 mg-3 mg-5 mg IV push, 3 min apart.
- High: **Epinephrine** 0.1 mg/kg IV push, every 3-5 min.

(d) **Sodium bicarbonate** (1 mEq/kg) is Class I if patient has known preexisting hyperkalemia.

(e) Continued delivery of shocks is acceptable here (Class I), especially when medications are delayed.

(f) Medications sequence:
- **Lidocaine** 1.0-1.5 mg/kg IV push. Repeat in 3-5 min to maximum dose of 3 mg/kg. A single 1.5 mg/kg dose in cardiac arrest is also acceptable.
- **Bretylium** 5 mg/kg IV push. Repeat in 5 min at 10 mg/kg.
- **Magnesium sulfate** 1-2 g IV in torsades de pointes, suspected hypomagnesemic state, or refractory VF.
- **Procainamide** 30 mg/min in recurrent VF (maximum total dose 17 mg/kg).

(g) **Sodium bicarbonate** (1 mEq/kg IV). Follow these indications:

Class IIa
- If overdose with tricyclic antidepressants
- To alkalinize the urine in drug overdoses
- If known preexisting bicarbonate-responsive acidosis

Class IIb
- If patient is intubated and arrest continues for long intervals
- If circulation restored after prolonged arrest

Class III
- Hypoxic lactic acidosis

Modified from Guidelines for Cardiopulmonary Resuscitation and Emergency Cardiac Care, *JAMA* 268:2217, 1992.

Pulseless Electrical Activity Algorithm

The term *pulseless electrical activity (PEA)* includes the following:

- Electromechanical dissociation (EMD)
- Pseudo-EMD
- Idioventricular rhythms
- Ventricular escape rhythms
- Bradyasystolic rhythms
- Post-defibrillation idioventricular rhythms

Continue Basic Life Support
Perform Secondary ABCD Survey:

- Intubate if needed
- Access ventilations
- Obtain IV access

Check for occult blood flow using Doppler ultrasound echocardiograph, end tidal CO_2 device

↓

Consider the differential diagnoses:
(Possible treatments shown in parentheses)

Five H's:

- Hypovolemia, includes anyaphylaxis (volume infusion)
- Hypoxia (oxygen and ventilation)
- Hypothermia
- Hyper-/hypokalemia (and other electrolyte abnormalities)
- Hydrogen ion (acidosis)

Five T's:

- Tension pneumothorax (needle decompression)
- Tamponade, cardiac (pericardiocentesis)
- Thrombosis, pulmonary (surgery, thrombolytics)
- Thrombosis, acute myocardial (thrombolytics, see p. 201)
- Tablets, drug overdoses (drug-specific interventions)

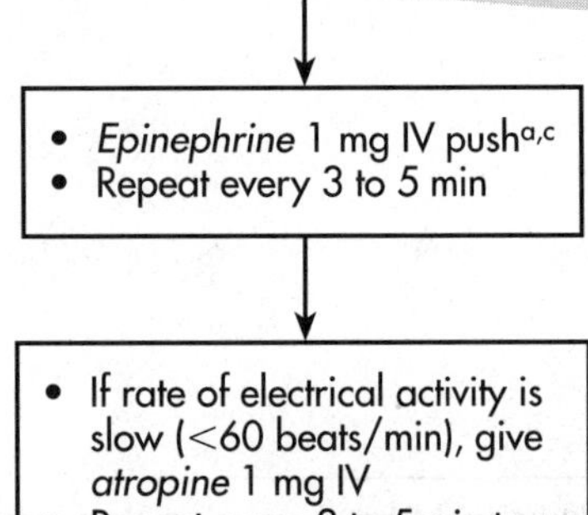

Class I: Definitely helpful

Class IIa: Acceptable, probably helpful

Class IIb: Acceptable, possibly helpful

Class III: Not indicated, may be harmful

(a) **Sodium bicarbonate** 1 mEq/kg is Class I if patient has known preexisting hyperkalemia.

(b) **Sodium bicarbonate** (1 mEq/kg) is given as follows:

Class IIa

- If known preexisting bicarbonate-responsive acidosis
- If overdose with tricyclic antidepressants
- To alkalinize the urine in drug overdoses

Class IIb

- If patient is intubated and arrest continues for long intervals
- If circulation is restored after prolonged arrest

Class III

- Hypoxic lactic acidosis (unventilated patient)

(c) The recommended dose of **epinephrine** is 1 mg IV push every 3 to 5 min. If spontaneous circulation does not return, consider several Class IIb dosing regimens:

- Intermediate: **Epinephrine** 2-5 mg IV push, every 3 to 5 min.
- Escalating: **Epinephrine** 1 mg-3 mg-5 mg IV push, 3 min apart.
- High: **Epinephrine** 0.1 mg/kg IV push, every 3 to 5 min.

(d) The shorter atropine dosing interval (3 min) is possibly helpful in cardiac arrest (Class IIb).

Modified from Guidelines for Cardiopulmonary Resuscitation and Emergency Cardiac Care, *JAMA* 268:2219, 1992.

Asystole Treatment Algorithm

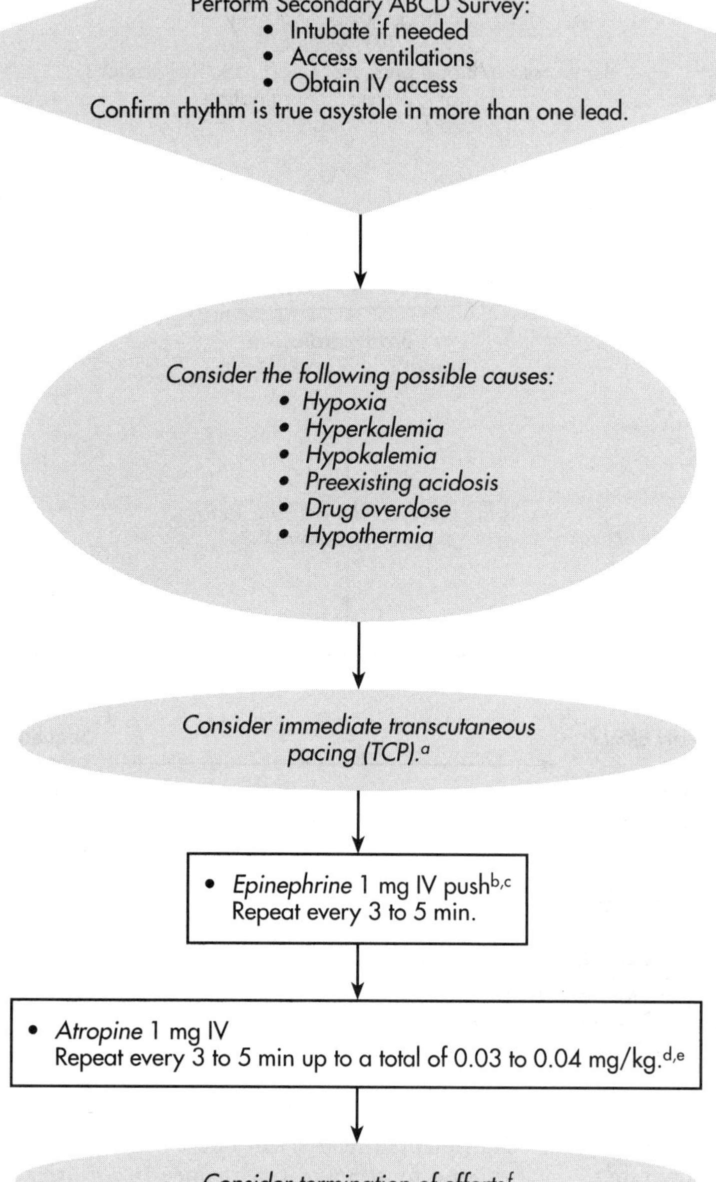

Class I: Definitely helpful

Class IIa: Acceptable, probably helpful

Class IIb: Acceptable, possibly helpful

Class III: Not indicated, may be harmful

(a) Pacing is an acceptable intervention (Class IIb). Perform TCP as early as possible, without waiting for the effects of medications. Not recommended as routine treatment for asystole.

(b) The recommended dose of **epinephrine** is 1 mg IV push every 3 to 5 min. If spontaneous circulation does not return, consider several Class IIb dosing regimens:
- Intermediate: **Epinephrine** 2 to 5 mg IV push, every 3 to 5 min
- Escalating: **Epinephrine** 1 to 3 mg to 5 mg IV push, 3 min apart
- High: **Epinephrine** 0.1 mg/kg IV push, every 3 to 5 min

(c) **Sodium bicarbonate** 1 mEq/kg is definitely indicated (Class I) if patient has known preexisting hyperkalemia.

(d) The shorter **atropine** dosing interval (3 min) is Class IIb in asystolic arrest.

(e) **Sodium bicarbonate** (1 mEq/kg) follow these indications:

Class IIa
- If known preexisting bicarbonate responsive acidosis
- If overdose with tricyclic antidepressants
- To alkalinize the urine in drug overdoses

Class IIb
- If patient intubated and arrest continues for long intervals
- If circulation restored after prolonged arrest

Class III
- Hypoxic acidosis (unventilated patient)

(f) Consider stopping resuscitative efforts when patient remains in documented asystole or other agonal rhythms for more than 10 minutes *after:*
- Patient successfully intubated
- Initial IV medications given
- No reversible causes identified
- Physician concurs

Modified from Guidelines for Cardiopulmonary Resuscitation and Emergency Cardiac Care, *JAMA* 268:2220, 1992.

Bradycardia Algorithm (For Patients not in Cardiac Arrest)

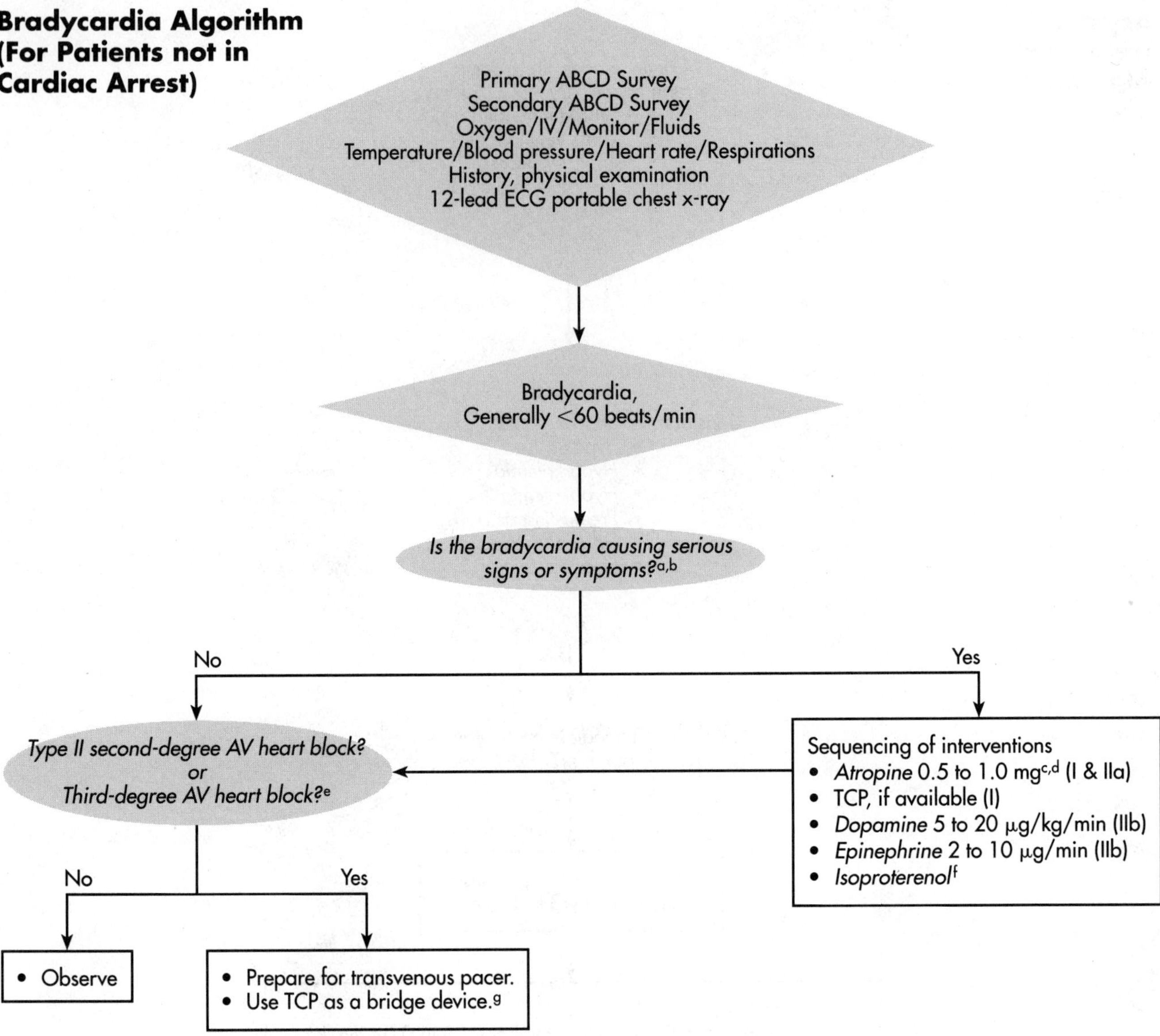

(a) the clinical signs or symptoms must be related to the slow rate. Clinical manifestations include the following:

- Symptoms (chest pain, shortness of breath, decreased level of consciousness)
- Signs (low blood pressure, shock, pulmonary congestion, congestive heart failure, AMI)

(b) Start TCP before atropine takes effect if patient is symptomatic.

(c) Transplanted hearts will not respond to *atropine.* Go at once to pacing, *catecholamine infusion,* or both.

(d) *Atropine* should be given in repeat doses every 3 to 5 min up to total of 0.03 to 0.04 mg/kg. Use the shorter dosing interval (3 min) in severe clinical conditions. *Atropine* is seldom effective in atrioventricular (AV) block at the His-Purkinje level (type II AV block and new third-degree block with wide QRS complexes) (Class IIb).

(e) A potentially fatal error is to treat third-degree heart block plus ventricular escape beats with lidocaine.

(f) Only use *isoproterenol* with extreme caution. At low doses it is Class IIb (possibly helpful); at higher doses it is Class III (harmful).

(g) Check that patients can tolerate TCP and that cardiac capture occurs. Use analgesia and sedation as needed.

Modified from Guidelines for Cardiopulmonary Resuscitation and Emergency Cardiac Care, *JAMA* 268:2221, 1992.

Tachycardia Algorithm

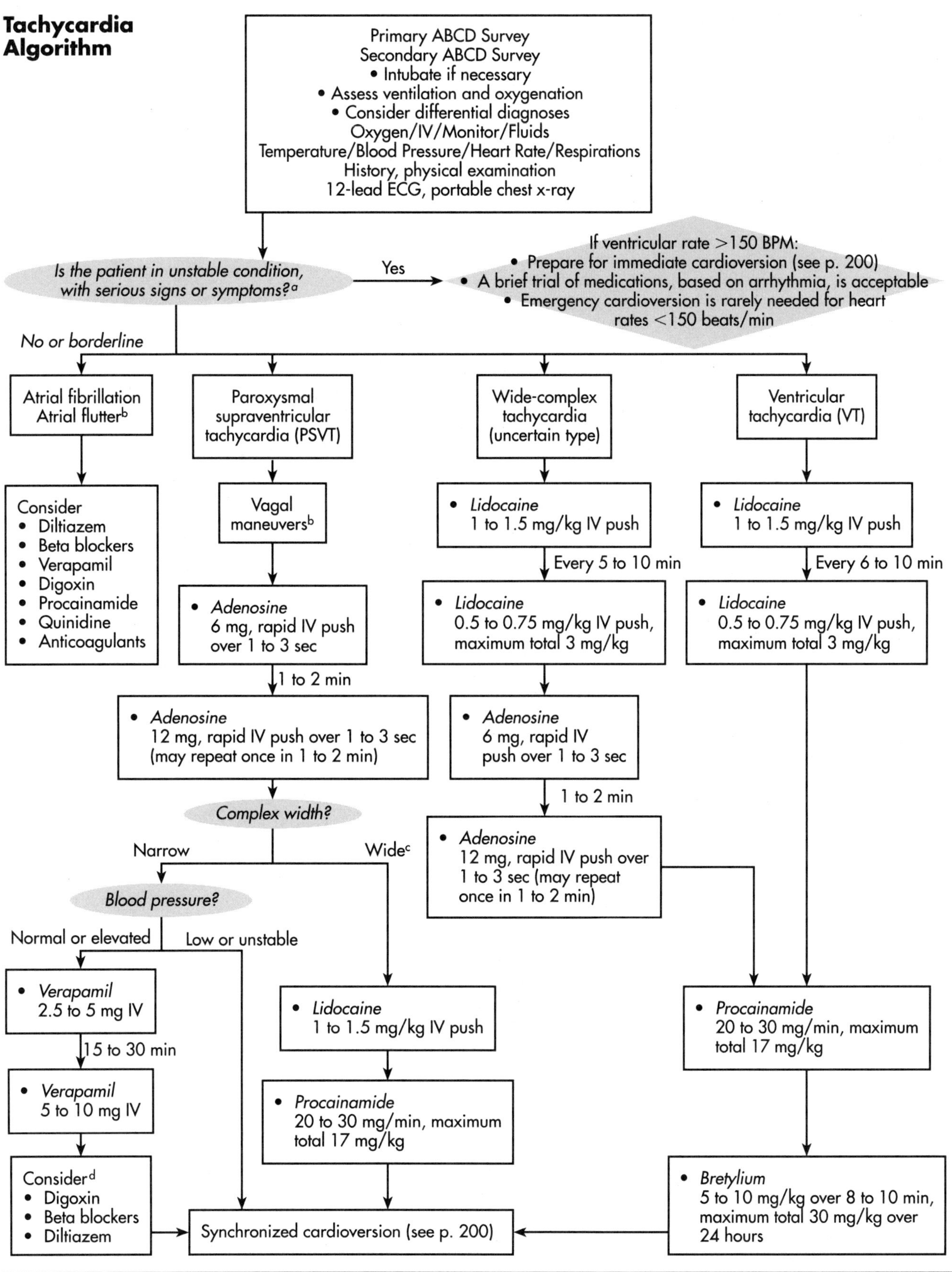

(a) A patient's unstable condition must be caused by the tachycardia. Clinical signs and symptoms may include chest pain, shortness of breath, decreased level of consciousness, low blood pressure (BP), shock, pulmonary congestion, congestive heart failure, and acute myocardial infarction.

(b) Avoid carotid sinus pressure in patients with carotid bruits; avoid ice-water immersion in patients with ischemic heart disease.

(c) Wide-complex tachycardia known with certainty to be PSVT and BP that is normal or elevated, can be treated with verapamil.

(d) Avoid beta blockers after verapamil.

Modified from Guidelines for Cardiopulmonary Resuscitation and Emergency Cardiac Care, *JAMA* 268:2223, 1992.

Electrical Cardioversion Algorithm (Patient Is Not in Cardiac Arrest)

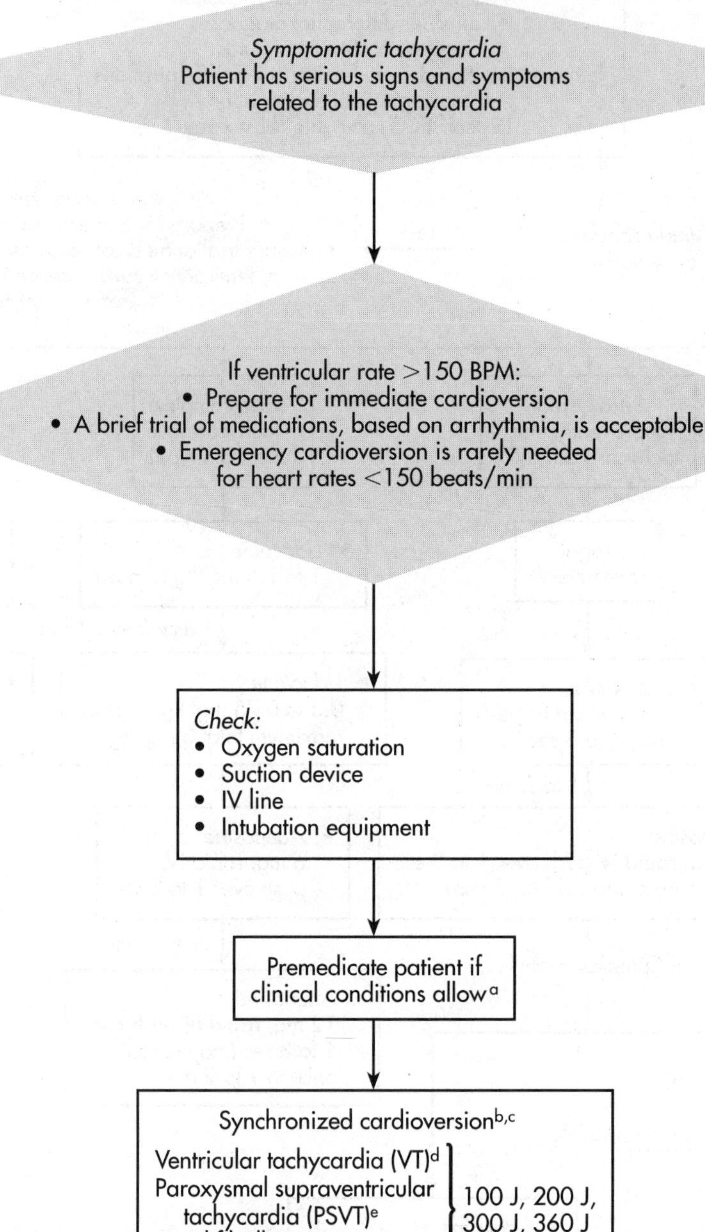

(a) Many experts recommend anesthesia if service is readily available. Effective premedication regimens have included a sedative (e.g., **diazepam, midazolam, barbiturates, etomidate, ketamine, methohexital**) with or without an analgesic agent (e.g., **fentanyl, morphine, meperidine**).

(b) You often need to resynchronize the defibrillator after each cardioversion.

(c) If synchronization is delayed and clinical conditions are critical, perform unsynchronized shocks.

(d) Treat polymorphic VT (irregular form and rate) like ventricular fibrillation: 200 J, 200 to 300 J, 360 J.

(e) PSVT and atrial flutter often respond to lower energy levels (start with 50 J).

Modified from Guidelines for Cardiopulmonary Resuscitation and Emergency Cardiac Care, *JAMA* 268:2224, 1992.

Acute Myocardial Infarction Algorithm

Early Management of Patients with Chest Pain and Possible Acute Myocardial Infarction (AMI) in Three Management Settings

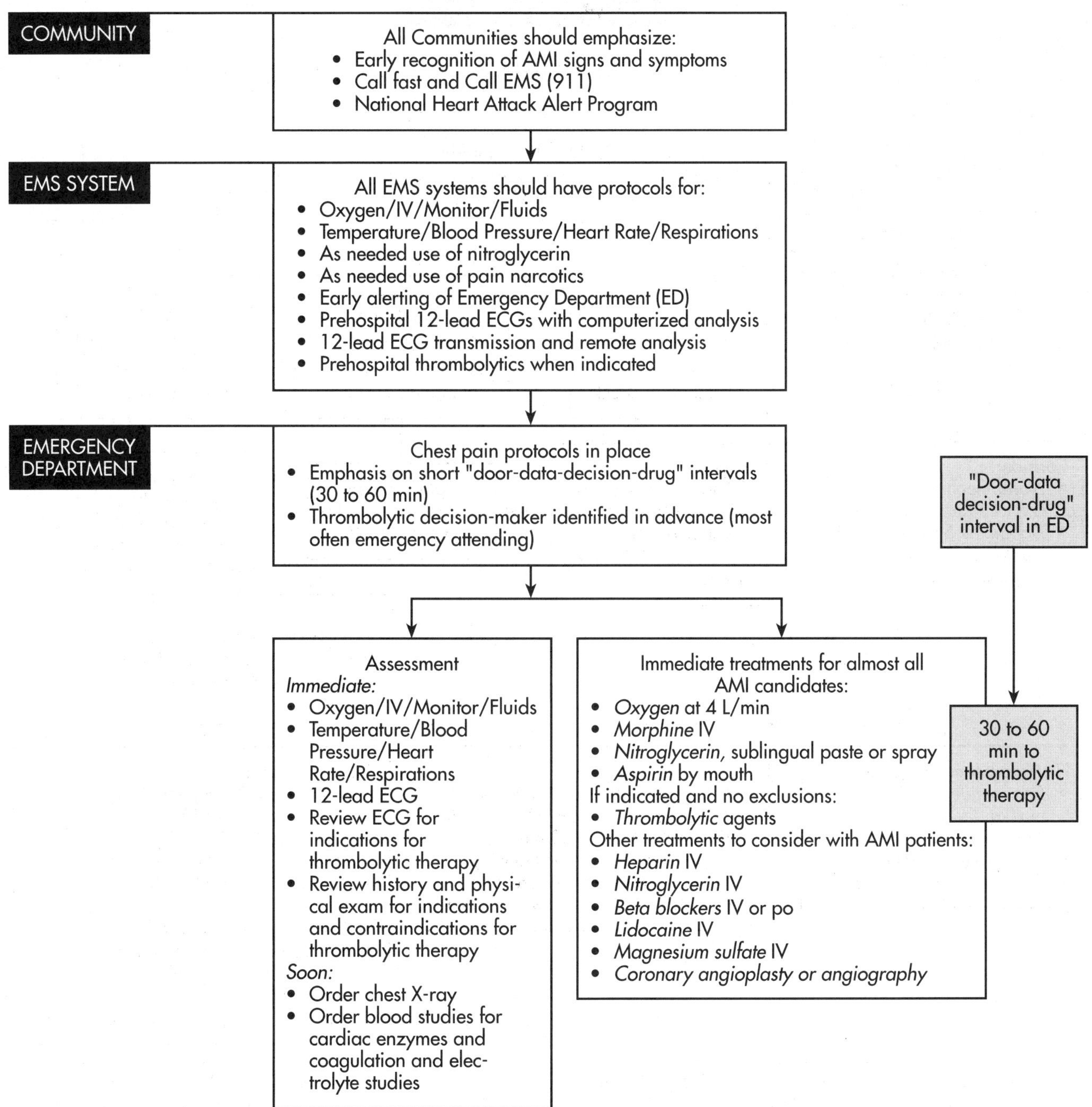

Modified from Guidelines for Cardiopulmonary Resuscitation and Emergency Cardiac Care, *JAMA* 268:2220, 1992.

Algorithm Approach to Problems of Acute Pulmonary Edema, Shock, and Hypotension

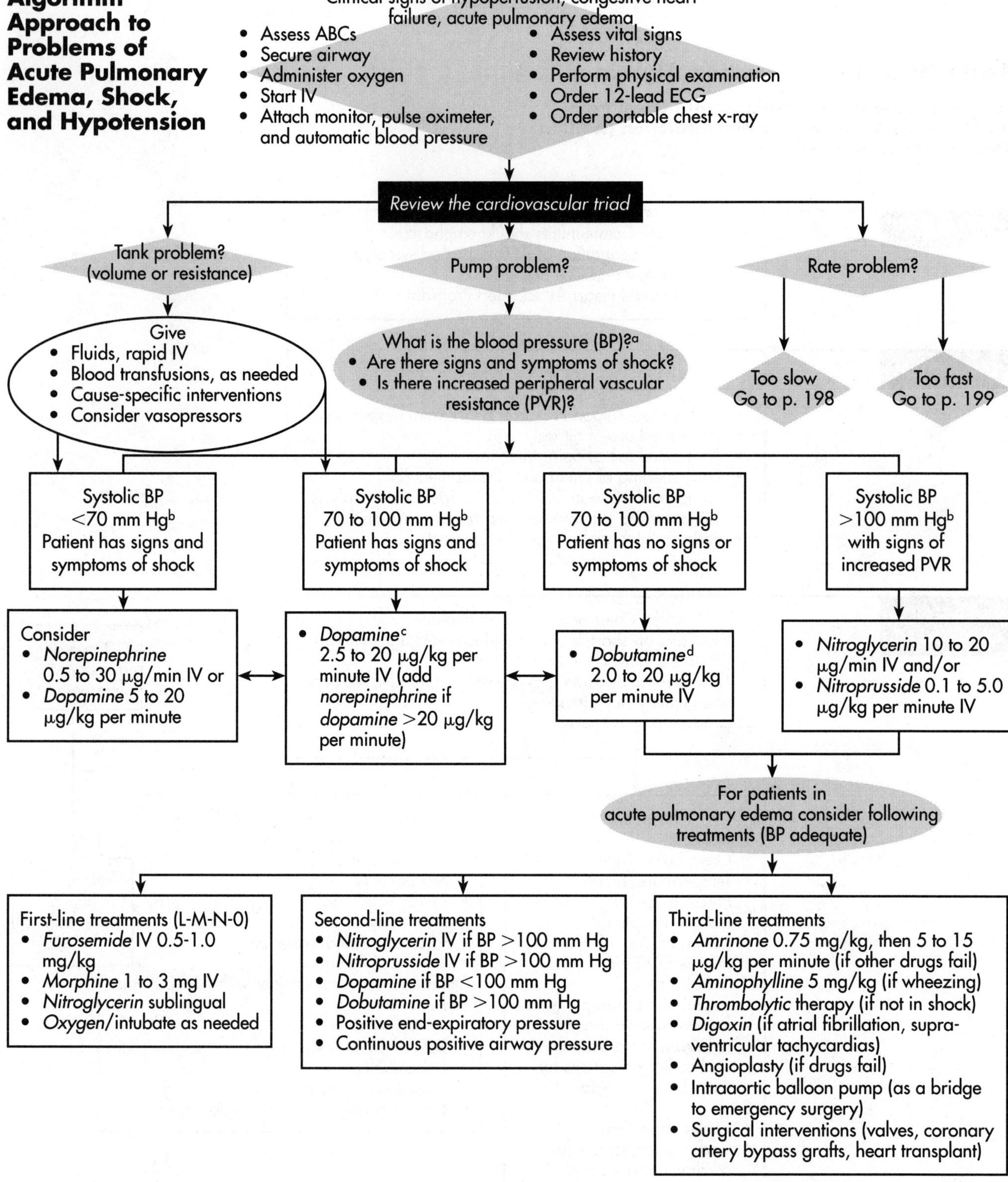

(a) Guide treatment after this point by invasive hemodynamic monitoring if possible. Guidelines presume clinical signs of hypoperfusion.

(b) Rapid fluid bolus of at least 250 to 500 mL normal saline should be tried. If clinical response is inadequate, consider sympathomimetics.

(c) Start dopamine and stop norepinephrine when profoundly low BP improves. Dobutamine is preferred over dopamine when there is a hypotension with no signs and symptoms of shock.

(d) If moderate hypotension treated with dobutamine does not respond, add dopamine and reduce or eliminate dobutamine.

Modified from Guidelines for Cardiopulmonary Resuscitation and Emergency Cardiac Care, *JAMA* 268:2227, 1992.

Pediatric Bradycardia Algorithm

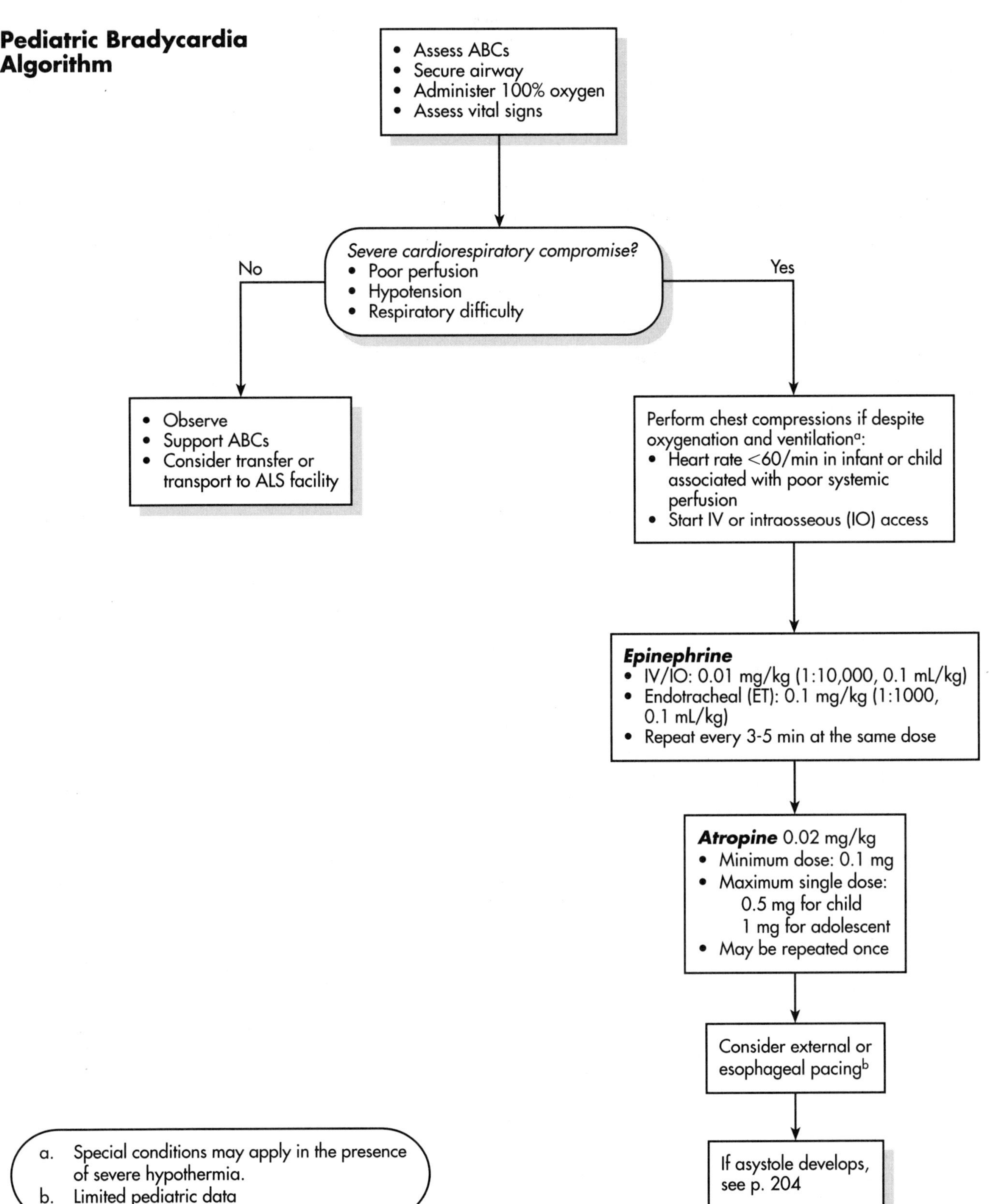

Modified from American Heart Association: *Pediatric advanced life support,* Dallas, Texas, 1997, The Association.

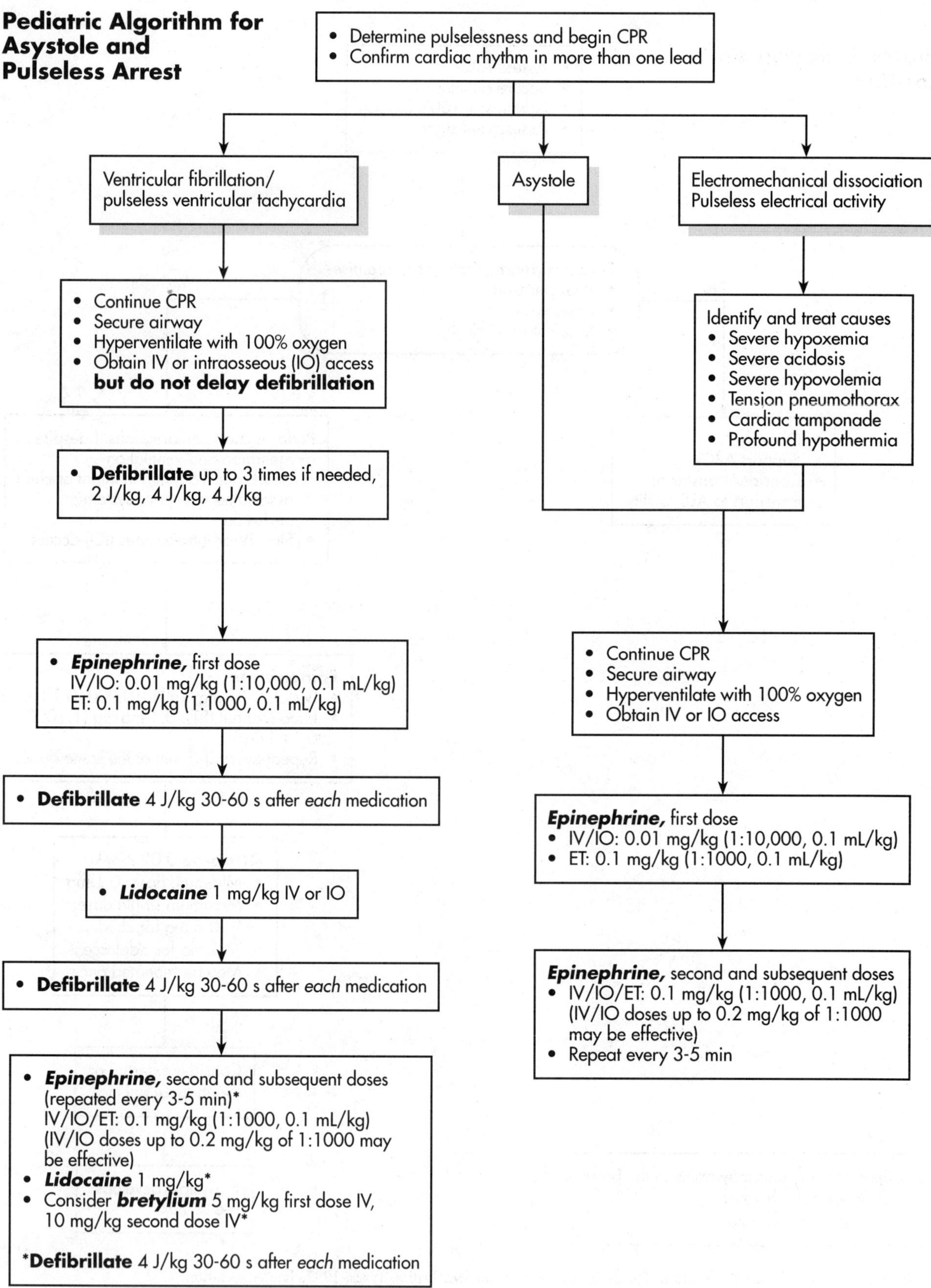

Modified from American Heart Association: *Pediatric advanced life support,* Dallas, Texas, 1997, The Association.

Appendix 2

NFPA 473

Standard for Competencies for EMS Personnel Responding to Hazardous Materials Incidents

1997 Edition

Chapter 1 Administration

1-1 SCOPE. This standard identifies the levels of competence required of Emergency Medical Services (EMS) personnel who respond to hazardous materials incidents. It specifically covers the requirements for basic life support and advanced life support personnel in the prehospital setting.

1-2 PURPOSE. The purpose of this standard is to specify minimum requirements of competence and to enhance the safety and protection of response personnel and all components of the emergency medical services system. It is not the intent of this standard to restrict any jurisdiction from exceeding these minimum requirements. *(See Appendix B.)*

Chapter 2 Competencies for EMS/HM Level I Responders

2-1 GENERAL.

2-1.1 INTRODUCTION. All EMS personnel at EMS/HM Level I, in addition to their BLS or ALS certification, shall be trained to meet at least the first responder awareness level as defined in NFPA 472, *Standard for Professional Competence of Responders to Hazardous Materials Incidents,* and all competencies of this chapter.

2-1.2 DEFINITION. EMS personnel at EMS/HM Level I are those persons who, in the course of their normal duties, might be called on to perform patient care activities in the cold zone at a hazardous materials incident. EMS/HM Level I responders shall provide care only to those individuals who no longer pose a significant risk of secondary contamination.

2-1.3 GOAL. The goal of the competencies at EMS/HM Level I shall be to provide the individual with the knowledge and skills necessary to safely deliver emergency medical care in the cold zone. Therefore the EMS/HM Level I responder shall be able to:

(a) Analyze a hazardous materials emergency to determine what risks are present to the provider and the patient by completing the following tasks:

1. Determine the hazards present to the Level I responder and the patient in a hazardous materials incident
2. Assess the patient to determine the risk of secondary contamination

(b) Plan a response to provide the appropriate level of emergency medical care to persons involved in hazardous materials incidents by completing the following tasks:

1. Describe the role of the Level I responder in a hazardous materials incident
2. Plan a response to provide the appropriate level of emergency medical care in a hazardous materials incident
3. Determine if the personal protective equipment provided is appropriate
4. Determine if the equipment and supplies provided are adequate

(c) Implement the planned response by completing the following tasks:

1. Perform the necessary preparations for receiving the hazardous materials patient and preventing secondary contamination
2. Treat the hazardous materials patient
3. Transport the patient as appropriate

(d) Terminate the incident

Chapter 3 Competencies for EMS/HM Level II Responders

3-1 GENERAL.

3-1.1 INTRODUCTION. All personnel at EMS/HM Level II shall be certified to the EMT-A level or higher and shall meet all competencies for EMS/HM Level I in addition to all the competencies of this chapter.

3-1.2 DEFINITION. Personnel at EMS/HM Level II are those persons who, in the course of their normal activities, might be called upon to perform patient care activities in the warm zone at hazardous materials incidents. EMS/HM Level II responder personnel might be required to provide care to those individuals who still pose a significant risk of secondary contamination. In addition, personnel at this level shall be able to coordinate EMS activities at a hazardous materials incident and provide medical support for hazardous materials response personnel.

3-1.3 GOAL. The goal of the competencies at EMS/HM Level II shall be to provide the Level II responder with the knowledge and skills necessary to perform and/or coordinate patient care activities and medical support of hazardous materials response personnel in the warm zone. Therefore the Level II responder shall be able to:

(a) Analyze a hazardous materials incident to determine the magnitude of the problem in terms of outcomes by completing the following tasks:

1. Determine the hazards present to the Level II responder and the patient in a hazardous materials incident

2. Assess the patient to determine the patient care needs and the risk of secondary contamination

(b) Plan a response to provide the appropriate level of emergency medical care to persons involved in hazardous materials incidents and to provide medical support to hazardous materials response personnel by completing the following tasks:

1. Describe the role of the Level II responder in a hazardous materials incident

2. Plan a response to provide the appropriate level of emergency medical care in a hazardous materials incident

3. Determine if the personal protective equipment provided to EMS personnel is appropriate

(c) Implement the planned response by completing the following tasks:

1. Perform the necessary preparations for receiving the patient

2. Perform necessary treatment to the hazardous materials patient

3. Coordinate and manage the EMS component of the hazardous materials incident

4. Perform medical support of hazardous materials incident response personnel

(d) Terminate the incident

Appendix B Training

This appendix is not a part of the requirements of this NFPA document but is included for informational purposes only.

B-1 GENERAL. The Emergency Medical Services (EMS) personnel responding to hazardous materials incidents should be trained and should receive regular continuing education to maintain competency in three areas: emergency medical technology, hazardous materials, and specialized topics approved by the authority having jurisdiction.

B-1.1 EMS TRAINING. Recognized US DOT, state, regional, or local training curricula should constitute the entry level EMS preparation for continuing hazardous materials training. At a hazardous materials incident it is desirable that all EMS BLS provider personnel be trained to the US DOT EMT-A level or equivalent.

B-1.2 HAZARDOUS MATERIALS TRAINING. The foundation for EMS response to a hazardous materials incident should be the competencies described in NFPA 472, *Standard for Professional Competence of Responders to Hazardous Materials Incidents.*

B-1.3 SPECIALIZED TRAINING. Following completion of approved EMS training and appropriate level of hazardous materials instruction described in this standard, the authority having jurisdiction should stipulate additional specialized instruction that the EMS personnel responding to hazardous materials incidents must complete.

B-2 TRAINING PLAN.

B-2.1 The authority having jurisdiction should develop a formal training plan and provide a program to train EMS personnel to the level being utilized.

B-2.2 A training plan should be developed and contain guidelines for the following functional categories:

(a) Program management
(b) Content development
(c) Instructor competencies
(d) Technical specialist competencies

B-2.3 The training plan should be criteria-based to maintain a consistent quality of curriculum and instruction.

B-2.4 The training plan should specify entry knowledge and skill levels, training, and refresher training for both students and instructors.

B-2.5 The training plan should define evaluation criteria for successful completion of knowledge and skill objectives of the training program.

B-2.6 The training plan should provide for supervised field experience for EMS hazardous materials responder and EMS hazardous materials coordinator training levels.

B-3 TRAINING PROGRAM. The training program should be a comprehensive competency-based guideline of the implementation and presentation of the required subject material. As a minimum it should address the areas discussed in this section.

B-3.1 PROGRAM MANAGER.

B-3.1.1 The program manager should have the authority and responsibility for the overall implementation of the program.

B-3.1.2 The program manager should be able to demonstrate knowledge of the following:

(a) The content of NFPA 472, *Standard for Professional Competence of Responders to Hazardous Materials Incidents;* NFPA 471, *Recommended Practice for Responding to Hazardous Materials Incidents;* and this standard
(b) EMS delivery systems
(c) Budgeting and financial planning
(d) Processes used to develop instructional materials

B-3.1.3 The program manager should demonstrate the skill and ability to perform the following tasks:

(a) Coordinate the training program
(b) Evaluate program effectiveness
(c) Identify instructors and technical specialists

B-3.2 CONTENT. The content of the training program should include the competencies of this standard as a minimum.

B-3.3 EVALUATION. In recognition of the need for technically sound curricula and instruction to meet the competencies outlined in this standard, careful evaluation of all instructors' training, background, and experience should be made.

B-3.3.1 The authority having jurisdiction should ensure that the training program meets the needs of the local area.

B-3.3.2 The program manager should ensure that the training program meets the needs of the hazardous materials response team and the EMS providers.

B-4 INSTRUCTION. The need exists for technically sound curricula and delivery to meet the competencies outlined in this standard.

B-4.1 INSTRUCTORS. The instructor should

(a) Have mastery of the material he/she presents
(b) Have an understanding of the training program objectives
(c) Have the ability to teach and evaluate

B-4.2 TECHNICAL SPECIALIST. The technical specialist is a person who has technical expertise and practical knowledge in a specific area. This category is intended to support training activities by allowing individuals not otherwise qualified at the instructor level to present an essential segment for which they do have expertise.

B-4.3 FINAL EVALUATION. Upon completion of the training program, the student should demonstrate competency in all prescribed content areas. This evaluation should include written and practical testing as specified by the program manager and instructors.

Index

A

B

D

Q

R

S